Geriatric Clinical Protocols

Linda Joan Pearson, B.S.N., M.S.N., F.N.P.
Assistant Professor, University of
Colorado School of Nursing

M. Ernestine Kotthoff, R.N., B.S., A.N.P.
Adult Nurse Practitioner, University of
Colorado Medical Center
Denver, Colorado

J. B. Lippincott Company
Philadelphia
New York   San Jose   Toronto

ISBN 0-397-54270-4
Library of Congress Catalog Card Number 79-12888

Printed in the United States of America
2 4 6 8 9 7 5 3 1

Library of Congress Cataloging in Publication Data

Pearson, Linda Buck.
  Geriatric clinical protocols.

  Includes bibliographies and index.
  1. Geriatric nursing. 2. Medical protocols.
3. Geriatric nursing—Study and teaching. I. Kotthoff,
Mary Ernestine, joint author. II. Title. [DNLM:
1. Geriatrics—Nursing texts. WY152 P361g]
RC954.P4   618.9'7   79-12888
ISBN 0-397-54270-4

Contributing Authors

Elsie M. Balint, R.N., B.A.
Geriatric Nurse Practitioner (University of Colorado). Currently works as a GNP in independent practice with physicians in extended care facilities, Eugene, Oregon.

Beverly J. Bakkum, R.N.
Family Health Practitioner (Montana State University), and Geriatric Nurse Practitioner (University of Colorado). Currently works as GNP in a nursing home, Livingston, Montana.

Colleen Broderick, R.N., B.S.
Geriatric Nurse Practitioner (University of Colorado). Currently works as a GNP in Bigfork, Montana.

Audrey P. Corson, R.N., M.S.
Adult Nurse Practitioner (University of Colorado). Currently works as an ANP at Denver General Hospital and is enrolled at the University of Colorado School of Medicine, Denver, Colorado.

Gail de la Cruz, R.N.
Geriatric Nurse Practitioner (University of Colorado). Currently Director of Nursing in nursing home, Santa Fe, New Mexico.

D. E. Farrell, M.A. CCC-A
M.A. in Speech Pathology and Audiology (Northeast Missouri State University). Currently a Ph.D. candidate in Audiology at the University of Colorado, and works as a clinical audiologist in Aurora, Colorado.

Joyce Gill, R.N.
Geriatric Nurse Practitioner (University of Colorado). Currently works as a GNP in a nursing home, Lewistown, Montana.

Kathleen Hynes, B.A., M.A.
Currently an Instructor teaching medical ethics in the Department of Preventive Medicine, University of Colorado School of Medicine, and completing her doctoral dissertation in Sociology at the University of Denver.

M. Ernestine Kotthoff, R.N., B.S.N.
Adult Nurse Practitioner (University of Colorado). Currently works as an ANP at the University of Colorado Medical Center, Department of Internal Medicine, Denver, Colorado.

Linda J. Pearson, R.N., M.S.
Family Nurse Practitioner (University of Washington). Currently works as FNP in private practice with Family Practice physicians, Englewood, Colorado, and is Assistant Professor at the University of Colorado School of Nursing, Denver, Colorado.

Dodie Russell, R.N., M.S.
Adult Nurse Practitioner (University of Minnesota). Currently an Instructor for the ANP/GNP Masters Program at the University of Minnesota School of Public Health, and is affiliated with a private Internal Medicine practice, Minneapolis, Minnesota.

Irene Suzuki, R.N., M.S.
Adult Nurse Practitioner (University of Colorado). Currently works as an ANP at the University of Colorado Medical Center, Denver, Colorado.

Acknowledgments

We would like to acknowledge the contributions to this book made by the following:

Robert ten Bensel, M.D., M.P.H., Professor, School of Public Health, University of Minnesota

William Bentley, M.D., Clinical Instructor in Neurology, School of Medicine, University of Colorado, Denver, Colorado

George T. Demos, M.D., Private practice in Otolaryngology in Aurora, Colorado

Robert E. Donohue, M.D., Associate Professor of Surgery (Urology), University of Colorado School of Medicine, and Chief of Urology, Denver VA Hospital

William C. Gentry, Jr., M.D., Associate Professor Department of Dermatology, University of Minnesota School of Medicine

Carolyn Hudak, R.N., M.S., A.N.P., Associate Professor of Nursing and Assistant Professor of Medicine, University of Colorado, Denver, Colorado

Mervyn L. Lifschitz, M.D., Instructor in Medicine, University of Colorado School of Medicine, Denver, Colorado

Herbert R. Markheim, M.D., Visiting Professor, Department of Orthopedics, University of Colorado Medical Center, Denver, Colorado

Robert McCartney, M.D., Private Practice in Internal Medicine, Denver, Colorado

Lawrence Robbins, M.D., Fellow in Department of Internal Medicine, University of Colorado

Richard P. Saucier, M.D., Clinical Instructor of Psychiatry, University of Colorado Medical Center; Private Practice and Psychiatric Consultation for several Denver agencies

John Woodward, M.D., Senior Resident in Neurology, University of Colorado, Denver, Colorado

Dedication

To my husband and son who have always supported me and have given me happiness.

L.J.P.

To my friends and support systems who assisted me during the preparation of this book—there were many trying times and their assistance was immeasurable. A special thanks is extended to my colleague Dr. Richard Byyny and my friend Dr. Richard Saucier.

M.E.K.

Both authors would like to thank Dr. Richard Saucier for his support and Lynn Kelly for her invaluable assistance through typing.

Preface

One of the striking results of registered nurses moving into expanded roles of nursing is their motivation for increased self-directed learning within their own specialty. Nurses, while accepting more responsibility for primary health care of specific populations, are recognizing that this widened scope of practice is also widening their scope of accountability. Many nurse practitioners are meeting this professional challenge through the use of clinical protocols. Protocols act as both an educational tool and a method for audit and peer review. In addition, the majority of the state nurse practice acts that have rules and regulations for expanded-role nurses are utilizing interdisciplinary protocols as a requirement for practice.

This popularity of protocols has been noticed by the authors, both statewide and nationally. It has been our observation that the book *Clinical Protocols: A Guide for Nurses and Physicians*, by Hudak and associates, has been widely utilized by nurses and physicians seeking to develop protocols for their own particular setting.

Published protocols are becoming very popular reading material for health care providers. However, the majority of the heretofore published protocols cover common clinical entities of the young and middle-aged. Very few have been written for the elderly.

This lack of protocols for common clinical entities seen in the elderly was brought to the authors' attention by the spring 1977 class of Geriatric Nurse Practitioner students at the University of Colorado School of Nursing. As a group, they had an average of 10 years experience in working with the elderly; their inability to find published protocols for problems *frequently* experienced in their geriatric settings was a beginning motivator for writing this book.

The field of geriatrics is a constantly expanding field in the United States. Each day over 1,000 more Americans turn 65. Today, about one person in 10 is over 65 (Davis, 1976). America's over-65 population is already about twice what it was in 1950; the Census Bureau predicts that between 1950 and 2030 the over-65 population will have quadrupled (Davis, 1978).

Partly because of the increasingly high percentage of Americans in the over-65 bracket, an increasing number of nurses have selected the elderly as their age specialty. When one recalls that protocols are not only a popular learning and audit tool, but also a growing legal requirement, it becomes evident that there is a demand for clinical protocols for the older age group.

This book has been written in order to help fill this need. The format is similar to the Hudak and associates book because of readers' comments on its readability and style. The contributing authors' expertise in the geriatric field has been invaluable in helping to write a book designed for nurses and physicians working with older Americans.

Each chapter of this book contains a clinical entity frequently encountered by health providers who care for the elderly. The format of each protocol chapter will include the following:

1. An overview section that speaks to the pathophysiology necessary for the reader to fully understand the age-related differences of the elderly.

2. A list of those conditions that cannot be missed when the patient's complaint is applied to the specific protocol.

3. A list of historical descriptors (subjective data) necessary to ensure a complete work-up of a patient's complaint.

4. A list of physical exam components (objective data) necessary to ensure the complete work-up of a patient's complaint.

5. A worksheet rationale section that takes each subjective and objective datum the reader was asked to collect and gives the rationale for why it is important. Obtaining the data and understanding the rationale will enable the reader to arrive at an accurate assessment of the patient's condition.

6. An assessment section that provides the reader with a quick, concise, and complete reference to the range of possible diagnoses applicable to each protocol's chief complaint.

7. A plan section that provides the reader with appropriate steps to take for each possible assessment. Where applicable, a patient education section is included.

8. A bibliography that will enable the reader to locate the best sources available should she or he desire a more indepth explanation of the clinical entity covered by the protocol.

L.J.P.
M.E.K.

REFERENCES

1. Richard H. Davis, ed. *Aging: Prospects and Issues*. Berkeley: University of Southern California Press, 1976.
2. ———. "Geriatrics: Youthful Enthusiasm Sparks a Boom," *Medical World News*, June 26, 1978, 38.

Introduction: Notes on Value Conflicts in Patient Care

The focus of this text is on protocols for managing the multiple clinical problems frequently seen in the elderly population. However, health care decisions rest on more than observable clinical data; they also involve substantive ethical and philosophical issues. It is within this context then that a comment should be made on the ethical problems that accompany clinical practice.

The first underlying assumption of this book: the quality of health care is enhanced when the health professional reflects on the value issues implicit in varying degrees in the delivery of health care. Ethical dilemmas in medicine arise when the clinical data are interpreted in light of the patient's human condition. Very few medical-ethical quandaries arise when the human element is omitted. A second assumption underlying this text is that value issues (as reflected in the provider's belief system and the patient's belief system) form a knowledge base which is of importance in conjunction with the clinical data gathered, and thus ought to be integrated into the planning for the daily delivery of health care.

DEFINING AN ETHICAL PROBLEM: A VALUE CONFLICT

An ethical problem is defined as a situation in which a value conflict exists. This conflict may arise within an individual over two or more personally held values, or the conflict may exist between an individual and societal mandates. A third area of conflict and the focus of the following discussion is on the value conflicts that exist between an individual patient and his or her health care provider.

Even prior to using the protocols contained in this book the health professional either assumes or directly clarifies with the patient the type of patient-provider relationship into which they both are entering. A decision about this relationship entails a value judgment for both.

Sissela Bok (1974) notes an overriding tendency for health professionals who care for the elderly to unwittingly enter into a paternalistic relationship with their clients.

> Since it is exceptionally difficult at times to know whether paternalism is justified with respect to chronically ill and aged persons, the mere fact of belonging to these groups greatly increases the vulnerability to control by others ... the ability to protect one's freedom of personal choice shrinks with weakness and prolonged illness and the incidence of such illness has greatly increased. At the beginning of this century, the major communicable diseases were the leading causes of death and the average life expectancy was 47 years. Now, the average life expectancy is around 70 years and chronic degenerative diseases cause most of the deaths at that age.

Accepting the reality of this paternalistic tendency, an ethical problem frequently arises from a conflict between the patient's value of remaining an autonomous decision-maker and the health provider's value of "making the decisions in caring for the patient."

RESOLVING A VALUE CONFLICT

The health professional can enhance his or her ability in resolving value conflicts by utilizing a decision-making process. The decision process is more useful when it reflects the professional's own values. Included in the process should be a selected series of questions (not too many extraneous questions or else the health professional will never reach a *decision*). In order to minimize biases, *these same questions should be asked in every patient-provider interaction and should be answered in every value conflict situation.*

The following approach has proven beneficial for a variety of health professionals. It is only an example of the types of questions one may wish to use while resolving each value issue that is part of the clinical situation.

1. What is most compatible with my beliefs? That is, what does "who I am" say I should do?
2. According to society, what is the "right" thing to do? That is, what does society expect of me?

3. In my judgment, what is the "good" thing to do? That is, what will produce the best consequences for the patient and for myself as provider?

If answers to the above screening questions identify a value conflict between the patient and provider, health care providers might want to further clarify their understanding of the value conflict. In so doing, they may wish to ask the following types of questions:

1. Which one of my values is in conflict with the patient's values in this patient-provider interaction? Can I specify my understanding of the patient's values?

2. Who is involved in handling the clinical problem and who is involved in resolving the ethical problem (e.g., patient, family, court, health care provider, etc.)?

3. Is it my role as a health care provider to make the clinical decisions? the ethical decisions? or both? The answers to these questions involve such considerations as: If it is my role to resolve the ethical decision, am I competent? Do I make the decision in isolation? Am I making the ethical decision because my role vis-à-vis the health profession allows me to assume responsibility in a wide variety of nonclinical areas? Or am I making the ethical decision because I assume my professional position implies my values have "more worth" or are "better than" the patient's?

4. What are the alternatives that may minimize the value conflicts for me as the health provider and for the patient? (The more realistic alternatives one can generate, the more likely the health provider will be able to resolve a value conflict.)

5. Does my decision seem to fit in with my overall value system—either personal or professional? And will it be acceptable to the patient's value system?

Any such series of questions obviously does not provide "right" answers, but it does offer a conceptual framework for handling the variety of value issues which accompany the clinical problems reviewed in these protocols.

These series of discriminating questions are more useful to the health provider if she or he can ask them in relation to very specific, narrowly defined values. Although personally held values may be vaguely stated, in resolving a value conflict, specification of the value under consideration is needed. For example, it would be relatively useless to say "I believe in informed consent." However, when the health professional more clearly defines this value as, "I believe in informed consent to the extent that the patient is able to understand

and utilize the clinical data," then the value becomes more precise. Clarifying the value at the outset of the ethical conflict should increase the likelihood of focusing the aforementioned questions; so although initially such a series of questions may appear cumbersome, health professionals can become as adroit with their own series of questions as they are with the process of differential diagnoses.

By alerting oneself to the value components that accompany these clinical protocols, health professionals are less likely to initiate a parternalistic relationship with their patients. Recognizing the patients' values in a clinical situation, health professionals are more likely to allow patients to participate in certain aspects of the treatment plan. By involving the patients and acknowledging the role of the patients' values in carrying out a treatment plan, compliance is improved. Moreover, to the extent that health professionals can acknowledge their own values and their patients' values, which are inherent in the patient-provider relationship, they are better able to provide high quality patient care.

REFERENCES

1. Bok, Sissela. "Commentary on Jerome Kaplan." In Tancredi, Laurence. *Ethics of Health Care*, Washington, D.C.: National Academy of Sciences, 1974, pp. 304–313.
2. Kuni (Hynes), Kathleen. "Application of Ethics." *Journal of Medical Education*, Vol. 50, 1975, 1000–1001.
3. Marshall, Becker. *The Health Belief Model*. Thoroughway, N.J.: Slack Company, 1976.

Contents

Contributing Authors   v

Acknowledgments   vii

Preface   xi

Introduction: Notes on Value
Conflicts in Patient Care   xv
KATHLEEN HYNES

Unit **I**   Protocols for Presenting Complaints in the Elderly   1

Chapter   1   **Acute Mono- and Polyarticular
Pain**   3
GAIL DE LA CRUZ

2   **Falls and Hip Injury**   64
COLLEEN BRODERICK, M. ERNESTINE
KOTTHOFF,
and LINDA J. PEARSON

3   **Hearing Deficit**   95
D. E. FARRELL

4   **Urinary Incontinence**   192
BEVERLY J. BAKKUM, M. ERNESTINE KOTTHOFF,
and LINDA J. PEARSON

5 Urinary Tract Infection 232
ELSIE M. BALINT

6 Peripheral Edema 270
JOYCE GILL

7 Skin Diseases 325
DODIE RUSSELL

Unit II Protocols for Chronic Conditions Common to the
Elderly 379

8 Constipation 381
COLLEEN BRODERICK, M. ERNESTINE
KOTTHOFF,
and LINDA J. PEARSON

9 Depression 410
M. ERNESTINE KOTTHOFF

10 Obesity 435
LINDA J. PEARSON

11 Dementia 469
AUDREY P. CORSON

12 Congestive Heart Failure 506
BEVERLY J. BAKKUM, M. ERNESTINE KOTTHOFF,
and LINDA J. PEARSON

13 Hypertension 540
IRENE SUZUKI

Index 584

Protocols for Presenting Complaints in the Elderly

Acute Mono- and Polyarticular Pain

OVERVIEW

Joint stiffness and pain are symptoms commonly associated with the aged population. These chief complaints are often erroneously attributed to degenerative joint disease, and little if any diagnostic or therapeutic intervention is instituted. The primary care provider must be alert to conditions that present in this manner and have a knowledge base of both normal and musculoskeletal physiology and an awareness of the various etiological agents of rheumatic disease.

Rheumatic diseases are defined as conditions associated with the presenting complaints of joint stiffness and/or pain. These disorders include conditions which affect the bone, ligaments, tendons, tendon sheaths, cartilage, fascia and periosteum. Rheumatic diseases may manifest 1) as an arthritis in which the joints themselves are inflamed, 2) a fibrositis in which the inflammation involves connective tissue structures around or near the joint or 3) a presentation of a systemic illness.

The disease processes may be either acute or chronic, have mono- or polyarticular involvement, or be secondary to known or unknown etiological agents. Thus, an accurate assessment of rheumatic disorders will depend on an adequate knowledge base of the types of connective tissue, the structure and function of joints and age-related changes pertinent to the elderly population.

There are three types of connective tissues important in rheumatic disorders: collagen, cartilage and bone. *Collagen* is a fibrous material that provides strength and support for tissues. It is a component part of bones and ligaments which hold bones together at the joints, and tendons which attach muscles to the bones. It also plays a role in tissue repair. *Cartilage* is the second type of connective tissue. There are two main types of cartilage: hyaline and fibrous. Cartilage, too, binds bones together or comprises structures (i.e., nose and larynx). *Bones* are the third type of connective tissue important in rheumatic disorders.

Joints are classified into three type fibrous, cartilaginous and synovial. Fibrous joints are attached by fibrous tissue, and very little if any motion occurs at this type of joint. Bones of a cartilaginous joint are united by hyaline cartilage or by fibrocartilage. Eventually hyaline cartilage joints are replaced by bone when growth ceases, for example cranial sutures. Examples of fibrocartilaginous joints are the intervertebral discs between the vertebrae. They provide stability and permit motion to the vertebral bodies.

Synovial joints are designed to permit free movement. They consist of rigid cartilage or cartilage covered bones united by a fibrous capsule that is lined by a synovial membrane. It is these joints that are most affected by arthritis. They are classified according to the shapes of the articular surfaces and the types of movement allowed. These are hinge, condylar, plane, pivot, saddle joints, and so on. During movement, synovial fluid circulates around the articular space and absorbs friction. These moving joints can, however, wear down with time and constant use or misuse; when joint lubrication becomes inefficient, articular cartilage will be quickly worn away due to the friction. Synovial tissue is a vascular connective tissue which contains blood vessels, lymphatic vessels, a few nerve fibers and a capillary network which is necessary in the production of synovial fluid. Thus, destruction in the site of a synovial joint is a serious problem.

In the aging process certain body structures lose their normal functioning capacity. Collagen, for example, loses resiliency and tends to calcify. Cartilage dries with age, loses elasticity, develops fissures, cracks and frays. Muscles may become flaccid and lose tonicity. In order to maintain normal joint function there must be adequate muscle contraction and joint mobility. This is a very important consideration in caring for the elderly patient who already, due to aging, has decreased muscle tone, decreased elasticity and resiliency of joint structures, decreased production of synovial fluid and probably impaired circulation.

Rheumatic diseases and the symptomatology associated with these disorders involve primarily the synovial joints and/or the periarticular structures that comprise joints. The common etiologic agents of rheumatic disease include infection, immune response, traumatic or neurogenic causes. The assessment section of this protocol has been divided into those conditions that predominantly present as mono- or polyarticular involvement, and some common periarticular entities seen in the elderly will be briefly discussed. However, the reader must remember that the classifications herein provided are done with the knowledge that some of the entities classified as either mono- or polyarticular *may* present as either, for there is no absolute classification system.

ACUTE MONO- AND POLYARTICULAR PAIN WORKSHEET

To be used for patients with pain in and around the joint(s).

> *What you can not afford to miss: monoarticular—septic arthritis, gout, episodic rheumatoid arthritis, mechanical tuberculous arthritis, osteoarthritis, pseudogout, neurogenic arthropathy, serum sickness, inflammatory intestinal disease, tumors, osteoporosis. Polyarticular—degenerative joint disease, psoriatic arthritis, acute rheumatic fever, collagen vascular diseases, cervical spondylosis, hypothyroidism.*

Chief Complaint: _____

SUBJECTIVE DATA:

Onset (sudden, gradual, date): _____

Location: _____

Frequency (number of episodes): _____

Duration of episodes: _____

Precipitated by: _____

Made worse by: _____

Relieved by: _____

Not relieved by: _____

Acute Mono- and Polyarticular Pain Worksheet

Course (constant, progressive, intermittent): _____

Describe previous episodes: _____

Quality of pain: _____

Time relationship (A.M., P.M.): _____

Associated with: _____

Describe Positive Responses Using the Proper Descriptors:

LOCAL SYMPTOMS:
YES   NO

_____ _____ Trauma: (date) _____ (type) _____

_____ _____ Swelling: _____

_____ _____ Stiffness: (time relationship) _____

                (A.M.) _____ (P.M.) _____

                (after rest) _____

_____ _____ Inflammation (i.e., redness, heat): _____

_____ _____ Discoloration: _____

_____ _____ Decreased range of motion: _____

_____ _____ Pain on motion: _____

SYSTEMIC SYMPTOMS:
YES   NO

_____ _____ Fever/chills: _____

(high grade)＿＿   (low grade)＿＿

(intermittent) ＿＿＿＿＿＿＿＿＿＿＿＿＿＿＿＿＿

＿＿ ＿＿ Sweats: ＿＿＿＿＿＿＿＿＿＿＿＿＿

＿＿ ＿＿ Fatigue:＿＿＿＿＿＿＿＿＿＿＿＿＿

＿＿ ＿＿ Weight loss: ＿＿＿＿＿＿＿＿＿＿＿

＿＿ ＿＿ Malaise:＿＿＿＿＿＿＿＿＿＿＿＿＿

＿＿ ＿＿ Skin/nails: ＿＿＿＿＿＿＿＿＿＿＿＿

(rashes)＿＿＿＿＿＿ (lesions) ＿＿＿＿＿＿

RESPIRATORY SYMPTOMS:
YES   *NO*

＿＿ ＿＿ Cough: ＿＿＿＿＿＿＿＿＿＿＿＿＿

＿＿ ＿＿ Sputum (color, amount, consistency): ＿＿＿

＿＿ ＿＿ Dyspnea: ＿＿＿＿＿＿＿＿＿＿＿＿

＿＿ ＿＿ Sore throat approximately three weeks previously: ＿

＿＿ ＿＿ Other: ＿＿＿＿＿＿＿＿＿＿＿＿＿

GASTROINTESTINAL SYMPTOMS:
YES   *NO*

＿＿ ＿＿ Abdominal pain/cramping: ＿＿＿＿＿＿＿

＿＿ ＿＿ Diarrhea (bloody):＿＿＿＿＿＿＿＿＿＿

＿＿ ＿＿ Nausea, vomiting: ＿＿＿＿＿＿＿＿＿

GENITOURINARY TRACT SYMPTOMS:
YES   *NO*

＿＿ ＿＿ Urethritis/dysuria:＿＿＿＿＿＿＿＿＿＿

_____ _____ Penile/vaginal discharge (color, amount): _____

_____ _____ Hematuria: _____

_____ _____ Polyuria: _____

PAST MEDICAL HISTORY:
YES   *NO*

_____ _____ Allergies (describe reaction and source): _____

_____ _____ Venereal disease (date, treatment, course): _____

_____ _____ Alcoholism: _____

_____ _____ Diabetes mellitus: _____

_____ _____ Rheumatic fever: _____

_____ _____ Urinary tract infections: _____

_____ _____ Endocrine disorder: _____

_____ _____ Tuberculosis (date, treatment, course): _____

_____ _____ Other diseases or infections (describe): _____

_____ _____ Hospitalizations (date, cause, treatment, outcome):
_____

_____ _____ Current medications (kind, how taken): _____

_____ _____ Recent injections (kind, site) (especially note intraar-

ticular injections) _____

_____ _____ Immunizations (tuberculin test): _____

(date)_____ (result)_____

(other)_____

NEUROLOGIC SYMPTOMS:
YES   NO

_____ _____ Numbness:_____

_____ _____ Paresthesia: _____

_____ _____ Paralysis: _____

_____ _____ Headache: _____

FAMILY HISTORY:
YES   NO

_____ _____ Gout, rheumatoid arthritis, diabetes mellitus:_____

_____ _____ Tuberculosis, ulcerative colitis, hypertension: _____

_____ _____ Cerebrovascular accident (CVA), cancer, psoriasis,

endocrine disorders: _____

_____ _____ Other: _____

OBJECTIVE DATA: (Describe All Positive Responses)
General appearance:_____

Vital signs: _____Temp. _____Blood pressure _____

Pulse _____Resp. _____Weight _____

Posture: _____

Gait:_____

Acute Mono- and Polyarticular Pain Worksheet

EXAMINATION OF INVOLVED JOINT(S):

*0−3+ scale for heat, swelling, tenderness and pain on motion (POM)

Joints	Heat		Swelling		Tenderness		POM	
	R	L	R	L	R	L	R	L
Temporomandibular								
Sternoclavicular								
Shoulder								
Elbow								
Wrist								
Metacarpophalangeal								
Proximal interphalangeal								
Distal interphalangeal								
Hip								
Knee								
Ankle								
Tarsal								
Metatarsophalangeal								
C spine								
T spine								
L spine								

*From C.M. Hudak, P.M. Redstone, N.L. Hokanson, I.E. Suzuki. Clinical Protocols: A Guide for Nurses and Physicians: Philadelphia: J.B. Lippincott Co., 1976, p. 433.

EXAMINATION OF INVOLVED JOINT(S):
YES   NO

_____ _____ Lesions/rashes: _____

_____ _____ Nodules: _____

_____ _____ Draining areas: _____

_____ _____ Cellulitis:_____

_____ _____ Tissue induration:_____

_____ _____ Deformity: _____

_____ _____ Crepitation: _____

_____ _____ Limitation of range of motion: _____

_____ _____ Immobility: _____

_____ _____ Atrophy of surrounding muscles: _____

_____ _____ Tenosynovitis: _____

_____ _____ Discoloration:_____

GENERAL PHYSICAL EXAMINATION: (DESCRIBE ALL POSITIVES)
YES   NO

_____ _____ Lymphadenopathy: _____

Thorax:

_____ _____ Abnormal breath sounds: _____

_____ _____ Abnormal fremitus: _____

_____ _____ Abnormal excursion: _____

_____ _____ Cardiac abnormalities (rubs, murmurs, thrill):_____

_____ _____ Tachycardia:_____

Abdomen:

_____ _____ Tenderness: _____

_____ _____ Masses: _____

Genitalia:

_____ _____ Discharge, foul odor:_____

_____ _____ Lesions, inflammation: _____

_____ _____ Tenderness on palpation of adnexae or cervix: _____

_____ _____ Tenderness on palpation of penis, epididymis, scrotum, testes: _____

Neurologic:

_____ _____ Cranial nerves (not intact):_____

_____ _____ Paresthesia: _____

_____ _____ Abnormal deep tendon reflexes (DTR's): _____

_____ _____ Paresis: _____

_____ _____ Pain (location): _____

Rectal:

_____ _____ Prostate (note size, tenderness, consistency): _____

_____ _____ Discharge: _____

_____ _____ Pain: _____

_____ _____ Blood in stool: _____

Skin/Nails:

_____ _____ Rashes, lesions, scales, nodules: _____

LAB DATA:

The following represents a list of the lab data that should be obtained on patients presenting with an undiagnosed joint pain. Additional tests may be necessary to complete a diagnosis; if a particular entity is suspect by the history and physical, obtain the appropriate additional studies as indicated in the assessment section.

LAB DATA FOR *MONOARTICULAR* PRESENTATION: (DESCRIBE RESULTS)

DONE   **NOT DONE**

_____ _____ Complete blood count (CBC) with differential:_____

_____ _____ Chest x-ray: _____

_____ _____ Urinalysis: _____

_____ _____ X-ray of involved joint: _____

_____ _____ Joint fluid analysis: _____

_____

_____ _____ Erythrocyte sedimentation rate (ESR):_____

_____ _____ Serum uric acid: _____

LAB DATA FOR *POLYARTICULAR* PRESENTATION: (DESCRIBE RESULTS)

SAME TESTS AS ABOVE, IN ADDITION ADD:

_____ _____ Thyroid function tests: _____

_____ _____ Rheumatoid factor and titer:_____

_____ _____ Antinuclear antibody (ANA) and titer: _____

The following lab tests should be added to the above if the history and/or physical exam have increased your suspicions for the following clinical entities:

_____ _____ ASO titer (to rule out rheumatic fever, history of strep infection): _____

_____ _____ Acid Phos (to rule out prostatic cancer metastasis to bone especially in elderly males with an abnormal prostate exam): _____

_____ _____ TB test, joint fluid/sputum for Acid Fast Bacilli (to rule out tuberculosis): _____

_____ _____ Gonococcal (GC) culture—urethral, cervix, rectum, pharynx, joint fluid—(to rule out gonorrhea): _____

_____ _____ Blood culture (to rule out systemic involvement of septic arthritis): _____

_____ _____ Nerve conduction tests (to confirm carpal tunnel):

ACUTE MONO- AND POLYARTICULAR PAIN WORKSHEET RATIONALE

SUBJECTIVE DATA:

Onset   Helps differentiate acute from chronic disease processes. Sudden onset may follow trauma or overindulgence in food or alcohol (as in the patient with gout), and rheumatoid arthritis usually has an abrupt onset. Gradual onset may be associated with rapid weight gain and obesity (osteoarthrosis).

Location

Be specific when indicating which joint is affected. It is important to note whether or not the pain is located in the joint or surrounding structures. *Note the presentation pattern* (i.e., migratory, symmetrical, assymmetrical). A migratory and monoarticular presentation is usually seen in arthritis associated with rheumatic fever. Symmetrical involvement (especially of the metacarpophalangeal (MCP) or proximal interphalangeal (PIP) joints of hand) is seen in rheumatoid arthritis. Asymmetrical involvement of the distal interphalangeal (DIP) joints of the hands and/or weight-bearing joints is seen in degenerative joint disease.

Frequency,

A good history about the frequency of episodes can give a good indication of the disease process. Discomfort may occur routinely after certain recreational or occupational activities as is common in osteoarthrosis, or after overindulgence in food or alcohol as is commonly seen in patients with gout. Episodic rheumatoid arthritis occurs frequently with immobilizing manifestations.

Duration

Note whether symptoms are intermittent and characterized by symptom free periods or constant and progressive. Stiffness that persists for several hours after awakening is usually associated with rheumatoid arthritis in contrast to the pain and stiffness of osteoarthritis which persists for a shorter time. Symptoms are constant and progressive in the presence of untreated septic arthritis, osteomyelitis, tuberculous arthritis, gonococcal arthritis and trauma. In gout the attack usually lasts three to five days; if untreated it may last for several weeks.

Precipitated By

Obtain a thorough history of activities, prolonged inactivity or trauma (even though the traumatic event may not be recent). Note also the administration of any medication to which the patient may be allergic (suspect arthritis associated with serum sickness), a diet history (may indicate gout), or previous illnesses (i.e., ulcerative colitis, psoriasis, etc.).

Made Worse By

Weather changes and activity tend to aggravate osteoarthritis, inactivity makes rheumatoid arthritis worse and a diet of highly seasoned foods and alcohol tends to aggravate gout.

Relieved By
Not Relieved By

Note those drugs or therapies used which have been beneficial or not helpful. Ask about drugs that are used for relief (e.g., salycilates, cortisone preparations). Be alert for any drug that may mask other symptoms (such as prednisone). Rest and heat relieve osteoarthritic pain. In addition, the patient's response to these questions will give a good indication of his or her cultural habits regarding self-treatment and compliance.

Course and Quality Of Pain	Note whether the patient's condition has worsened since the first attack or remained the same.
Previous Episodes	Describing previous episodes may act as a "cross reference" for the patient to remember when these symptoms previously occurred, what they are associated with and what precipitates them.
Quality	Sudden, severe pain in the thoracic or lumbar spine indicates a more severe problem such as a herniated disc, malignancy or osteoporosis with collapse.
Time Relationship	Pain not related to time indicates an infectious etiology. Pain that is worse after awakening in the A.M. indicates rheumatoid arthritis. Pain that is worse during certain seasons could be caused by allergies, allergy medications or serum sickness.
Associated With	Joint pain can be associated with gastrointestinal symptomatology in inflammatory bowel disease (e.g., ulcerative colitis, regional ileitis and Whipple's disease). Joint pain in association with the complaint of vaginal discharge, abdominal pain or fever or chills could indicate gonorrhea. A complaint of joint pain associated with weight loss, cough, hemoptysis and night sweats may indicate tuberculosis as the etiology. Joint pain associated with a petechial rash, fever and hematuria may indicate a diagnosis of serum sickness. There is an increased in-

cidence of pseudogout associated with diabetes. In addition, some rheumatic diseases have an increased incidence when endocrine disorders are present (e.g., patients with hyperparathroidism and diabetes have a higher incidence of pseudogout).

Local Symptoms

Trauma

The patient may not give a recent history of trauma. He or she may not remember to look for signs noted later in the physical exam. Pathologic fractures can occur without significant pain in the elderly when osteoporosis or malignancy exists.

Swelling

Describe the exact location of the swelling, and swelling in any other involved structures. Ask the patient to describe the consistency of the swelling: filled with fluid, hard, etc.

Stiffness

This may be confused with a *reluctance* to move the joint(s) due to pain. Establish the presence of pain *versus* stiffness or pain *and* stiffness or deformity. Stiffness with associated pain may also be secondary to spasms of surrounding muscles.

Inflammation

Usually does not occur with osteoarthritis, cervical spondylosis, neuropathic arthropathy or serum sickness.

Discoloration

Discoloration may be helpful in determining a traumatic event or bleeding, although it may be difficult to see on a dark-skinned patient. Erythema is seen in traumatic or inflammatory arthritis (e.g., septic joints).

Immobilizing

Immobilization may occur as a result of stiffness after prolonged rest as in rheumatoid arthritis. Osteoarthritis pain is increased with activity and decreased by rest. Immobilization due to deformity is seen in far advanced chronic diseases. If the pain is severe the patient may *voluntarily* immobilize the part. If this occurs for a prolonged period it may cause atrophy of the involved muscles and weakness.

Decreased and/or pain on range of motion (ROM)

Describe type, quality, location, etc. Describe limitation of movement (LOM) and if the limitation is associated with pain. Describe the type of activity that causes pain: flexion, extension, rotation, etc.

Systemic Symptoms
Fever, chills

The pattern of fever or chills will help in diagnosing a bacterial infection. Unfortunately, this sign may be minimal or absent in the elderly. Fever/chills may be seen in acute rheumatic fever, polymyalgia rheumatica, inflammatory bowel disease, suppurative arthritis, or tuberculosis.

Sweats

Although sometimes absent in the elderly, sweats may indicate an extraarticular systemic problem.

Fatigue

It is important to elicit possible causative factors (e.g., overactivity, pain, underlying disease, known existing chronic disease, etc.).

19

Weight loss
Malaise

Weight loss and/or malaise are prodromal symptoms which may indicate a systemic problem. It may be seen in arthritis associated with inflammatory bowel disease or tuberculosis.

Skin/nails:
rashes, lesions

Rashes or lesions frequently accompany arthritic conditions such as psoriatic arthritis, rheumatoid arthritis, serum sickness or disseminated gonorrhea.

Respiratory Symptoms
Cough
Sputum
Dyspnea

Symptoms of an underlying respiratory disease are associated with tuberculosis or pneumonia. The causative organism of a lower respiratory infection may cause bacteremia in the elderly. Hypertrophic osteoarthropathy has a 5 to 10 percent rate of incidence in patients with bronchogenic cancer and pleural tumors.

Sore throat

A previously undiagnosed "strep throat" can progress into an undetected bacteremia in the elderly; the joint affliction usually has a migratory pattern (rheumatic fever).

Gastrointestinal Symptoms
Abdominal pain/
cramping

Abdominal pain may accompany serum sickness and intestinal disorders (e.g., ulcerative colitis).

Diarrhea

Diarrhea can be seen in suppurative arthritis secondary to salmonella or inflammatory bowel diseases (e.g., regional enteritis, ulcerative colitis). Bloody diarrhea and arthritis can be present in association with ulcerative colitis.

Nausea and vomiting	Nausea and vomiting associated with joint pain can indicate serum sickness.
Genitourinary Symptoms Urethritis with dysuria Penile/vaginal discharge	Urethritis (inflammation) and dysuria secondary to the underlying infection and/or inflammation may be seen in gonorrhea or Reiter's syndrome. However, Reiter's is commonly associated with the triad of symptoms: urethritis, conjunctivitis, and arthritis. Penile or vaginal discharge in association with joint pains may be indicative of a disseminated gonococcal infection.
Hematuria	Hematuria may be indicative of an underlying collagen vascular disease or serum sickness.
Polyuria	Polyuria may indicate an endocrine disturbance. Diabetes mellitus is associated with an increased incidence of pseudogout as well as an increased incidence of neuropathic joints.
Past Medical History Allergies	Medical records from previous treatment may be available which would help facilitate future therapy in case the patient is having any allergic manifestations. Serum sickness and its associated arthritis is an immune complex (allergic reaction) phenomenon.
Venereal disease	Inadequate therapy, resistant organisms or noncompliance to a treatment plan for gonorrhea could result in a progression of the disease

to a bacteremia with arthritis being the presenting symptom.

Alcoholism

A general debilitating condition predisposes the elderly person to an infectious process. In addition, alcoholics may have neurogenic arthropathy.

Diabetes mellitus

Diabetes mellitus, if uncontrolled, can be a predisposing factor to other diseases such as osteomyelitis, infectious arthritis, pseudogout, gout and neuropathic arthropathy.

Rheumatic fever

Rheumatic fever associated with streptococcal pharyngitis may be confused with rheumatoid arthritis because of polyarthritic symptoms. One distinguishing factor of rheumatic fever is that the joints are usually involved one at a time and follow a migratory pattern.

Urinary tract infections

Urinary tract infections are a predisposing factor in the elderly for bacteremia, osteomyelitis or infectious arthritis. Symptoms of a urinary tract infection (e.g. dysuria, frequency, etc.) may be the presentation of a gonococcal infection.

Endocrine disorder

Hyperparathyroidism and diabetes are endocrine disorders associated with an increased incidence of pseudogout. In addition, hypothyroidism may present as joint pain.

Tuberculosis

Tubercular infection of the skeletal system is spread from a primary lesion located in the respiratory or gastrointestinal tract. Tubercular infections of the musculoskeletal system may be seen in the debilitated geriatric patient.

Other diseases and infections

Renal disease or manifestations of kidney insufficiency may be more readily observed in the older individual because renal function declines with advancing age causing fluid or electrolyte imbalance. Nephropathy and neuropathic arthropathy are common complications of diabetes.

The clinical complications of ulcerative colitis may include polyarthritis, which may increase with an exacerbation of gastrointestinal symptoms.

Regional ileitis may take various clinical patterns including arthralgias. Whipple's disease may rarely include polyarthritis.

Hospitalizations

Knowledge of hospitalizations will give insight into the patient's general health and any chronic problems that may presently affect him or her.

Current medications injections, immunizations

The history of current medications is necessary when establishing therapy to prevent drug interaction and overdosing. This will also give an indication of possible causes of serum sickness if this is suspected. Iatrogenic lupuslike syndromes are caused by high doses of certain antihypertensive agents. If tuberculous arthritis is suspected obtain results of a recent or previous TB skin test. Other immunizations (e.g., tetanus or diptheria) may be cause of serum sickness. Neuropathic joints may occur secondary to injudicious use of intraarticular steroid injections.

Neurologic Symptoms

Numbness

Numbness in an extremity indicates nerve root compression or direct cord compression. Numbness may be seen in: 1) carpal tunnel syndrome secondary to median nerve compression, 2) degenerative joint disease secondary to osteophyte compression or 3) rheumatoid arthritis secondary to synovitis.

Paresthesia

Hypersensitivity of the dermatomes indicating direct cord or nerve root compression may be seen in carpal tunnel syndrome, degenerative joint disease and rheumatoid arthritis.

Paralysis

Central paralysis affects the movement of the limb as a whole and is produced by damage to the spinal cord. Peripheral paralysis affects individual muscles or groups of muscles. Peripheral paralysis can be produced by a physical or chemical neuritis or a diseased state of a nerve. Paralysis may be secondary to osteoporosis with collapse or disc disease.

Headache

Ninety percent of headaches in the elderly are muscle tension headaches; however, cervical arthritis and polymyalgia rheumatica are common causes of such headaches.

Family History

Some of these diseases appear to be genetically transmitted or have familial tendencies: endocrine disorders (e.g., diabetes mellitus), psoriasis, pseudogout, gout and hypertension. A family history can indicate a patient's tendencies toward that disease.

OBJECTIVE DATA:

General Appearance

Begin the survey upon meeting the patient. Assess the apparent state of health, any signs of distress, stature and posture. In cases of severe debilitation or obvious systemic infection it is necessary to assess the patient quickly in order to initiate treatment promptly.

Vital Signs

Vital signs are very important indicators of infectious processes or the presence of pain. The determination of a baseline is important. Vital signs may be altered due to medications that the patient may have been taking.

Weight

Note the norms for the patient's age group. Obesity complicates many diseases. Being underweight may indicate a metabolic disorder, a poor appetite or a socioeconomic problem.

Posture

Differentiate between changes in posture secondary to the normal aging process or improper posture due to pain, infection or deformity from disease, etc. Some age-related skeletal changes which may be observed are kyphosis and an increased prominence of bones due to muscle atrophy. Various peripheral nerve injuries produce characteristic postural changes such as wrist drop, claw hand, ape hand, winged scapula and shoulder drop.

Examination of
Involved Joint(s)
0–3+ Scale for heat swelling, tenderness and POM

This critical elicitation will aid in classifying and diagnosing the rheumatic syndrome as inflammatory or degenerative.

Lesions/rashes
Nodules—draining areas
Cellulitis

Describe according to anatomic distribution, configuration of groups and the morphology of lesions. Lesions or rashes may be seen in psoriasis, gonorrhea and serum sickness. The inflammation associated with gout and pseudogout resembles cellulitis with superficial desquammation and a tense, shiny appearance.

Tissue induration

There may be tissue induration present in arthritis. In arthralgias there will be no induration.

Deformity

May be characteristic of certain chronic rheumatic diseases. For example, subluxation of metacarpophalangeal joints with ulnar deviation of digits are hand deformities characteristic of rheumatoid arthritis. Deformities can be the result of a long-standing, progressive disease as in degenerative joint disease. Kyphosis may be present in osteoporosis, or may be seen as a result of the normal aging process.

Crepitation	A dry, crackling sound or sensation such as that produced by grating of ends of bone fragments may indicate joint damage. Crepitation is seen frequently with joint pain from an old injury. It may or may not be associated with pain.
Limitation of ROM	Assess the function of the musculoskeletal system through a thorough evaluation of the patient's ability to perform activities of daily living, for example, the ability to lean over, grasp, pinch, sit down, rise, etc. A passive ROM test of all joints should also be done.
Immobility	Evaluate by inspection and palpation while going through ROM and note the presence of stiffness or fixation of a joint (ankylosis). Also note instability of a joint.
Atrophy of surrounding muscles	Muscles will atrophy from disuse or a decrease in nerve conduction. Notice areas that appear retracted with prominent tendons; this indicates the extent of disuse of the part. Atrophy of muscles may be seen in tuberculous arthritis and carpal tunnel syndrome. Note that some atrophy in muscle groups occurs as a result of aging.
Tenosynovitis	Extreme tenderness or pain may be elicited by palpation of involved tendons of patients who have gonococcal arthritis; they usually experience tenosynovitis of the hand and foot. Shaking chills may often precede or accompany the synovitis. Tenosynovitis may also be seen

27

in tuberculous and rheumatoid arthritis.

Discoloration

Discoloration may be from bruising, secondary to trauma or redness from inflammation of infection.

General Physical Examination
Lymphadenopathy

Lymph node enlargement is a sign of infection in the area which is drained by the lymph system. Regional lymphadenopathy is seen in tuberculosis, GC and suppurative arthritis.

Thorax

Look for signs of a lower respiratory infection such as pneumonia. Note that in the older patient breath sounds may be distant due to kyphosis; excursion may be reduced because of poor muscle expansion. Listen for cardiac rubs and murmurs, which may be heard in patients suffering from rheumatic fever. Tachycardia may occur with fever and may be indicative of an underlying infectious process.

Abdomen

Abdominal pain can be a symptom of osteomyelitis of the vertebrae or a referred pain from cancer of the bone or spine. Abdominal pain can also be present with serum sickness.

Genitalia

Tenderness or inflammation are signs of an infection which may be the primary cause of the joint pain.

Neurologic

If neurologic responses of the upper extremities are abnormal, consider nerve root compression in area of C1–7 and thoracic vertebrae. Deep tendon reflexes of the lower extremities may be more difficult to elicit from the elderly individual normally but particularly in the diabetic or the patient with degenerative joint disease, neuropathic arthropathy and others. Ankle reflexes are frequently absent in the elderly. Paresthesis is sometimes noted in patients in the early stages of rheumatoid arthritis, carpal tunnel, or degenerative joint disease caused by a nerve root encroachment.

Rectal

Prostatitis may be acute or chronic. Prostatitis may be caused by gonorrhea (especially secondary to rectal intercourse). Chronic prostatitis may include symptoms of lumbosacral backache. Cancer of the prostate frequently metastasizes to bone; the patient may present with backache and/or a pathological fracture. Rectal pain or discharge may be a sign of infection (e.g., gonorrhea). Rectal bleeding may be seen in rectosigmoid malignancy, fissures or colitis.

Skin/nails

Nail pitting is seen in psoriasis. Nodules on the bony prominences are seen in rheumatoid arthritis, gout (tophi) and degenerative joint disease (Herberden's or Bouchard's nodes). Cutaneous lesions may be seen in disseminated gonorrhea. Rashes are seen in psoriasis and purpuric lesions are seen in serum sickness.

Lab Data

CBC with ·differential

Helps to determine the presence of infection. *Leukopenia*: Found in the presence of viral infections, overwhelming bacterial infection, septicemia or miliary tuberculosis (due to a poor immunologic response). Leukopenia may also be found in the presence of certain types of drugs (sulfonamides, antibiotics, analgesics, marrow depressants, antithyroid drugs and others).

Leukocytosis: Found in acute bacterial infections (e.g., pneumonia, abscess formation), metabolic disturbances (acute gout), serum sickness and in acute generalized infections (e.g., rheumatic fever).

Monocytosis: Seen in tuberculosis.

Eosinophilia: Allergic diseases and occasionally collagen vascular diseases.

Chest x-ray

Review reports of old films as well as recent ones in order to rule out the presence of pneumonia, tuberculosis, pleural effusion, abscesses and mass lesions and to monitor the course of the underlying disease that may present as joint pain.

Urinalysis

A urinalysis is done to detect bacteruria, sugar, protein and other indicators of kidney diseases including red blood cells, casts and crystals.

X-ray of joint(s)

All patients presenting with acute arthritic symptoms need radiologic studies to detect bone abnormalities. In cases where a metabolic disorder is suspected, a more thorough bone survey may be needed.

Joint fluid analysis

Analysis of the synovial fluid includes a culture and sensitivity, white blood cell count, cellular count, crystal exam and an exam for blood.

Erythrocyte sedimentation rate (ESR)

The ESR is a nonspecific test that is elevated in any inflammatory process. It can be a useful test to assist in the differentiation between osteoarthritis (no elevation) and other rheumatic diseases (i.e., an elevation is seen in collagen vascular diseases, rheumatoid arthritis, etc.).

Serum uric acid

The uric acid level is important to know; it is elevated in gout and psoriasis. Knowing the patient's level can help in the differential diagnosis. Other conditions in which the uric acid is elevated are malignancies, renal disease or polycythemia.

Thyroid function test

Low thyroid function tests may indicate hypothyroidism as a potential cause of joint pains.

Rheumatoid factor and titer

Gives useful objective evidence of rheumatoid arthritis; however, a negative rheumatoid factor test does not rule out rheumatoid arthritis. It is positive in 5 percent of rheumatoid variants (arthritis associated with psoriasis, ulcerative colitis, regional enteritis). It is negative in approximately 15 percent of patients with definite rheumatoid arthritis. The level of the titer is not a good indication of the severity of the disease; however, it has been shown that in patients with very high titers the outlook is bleaker than for those patients who are seronegative.

ANA

The ANA is positive in rheumatoid arthritis and collagen vascular diseases (e.g., lupus).

ASSESSMENT:

Rheumatic diseases can be classified into the monoarthritic group and the polyarthritic group. This classification has been made based on the entity's most common presentation.

Monoarticular

Monoarticular diseases affect only one joint but may eventually migrate to other joints or affect only one joint at a time. Some of the more common conditions in this group that often affect the elderly are septic (infectious) arthritis, gout, episodic rheumatoid arthritis, mechanical injury (trauma), tuberculous arthritis, pseudogout, neurogenic arthropathy, serum sickness, inflammatory intestinal diseases, tumors, osteoporosis.

Septic (infectious) arthritis

This is a medical emergency; if not treated rapidly septic arthritis will increase in severity, causing destruction of the joint (the purulent matter causes a release of proteolytic enzymes that destroy the joint). Elderly persons are particularly

susceptible to septic arthritis because they have more than one predisposing factor. Some predisposing factors are 1) underlying chronic
disease such as diabetes mellitus,
malignancy, alcoholism, uremia, 2)
extraarticular infections such as
pneumonia, bacterial endocarditis,
urinary tract infections, osteomyelitis and skin infections, 3) use of
immunosuppressive drugs and corticosteroids (high incidence in people with rheumatoid arthritis).

The most common mode of infection is from hematogenous spread.
The onset of joint manifestations
usually occurs within several days
after the introduction of the causative organism, which in some cases
may result from joint aspiration, injection, or contiguous osteomyelitis.
Joints commonly affected are large
joints, i.e., hip, shoulder, knees; occasionally the ankles, elbows, ster-
nocleidomastoid, and other joints
may be affected. When the hip is
affected the pain may be referred to
the knee; the patient may hold the
leg in adduction and internal rotation. The patient may guard the affected joint and the surrounding
muscles may have spasms. The onset is usually abrupt. The patient
will usually present with pain, heat,
swelling, redness and tenderness in
a joint; however, these symptoms
may be masked in an individual
who is taking adrenocorticosteroids
or immunosuppressive agents. Also,
joints such as the hip may not present with signs of inflammation as

evident as in those closer to the skin surface.

A diagnosis is made by joint aspiration and by isolation of the causative microbe which aids in differentiating between suppurative and nonsuppurative joint diseases. In suppurative arthritis the patient will have fever, usually high grade; a high grade fever is rare in noninfectious joint diseases. Microorganisms commonly responsible for infectious arthritis are staphylococcus, streptococcus, gonococcus, and a variety of gram negative organisms.

Joint aspiration must be done in acute monoarticular arthritis to rule out a septic arthritis, to decrease pressure, and to remove purulent matter. An examination of synovial fluid should include culture and sensitivity, gram stain, and a crystal exam.

Initial laboratory studies may show the patient has a leukocytosis with immature leukocytes being elevated on the differential. The ESR will be elevated.

Gout

Gout is a paroxysmal, metabolic disease characterized by hyperuricemia. The hyperuricemia is caused by one or a combination of the following: increased absorption, decreased metabolism, decreased excretion or increased biosynthesis of uric acid which is the end product of purine metabolism. Gout, therefore, is classified into metabolic gout (excessive synthesis) and renal gout (reduced clearance or iatrogenic gout secondary to such drugs as thiazides or aspirin).

While clinical gout can be divided into four categories (acute gouty arthritis, tophaceous gout, uric acid nephrolithiasis, and gouty kidney), acute gouty arthritis is the most common. The peak incidence of clinical gout occurs in men in the fifth decade, with the incidence in women rising after menopause. Gouty arthritis is an inflammatory reaction to the precipitation of microcrystals of sodium urate in the joint. The exact mechanism by which sodium urate crystals initiate inflammation has not been established. The first attack is usually monoarticular. The acute onset develops over several hours; the average attack lasts three to five days, but if untreated may last several weeks. Signs and symptoms include severe pain and tenderness, periarticular swelling, erythema and low grade fever. After the initial attack subsides most patients will have a recurrence within the first year; subsequent attacks will occur more frequently if underlying hyperurecemia is untreated.

An acute attack may occur after taking diuretics for cardiac or renal disease. It may occur following minor trauma, overindulgence in food or alcohol or after surgery. It exhibits a predilection for the larger joints, particularly in the feet and ankles. The picture classically involves the

metatarsal phalangeal articulation
of the great toe.

Diagnosis is made from observation
of the acute symptoms and signs
and from the dramatic relief obtained from the administration of
colchicine and indomethacin. Examination of the synovial fluid will
demonstrate the needlelike crystals
of sodium urate.

Lab: Leukocytosis and an increased
serum uric acid level are usually
present; however, uric acid may not
be elevated if the patient is on a
therapeutic regimen of ACTH, high
doses of salicylates, cortisone or
coumarins.

**Episodic rheumatoid
arthritis**

Monoarticular attacks of rheumatoid arthritis, while not common,
occur sufficiently frequently to be
sometimes confused with other diseases affecting the joints. The differentiation must be made by elimination of other possibilities and a
documentation of definitive signs
and symptoms of rheumatoid arthritis.

In episodic rheumatoid arthritis the
onset is usually abrupt with immobilizing joint manifestations developing over a period of 12 to 20
hours; however, the onset more
often develops over a period of
days. Clinical symptoms include
stiffness (particularly noticeable on
awakening in the morning), fever,
sweats, fatigue, articular pain,

swelling, redness, warmth and tenderness.

Patients with chronic rheumatoid arthritis usually manifest symmetrical polyarthritis in the course of their disease whereas patients with episodic rheumatoid arthritis may have inflammation limited to only one or two joints. Occasionally the monoarthritis may persist for many weeks or months.

Muscle atrophy of the affected extremity may be evident within weeks of onset. Deformities are seen as a result of the sustained chronic disease.

Lab: Mild anemia is common. Leukocytosis may be present. In addition, an eosinophila or a thrombocytopenia are occasional laboratory features. The ESR is increased above the normal range during the active phase. The rheumatoid factor is usually positive. The ANA test is positive in 60 to 70 percent of patients. An examination of synovial fluid will show a low viscosity and decreased glucose. Refer to rheumatoid arthritis under the polyarticular pain section for further information.

Mechanical injury

In the absence of a known direct trauma, diagnosis may be made by the exclusion of other findings and the presence of bloody or xanthochromic synovial fluid. An x-ray film will usually reveal joint effusion.

The joint fluid will contain a lowered white count and normal viscosity. The ESR will be normal.

Tuberculous arthritis

One of the most serious diseases of the articular tissues, tuberculous arthritis, is curable if diagnosed rapidly and treated. If untreated, the condition may lead to complete destruction of the joint.

The onset is usually insidious with a monoarticular presentation; however, in rare cases the initial manifestation may be that of a transient migratory polyarthritis. The joints most often affected are the thoracic spine, hips and knees. Usually, the primary site of the tuberculosis is pulmonary. Infection of the spine may lead to destruction of bone and vertebral collapse.

Frequent associated findings are a positive tuberculin skin test, previous history of a pleural effusion and/or a family history of tuberculosis.

Systemic signs and symptoms include fever, chills, weight loss, night sweats, cough and hemoptysis. Local symptoms include pain, stiffness, swelling, atrophy of surrounding muscles, tenderness to palpation and joint effusions. The joint may be boggy or have a doughlike consistency because of hypertrophy of the synovium.

In the absence of a proven associated tuberculosis, diagnosis may require tissue biopsy of regional lymph nodes, synovial fluid cultures for acid-fast bacilli, TB skin test and x-rays. The course of the untreated disease is usually marked by destruction of the joint, but spontaneous remissions sometimes occur.

Chondrocalcinosis (pseudogout)

Pseudogout is most often seen in persons 60 years of age or older; there is no sexual preference. Chondrocalcinosis refers to the presence of calcium-containing salts in the articular cartilage; it is usually diagnosed through radiologic studies showing classic calcification of the articular surfaces. Blood and urine findings are normal.

The most commonly affected sites are the knees, the hips and infrequently the great toe. It is commonly associated with metabolic disorders such as diabetes mellitus, and hyperparathyroidism.

The onset is typically acute; it may involve only one joint or it may progress to involve several joints. The affected joints will be painful, reddened and swollen. Aspiration of joint fluid reveals calcium pyrophosphate crystals.

The acute episode usually subsides in one to two weeks; between attacks the affected joint is normal. In subsequent attacks the same joint is usually involved.

Neurogenic arthropathy

Neurogenic arthropathy (also known as Charcot joints) is joint destruction resulting from a loss of proprioception and pain. It is frequently seen in the diabetic, in patients with spinal cord injuries, pernicious anemia, and peripheral nerve injury. Frequent administration of hydrocortisone by the intraarticular route can also cause a neurogenic arthropathy.

The patient will sometimes complain of pain, but the degree of pain is usually disproportionate to the destruction that has taken place in the joint. As the degeneration of the joint structures ensues, the results are a boggy, painless joint with extensive erosion of cartilage, osteophyte formation and loose joint bodies. Normal muscle tone and protective reflexes are lost.

The onset of the arthritis may be either insidious or acute. The joints most affected are the large weight-bearing joints. The affected joints may be reddened and swollen.

The patient may cause increased destruction in the joint because the decreased pain sensation from an underlying disease predisposes the patient to increased trauma.

Serum sickness

Serum sickness is one of the immune complex diseases which may occur after injection or ingestion of any foreign protein or serum. Serum sickness most commonly presents as monoarticular pain. It is a systemic reaction characterized by fe·

ver, arthralgia, skin eruptions and edema. Symptoms usually appear within one to two weeks after the injection. The skin eruptions may be patchy or generalized; other symptoms include nausea and vomiting and abdominal pain. In addition, neurologic manifestations may appear as weakness of an extremity or a sensory deficit. Lymphadenopathy at the area of injection is often found on physical exam. Occasionally there is a cardiac arrhythmia or a pericardial friction rub. The affected joints will be painful, swollen, with an accumulation of fluid. Lab: Examination of the blood may reveal a mild leukocytosis and an increase in circulating plasma cells. The ESR is usually elevated. Urine may show some proteinuria, a few red cells and occasionally some casts. The course is usually self-limited from one to several weeks; the patient usually recovers without a residual problem.

Inflammatory bowel diseases

In inflammatory bowel diseases, arthritis is a common complication of regional enteritis, colitis (ulcerative) and Whipple's disease; it is sometimes mistaken for rheumatoid arthritis and may occur coincidentally with it. Associated with inflammatory intestinal disease, it is asymmetric, affects large joints, may or may not parallel the course of the bowel disease and rarely results in residual deformity. The arthritis may be severe, migratory and accompanied by synovial swelling affecting knees, elbows and ankles.

The onset is typically acute, most often monoarticular; but involvement of other joints with symmetry may follow. The joint (most commonly knee and ankle, followed by PIP, elbow, shoulder and wrist) is usually red, swollen and painful. The course may subside in several weeks or may last for months.

The laboratory findings include anemia, increased sedimentation rate and a negative rheumatoid factor.

Tumors

Occult tumors, particularly of the prostate, breast, lung, thyroid, kidney and bladder, may metastasize to bone causing the patient to have presenting signs and symptoms of pain. The pain may get progressively worse and increase at night. The signs and symptoms that present will depend on the extent of the bony involvement. The lab and physical findings will be dictated by the degree of tumor involvement.

Osteoporosis

Osteoporosis is a disease process characterized by a decrease in skeletal mass without a change in bone chemical composition. It occurs more commonly in females, particularly after menopause. The onset is insidious, usually occurring after the age of 50. The following are associated with an increased incidence of osteoporosis: systemic steroids, immobilization, a decreased dietary intake of calcium or increased calcium excretion, certain metabolic diseases (e.g., diabetes mellitus) thyroid or women who have had bilateral oophorectomies without estrogen replacement. The most common problems associated with it are a collapse of the vertebrae causing back pain.

Osteoporosis causing a collapse of the vertebrae causes subjective symptoms of back pain radiating to the legs; increased pain with such movements as coughing, sneezing, etc.; weakness of extremities; numbness and paraesthesias. Objective findings include pain and tenderness on ROM of spine, absent or decreased DTR's, decreased sensation and muscle weakness.

The x-ray may show characteristic changes and the other lab is consistent with the underlying etiology.

Polyarticular

Polyarticular diseases include: degenerative joint arthritis, rheumatoid arthritis, psoriatic arthritis, polymyalgia rheumatica, gonococcal arthritis, acute rheumatic fever and collagen vascular diseases. Cervical spondylosis will also be considered here because the symptoms may be localized in the neck or referred to other joints of the upper extremities. Hypothyroidism will also be discussed under this heading.

Degenerative joint arthritis (osteoarthrosis)

Degenerative joint disease can occur as a "normal" response to aging; 90 percent of persons by the age of

40 are affected by this disease, the most common cause of chronic disability. It is not confined to the elderly, but approximately 87 percent of females and 83 percent of males between 55 and 64 years of age have had radiologic evidence of osteoarthrosis.

Osteoarthrosis may be classified as primary or secondary. In primary there is no abnormal wear, stresses or mechanical joint disturbance. Damage to the joint is probably caused by biochemical abnormalities of a genetic link that impairs cartilage metabolism. Secondary degenerative joint disease is caused by abnormal stresses to the joint caused by injuries, obesity and mechanical joint disturbances.

Degenerative joint disease may be monoarticular or polyarticular, although most studies indicate that most people have symptoms in no more than two joints. The most frequently affected sites are the distal interphalangeal joints of the hands and the large weight-bearing joints. When the joint involvement is monoarticular, it is usually secondary to a traumatic event.

Degenerative joint arthritis has an increased incidence in hyperparathyroidism, diabetes mellitus, acromegaly and hypothyroidism. The onset is usually insidious and is associated with joint pain and stiffness. The pain is usually aching, mild and relieved by rest while exacerbated by activity. There is no redness or warmth, but there may be a decrease in ROM. The rheumatoid arthritis factor is negative and there are no specific lab abnormalities. There are no systemic manifestations.

On physical examination one may find crepitation on joint motion, spasm or atrophy of the surrounding muscles. There will usually be limitation of motion and changes in the shape of the bone. Muscle pain and weakness may be secondary to stresses generated by an abnormal gait resulting from the disease.

Local pain, tenderness and swelling may be present at the base of the distal phalanx; there may be Heberden's nodes present at joint margins with flexion and angulation of the distal phalanx. Similar lesions occur in the proximal interphalangeal joints and are called Bouchard's nodes.

When the hip is involved there may be hip pain on motion and weight bearing with referred pain to the groin and knee. In addition, loss of motion, especially on extension and internal rotation, and loss of abduction are also common.

When the knee is involved, the patient may have pain, loss of full range of motion at the knee and sometimes atrophy of quadriceps. Damage is usually caused in the area of greatest physical stress (the posterior surface of the patella and the weight-bearing surface of the femoral and tibial condyles).

Degenerative joint disease may occur at any site along the spine (cervical and lumbar areas are common sites). Symptoms may be mild (e.g., headaches or backaches), but if the symptoms are more severe consider a herniated disc, malignancy, or osteoporosis with collapse. The pain may be local or referred. There may or may not be a neurologic deficit present.

Rheumatoid arthritis

Rheumatoid arthritis is the most common form of inflammatory arthritis. It is characterized by morning stiffness, joint pain and swelling which is more often symmetrical than asymmetrical. Subcutaneous nodules may develop over bony prominences and around the extensor aspects of the joints.

The onset of rheumatoid arthritis is usually in the thirties for females, but may occur at any age. Rheumatoid arthritis is two to three times more common in females; with increasing age, the female to male ratio declines. The etiology is unknown. Systemic symptoms include low grade fever, weakness, easy fatigability and poor appetite. Extraarticular manifestations are usually seen in patients with high titers of rheumatoid factor in their serum; these include rheumatoid vasculitis of the small and medium sized vessels (telangiectasia, skin ulcerations, neuropathy, digital gangrene) and a variety of visceral, cardiac and pulmonary changes. Muscle atrophy of the affected extremities may be evident within weeks of onset. Other complications which have been found in the elderly with cervical spine involvement are: 1) atlantoaxial subluxation (which at times has resulted in quadriparesis or sudden death), 2) cricoarytenoid arthritis (which may cause hoarseness and upper respiratory tract obstruction), and 3) carpal tunnel syndromes (the result of nerve compression).

The joints in rheumatoid arthritis are usually the metacarpophalangeal (MCP) and PIP joints of the hands and feet. As more joints become involved, the original ones also remain inflamed. This is in direct contrast to arthritis associated with acute rheumatic fever in which there is a monoarticular and migratory involvement. The course is extremely unpredictable in that the patient may have remissions and exacerbations, or the course may lead to progressive joint destruction. Refer to episodic rheumatoid arthritis for lab characteristics.

Psoriatic arthritis

Arthritis occurs in 2 percent of patients with psoriasis. There is no correlation between the activity of the skin and joint manifestations; either one may precede the other. The most common sites of involvement are the distal interphalangeal joints, which are almost always associated with psoriasis of the nails. Joint manifestations occur more frequently with a generalized psoriasis than with the local manifestations. Any peripheral joint may be affected with the distribution of involvement being usually asymmetric.

Psoriatic arthritis can easily be mistaken for rheumatoid arthritis; however, in contrast to rheumatoid arthritis, psoriatic arthritis is not associated with rheumatoid nodules, ulnar drift, subluxation or a generalized symmetrical joint involvement.

The joints are warm, swollen and tender and there is an evidence of increased synovium. X-ray evidence of sacroiliac involvement is seen in 25 to 35 percent of patients. Hyperuricemia may be present. The patient may or may not have a positive rheumatoid factor. The CBC may show a mild anemia. The ESR is increased.

Gonococcal arthritis

Gonococcal arthritis is almost always secondary to infection of the genitourinary tract in males. It is found more frequently in women who have vaginal or cervical infections. If the disease goes untreated, musculoskeletal symptoms will usually occur during the third week of the infection.

Large weight-bearing joints are most affected; eventually all joints are affected in untreated cases, before settling into one or two joints. Tenosynovitis is an associated symptom, especially of the hand and foot. Chills often accompany the synovitis. Papular, vesicular, or hemorrhagic pustular skin lesions are a common occurrence in gonococcal infections.

The diagnosis is made by isolating the organism from the involved joint by culture and a stained smear.

Lab results may show an increased white blood cell (WBC) count and bacteria in the urinalysis. A positive GC culture can be obtained from either the primary site or the joint fluid.

Cervical spondylosis

Degeneration of the cervical disks increase in frequency after age 40. Spondylosis usually affects several levels; it is confined to a single level in only one-fifth of the cases. There may be decreased or absent reflexes in the upper extremities. Paresis, dysesthesia and numbness of the upper extremities as well as fasciculations, atrophy and weakness of the affected upper limbs and gait disturbances may also be found in more severe cases. Diagnosis is made upon information gained from the history and x-rays.

Arthritis of acute rheumatic fever

Though arthritis associated with acute rheumatic fever is uncommon in the aged population, the infection can occur at any age. The symptomatology usually involves carditis, arthritis, skin rash and/or subcutaneous nodules. The arthritis usually affects one joint at a time, in a migatory pain pattern. Diagnosis can be made with evidence of a change in the ASO titer or a previous history of a documented untreated pharyngeal streptococcal infection. The joints most often affected are knees and ankles; less often affected are the elbows, wrists and hips.

Objective findings may include: redness, warmth, pain on ROM of the affected joint, pericardial rubs and rashes.

Polymyalgia rheumatica

Polymyalgia rheumatica is secondary to giant cell arteritis (inflammation of the arteries). It affects both males and females equally. The patient is usually over the age of 60.

The patient may complain of headache and/or symmetrical pain and stiffness of the shoulders or pelvic girdle. The spine (cervical and lumbar) may also be the site of pain. The pain is worse at night and may be associated with systemic symptoms such as weight loss. Objective findings include pain and decreased ROM of the joints, increased ESR, calcification of arteries and muscle tenderness and/or atrophy (as a result of disuse).

Collagen vascular disease

The diseases of systemic lupus erythematosis and scleroderma may initially present in younger age populations with arthralgias. However, joint pain as an initial sign of a collagen vascular disease is not a common occurrence in the elderly; the initial diagnosis is usually made much earlier in life.

Hypothyroidism

It is not uncommon for a patient with hypothyroidism to initially present with joint pain. This is particularly true in the elderly since hypothyroidism in this age group may not present with the common symptoms (e.g., course hair, amenorrhea, dry skin, etc.), but instead as polyarthralgia. Once the patient is restored to a euthyroid state, the joint pains disappear without any residual problems.

Periarticular Rheumatic Disorders
Shoulder hand syndrome (reflex neurovascular dystrophy)

The clinical shoulder hand syndrome may follow a Colles' fracture of the wrist, trauma, a myocardial infarction, CVA's, diabetes mellitus, pulmonary tuberculosis or bronchogenic cancer. The onset of pain may be acute or insidious. The etiology is unknown, but felt to be caused by reflex sympathetic stimulation.

The patient may complain of pain and stiffness in the hand and may have a decreased grasp or motor function, tenderness or vasomotor reactions.

Carpal tunnel

Carpal tunnel is the most common entrapment entity; it affects females most often and usually occurs in the 50-to-60 age group. The onset is insidious. It may occur secondary to old injury, edema, trauma, rheumatoid arthritis, fibrotic processes or diseases such as tuberculosis, diabetes or myxedema.

Symptoms include pain, tingling and paresthesias (particularly at night). The pain may radiate up the arm. Objectively, the patient may have a decrease in nerve conduction, thenar wasting and a decrease in hand sensation.

Monoarticular X-ray Changes
Septic arthritis

X-ray changes can go from early to an advanced state in 24 hours. *Early,* the joint can be either normal, or there may be a distension of the joint space and soft tissue swelling; in the *advanced* state, bony destruction is evident. Other *late* changes include osteoporosis, joint space narrowing and fusions (secondary to cartilage destruction and bony erosions).

Gout

Early there are no changes. *Later* there is bony erosion in approximately one-third of all cases. In the advanced stage there are punched-out areas of bone from repeated attacks.

Episodic rheumatoid arthritis

Early, the joint may be normal or show a soft tissue swelling and/or systemic decalcification. *Later* it may show punched-out bony areas or joint space narrowing. *Advanced,* there is bony ankylosis.

Trauma

Effusion into the joint, soft tissue

swelling and possible fractures may be seen.

Tuberculous arthritis	*Early*, joint may appear normal or weight-bearing joints may show a marked decalcification of the bone away from the joint surfaces, or there may be a destruction of the joint capsule. *Later*, changes include bony erosions, joint space narrowing and subchondral destruction of the bone. *Advanced*, there are large bilateral areas of necrosis which may occur at opposing points in the bones. *Far advanced*, there is widespread destruction of the bone and joint surfaces with a complete disorganization of bony structure.
Pseudogout	*Early*, there is symmetric calcification of cartilaginous structures. These changes are commonly seen in the meniscus of the knee. *Late*, there may be signs of advanced degenerative joint disease.
Serum sickness	Joints appear normal except for occasional effusion (an accumulation of fluid in the spaces).
Inflammatory intestinal disease	The joints may appear normal except for a soft tissue swelling; a few patients may have bony erosions and/or a joint space narrowing.
Tumors	In prostatic cancer that has metastasized to the bone, you can see characteristic lesions of increased bone density. Tumors of the bone may be detected on x-ray by 1) bony

deformities, 2) the presence of a soft tissue or mass or 3) evidence of a pathological fracture.

Osteoporosis

There is osteopenia (a decrease in bone density); however, this finding is also present in osteomalacia, so the diagnosis of osteoporosis is made on the basis of all clinical and lab data.

Polyarticular X-ray Changes
Osteoarthrosis

Early findings may be normal or show a narrowing of the joint space or a sharpening of the articular margins. *Later* changes may include a cartilage destruction with osteophyte formation and/or a characteristic lipping of the bone.

Rheumatoid arthritis

Early there is soft tissue swelling, osteoporosis around the involved joint and erosion of the peripheral bare space of bone surface which is not covered by cartilage. *Later* there is extensive erosion of cartilage causing joint space narrowing. Bony cysts may result. *Advanced,* there is destruction of cartilage and bone.

Psoriatic arthritis

Early there is a normal appearance. *Later* changes may include a joint destruction, ankylosis and/or a whittled appearance of the bones at the distal phalanges.

Gonococcal arthritis

(See Infectious arthritis.)

Cervical spondylosis

Early there is loss of the normal curve of the cervical spine. *Later* there is osteophyte formation anteriorly adjacent to the disk with joint space narrowing.

Rheumatic fever, polymyalgia rheumatica, hypothyroidism, carpal tunnel and shoulder hand	There are no specific diagnostic roentgen findings specific to these entities that would aid specifically in the differential diagnosis.

PLAN:

The following are *overall* guidelines for management of the patient with joint pain diagnosed as one of the monoarticular, polyarticular or periarticular diseases. The patient should be educated and counseled on the following:

Systemic Rest	Intermittent rest is more valuable when the patient has rheumatoid arthritis, osteoarthrosis, psoriatic arthritis or inflammatory intestinal disease.
Diet	Counseling should be done concerning the dietary allowances and restrictions in inflammatory bowel disease and gout. Weight reduction is essential for the obese patient.
Physical Activity	The type and duration of the rest program depends upon the type and course of the disease. The increase of physical activity must proceed gradually and with appropriate supply for any involved weight-bearing joints.
Exercise	Rest and therapeutic exercise should always be in proper balance. Therapeutic exercise should be designed to preserve joint motion and muscular strength, and to prevent contractures.

Posture and Body Alignment

Counsel regarding a firm mattress for back support, crutches or a cane for walking, correction of abnormal posture if possible and proper fitting shoes.

Physical Therapy
Occupational Therapy
Consults

Obtain consultation as needed to prevent avoidable disabilities, prevent progression of the disease process and to prescribe the correct exercise and activity.

Explanation to the Patient About His or Her Disease

The patient should understand the disease process and the importance of complying with the therapeutic regimen. He or she should know the names of the medications being taken and understand what the side effects are and the frequency of their administration.

Elevation of Affected Patient

To decrease swelling and aid circulation.

Splints or Braces

To support the impaired joint and prevent further stress on the joint structures.

Force Fluids

To hydrate the patient who is septic and to decrease fever. Fluids also enhance absorption and excretion of drugs.

Heat/Cold

Apply heat to muscle spasms and cold for inflammation: recent studies have shown that heat application to an inflamed joint further decreases oxygen to the joint thus predisposing to more extensive joint damage. Therefore, for inflamed joints use only ice. However, heat may be used to decrease muscle spasms in a *noninflamed* joint.

Immobilization

Immobilize any acutely inflamed joint in the functional position. This will reduce pain, slow down the infectious and/or degenerative process and minimize destruction.

ADDITIONAL PLAN FOR SPECIFIC ENTITIES:

Septic Arthritis

Refer to physician for appropriate antibiotic treatment and joint aspiration. The joint should be splinted, rested, followed by physical therapy if necessary.

Gout

The patient should be taking uricosuric agents (e.g., probenecid, sulfinpyrazone) after the initial attack. The treatment may also include the administration of agents that decrease the production of uric acid. Colchicine, indomethacin and phenylbutazone are used in acute attacks. The patient should avoid alcohol and/or highly seasoned foods. Obtain a serum uric acid level at intervals to follow the course of the disease. Patients with gout should also increase their daily fluid intake to prevent the possibility of dehydration resulting in an increased likelihood of stone formation.

Episodic Rheumatoid Arthritis

See plan for rheumatoid arthritis.

Trauma

If there is a fracture evidenced on x-ray, refer for treatment. If no fracture, treat the joint with elevation, splint, rest and cold for the first 24 hours and reevaluate the joint in 18 to 24 hours. If no improvement in symptoms, consult or refer the patient to a physician.

Tuberculosis

Refer to physician for appropriate treatment with antimicrobials.

Pseudogout

Refer the patient to his or her physician. Anti-inflammatory agents (e.g., ASA or nonsteroidal agents) and aspiration (to decrease the joint pressure) may be helpful.

Neurogenic Arthropathy

The management of neurogenic arthropathy usually consists of conservative measures (i.e., rest and decreased weight bearings to prevent joint destruction) and treatment and management of the underlying disease.

Serum Sickness

The patient should be referred; treatment may include ASA for joint pains, therapeutic agents for the relief of urticaria and occasionally the use of systemic steroids is warranted.

Inflammatory Intestinal Disease

Consult with and/or refer to the patient's physician; treatment may include anti-inflammatory agents (ASA and/or nonsteroidal anti-inflammatory drugs) and physical therapy.

Tumors

Refer the patient for treatment of the underlying cause.

Osteoporosis

Treatment involves a number of modalities: 1) discontinuance of any drugs contributing to osteoporotic disease (i.e., steroids), 2) dietary supplements of calcium or vitamin D if the disease is secondary to nutritional deficiencies, 3) physical therapy, estrogen replacement, 4) avoidance of immobilization, 5) correction of underlying cause, 6) exercise and 7) no bending or lifting of heavy objects (including opening windows).

Polyarthritic
Degenerative joint arthritis (DJD)

Aspirin or Acetominophen (since there is no need for anti-inflammatory action) is necessary for pain. If the patient is obese, strongly encourage weight loss. Physical therapy and adequate rest for the involved joint are also important.

Rheumatoid arthritis

Obtain adequate rest while striving for the goal of maintaining as much normal activity as possible and preventing joint deformities. The therapeutic range includes a baseline prescription of ASA. Later, therapy may include nonsteroidal anti-inflammatory agents, gold salts, steroids, immunosuppressives, etc. For specific guidelines see protocol for rheumatoid arthritis in *Clinical Protocols*, Hudak and associates, Lippincott.

Psoriatic arthritis

The treatment for psoriatic arthritis is the same as for rheumatoid arthritis with the exception of *not* using antimalarials. Therapy also includes adequate control of the associated dermatitis.

Gonococcal arthritis	Refer to physician for treatment; therapy usually includes IV antimicrobials, hospitalization, rest to the affected joints and repeated follow-up cultures.
Cervical spondylosis	Advise the use of a small, round cervical pillow with cervical spondylosis; an external cervical support with a nonrigid surgical collar or a neck brace may also be helpful. Consult with a physician and/or refer the patient for appropriate therapy, including anti-inflammatory agents.
Rheumatic fever arthritis	Refer the patient for treatment to a physician.
Polymyalgia rheumatica	If this entity is suspected, refer the patient. There is usually a dramatic improvement with steroids.
Collagen vascular diseases	Refer to appropriate protocol treatment plan for the specific entity.
Hypothyroidism	Consult with and refer the patient to his or her primary care physician; the therapy goal should be to return the patient to a euthyroid state.
Periarticular Shoulder hand	Aggressive physical therapy is essential to ensure an active exercise program with analgesics. Systemic corticosteroid therapy may be necessary in intractable pain (obtain physician consultation and/or referral).
Carpal tunnel	Carpal tunnel syndrome may be relieved by splinting, steroid injec-

tions or medications to decrease any inflammation and/or surgery. Consult with a physician and/or refer the patient.

Look for hypothyroidism, acromegaly, rheumatoid arthritis or diabetes mellitus; these entities have an increased incidence of carpal tunnel.

REFERENCES

1. American Rheumatism Association. *Primer on Rheumatic Disease*. Reprinted from *Journal of American Medical Association*.
2. _____. *Arthritis and Rheumatism*. Health Statistics Series B, No. 20, U.S. Department of Health Education and Welfare, 1960.
3. _____. *Arthritis Source Book*. Washington, D.C.: U.S. Public Health Service Division of Chronic Disease, Public Health Service Publication No. 1431, 1976.
4. Bates, Barbara. *A Guide to Physical Examination*. Philadelphia: J. B. Lippincott Co., 1974.
5. Beeson, Paul B. et al. *Textbook of Medicine*. Philadelphia: W. B. Saunders Company, 1975.
6. Boyle, James A., and Buchanan, Watson W. *Clinical Rheumatology*. Oxford and Edinburgh: Blackwell Scientific Publications, 1971.
7. _____. *Chronic Conditions Causing Limitation of Activities*. Health Statistics, Series B, No. 36, U.S. Department of Health, Eduation and Welfare, 1962.
8. Chusid, Joseph G. *Correlative Neuroanatomy and Functional Neurology*, 16th ed. Los Altos, Calif.: Lange Medical Publications, 1976.
9. Friedman, Sandor A., and Steinheber, Francis U. *The Medical Clinics of North America*. November, 1976, Vol. 60, No. 6, pp. 1141–1225.
10. Hollander, Joseph G., and McCarty, Daniel J. *Arthritis and Allied Conditions*, 8th ed. Philadelphia: Lea & Febiger, 1972.
11. Hudak, Carolyn M., Redstone, Paul A., Hokanson, Nancy L., Suzuki, Irene E. *Clinical Protocols*. Philadelphia: J. B. Lippincott Co., 1976.
12. Krupp, Marcus A. and Chatton, Milton J. *Current Medical Diagnosis and Treatment*. Los Altos, Calif.: Lange Medical Publications, 1977.

13. Pearson, L. B. "Protocols: How to Develop and Implement Within the Nurse Practitioners' Setting," *The Nurse Practitioner*, September/October, 1976.

14. _____. *Primer on Rheumatic Disease*. American Rheumatism Association, New York Arthritis Foundation, 1964.

15. Wallach, Jacques. *Interpretation of Diagnostic Tests, A Handbook Synopsis of Laboratory Medicine*. 2nd ed. Boston: Little, Brown and Co., 1974.

Chapter 2

Falls and Hip Injury

OVERVIEW

Accidents specifically involving falls have a very high incidence in the elderly population. In those over 65, accidents are as important a cause of death as pneumonia and diabetes (Rodstein, 1973). The fatality of the accident is at times related to the injury caused by the fall, but at other times the aged patient will succumb from the complications associated with the immobility necessitated by the injury. Hip fractures resulting from falls are one of the most common injuries in this age group. In recent years there has been much progress in the treatment of these injuries, resulting in earlier ambulation.

Initially, when an elderly patient is found on the floor there are assessments that the primary care provider must make to evaluate the extent of injury and need for referral. Once the acute treatment has been provided, the cause of the fall must be identified. Primary care providers must also seek to prevent falls through treatment of underlying conditions and providing staff and patient education in how to prevent them.

Prevention involves 1) understanding physiological variances in the aged that render them at a higher risk; 2) providing for early identification of metabolic diseases (i.e., Paget's, osteoporosis, osteomalacia), neurologic problems, cardiovascular problems associated with syncope or confusion (i.e., sick sinus syndrome, heart block, Stokes-Adams, arrhythmias), metastatic disease to bone, vestibular problems, and side effects of medications; and 3) the identification of environmental factors that may precipitate a fall.

There are several physiological variances in the aged that predispose them to falling. Not only is there less collagen formed, but that which is present loses some elasticity and resiliency rendering the supportive structures of the joints (ligaments, tendons, etc.) less effective. This decrease in collagen, with the increased incidence of degenerative joint disease and other rheumatic conditions, may result in joint instability. In addition, the aged person has some generalized muscle wasting and atrophy which further compromises joint stability.

Other physiologic variances that predispose the elderly to falling are 1) sensory changes (decreased visual acuity, hearing and smell), 2) decreased muscle tone and coordination, 3) a longer reflex response time (which alters the person's ability to perceive environmental hazards), 4) changes in the lumbar spine and/or disease processes that result in a shuffling gait, and 5) the multiplicity of chronic diseases in the aged population (which renders them less responsive to stress).

This protocol has been divided into three specific components: *Part A* is to be used for patients with an acute onset of hip pain or pain in the lower extremities secondary to a fall, *Part B* is to be used in patients with a history of falls in the recent past for which the etiology of the fall has not been identified, and *Part C* is to be used for all elderly patients with the goal of preventing falls by increasing patient and staff awareness.

PART A WORKSHEET

To be used for patients with acute onset of hip pain secondary to trauma.

What you cannot afford to miss: hip fracture, hip dislocation.

Chief Complaint: _____

SUBJECTIVE DATA:

If the patient is conscious proceed with these questions: Describe

the pain. (location, quality, radiation, etc.) _____

_____

_____

Describe all positives
YES   NO

_____ _____ Can you move your hip without pain?_____

_____ _____ Do you remember how you fell? (If yes, describe) _

_____

_____ _____ How did you land? (Describe) _____

_____

_____ _____ Was the pain present prior to falling? _____

_____ _____ Was the pain present only after falling?_____

_____ _____ Did you stumble or trip over something? (Describe

events preceding fall and prior to fall.) _____

_____

_____

_____ _____ Were you conscious prior to the fall?_____

_____ _____ Did you suddenly lose consciousness prior to fall-

ing?_____

_____ _____ Were you dizzy or lightheaded? _____

_____ _____ Had you just changed positions rapidly? (i.e., standing, sitting, lying to sitting, reaching up, looking up-

ward or sideways) _____

_____ _____ Any previous episodes like this?_____

_____ _____ What medications are you taking?_____

_____   _____   Are you a diabetic? _____

OBJECTIVE DATA:

Vital Signs: _____Pulse _____Blood pressure
Have the patient remain in the same place if safe (i.e., no fire, etc.).
Do not attempt walking.

(A "yes" response indicates a need for immediate referral)
YES   NO

Note the position the extremity is in:

_____   _____   Is the leg externally rotated, abducted, flexed?_____

_____   _____   Is the leg internally rotated, adducted, flexed? _____

_____   _____   Is the leg externally rotated with shortening?_____

_____   _____   Is the leg adducted, externally rotated with short-

ening? _____

·If the leg is not in an abnormal position, note:

_____   _____   Does moving extremity cause pain? _____

_____   _____   Limited range of motion of hip? _____

_____   _____   On palpation of hip joint is there pain or tenderness?

_____

_____   _____   Evaluation of the extremity abnormal? _____

_____

_____   _____   Skin not intact: _____

_____   _____   Peripheral pulses absent or unequal bilaterally: ____

_____

_____   _____   Bone (any crepitus)): _____

_____   _____   Tendons, ligaments (abnormal motion or instability):

_____

_____   _____   Motor strength, range of motion unequal bilaterally:

_____

_____   _____   Sensory not intact: _____

When patient is to be moved, immobilize the part by splinting one leg to the other or use a leg splint and transfer to flat area (bed, ambulance, pram, etc.). Refer for x-ray and thorough examination.

PART A WORKSHEET RATIONALE

SUBJECTIVE DATA:

Quickly make an assessment as to whether the patient is conscious or unconscious. If the patient is unconscious, quickly feel for carotid pulses and note respiration; if absent, institute CPR.

Description of fall and pain

Evaluation of a potential hip injury can rarely be completed without x-rays and physician evaluation. Data obtained at the time of the injury are essential to the assessment. If the patient can recall how he or she fell and landed, this may provide clues to anatomical injuries. It will also give some feeling as to whether the fall came first and then the injury, or if some precipitating event caused the fall (i.e., syncopal episodes, pathologic fractures, etc.) Some falls are precipitated by a bone that pathologically fractures, which subsequently results in a fall.

In this case, the patient will describe the pain, then the fall. If the patient was pain-free prior to the fall, one must think of accidental falling or other underlying etiologies (e.g., cardiovascular, neurological, or manifestations of systemic diseases).

Were you conscious?
Did you suddenly lose consciousness?

Arrhythmias, seizures, heart block, Stokes-Adams attacks, or any cerebral hypoxic episode can cause loss of consciousness and lead to a fall. These data are essential to obtain at the time of the injury—immediate attention might need to be directed to the neurologic or cardiovascular system if the answer was yes.

Dizzy, lightheaded

Identification of the precipitating event will be useful information for evaluation by the physician. Dizziness could be secondary to hypoxia, vestibular or cerebellar disease, side effects of medications, hypoglycemic episodes, seizures, anemias, or gastrointestinal (GI) hemorrhage.

Changed positions rapidly

Again these data are very important information that should be presented to the physician to whom the patient is being referred. Postural hypotension can be secondary to medications (i.e., hypertensive agents) or the result of a pooling of blood in the extremities. Other contributing causes of orthostatic hypotension are large varicosities, diabetic neuropathies, and/or poor cardiovascular compensatory mechanisms. Turning the head from side to side or a hyperextension of the neck when osteoarthritis with osteophyte formation of the cervical spine is present can cause compression of the vertebral arteries leading to cerebral hypoxia; a sideways motion can compress the carotids also causing cerebral hypoxia.

Previous episodes, medications These data are important to know so that they can be presented to the physician to whom the patient is referred; the data aid in the differential diagnosis of why the patient fell.

Diabetes It is essential to know if the patient is a diabetic so that insulin reactions causing the fall can be immediately remedied.

OBJECTIVE DATA:

If the patient is conscious proceed with the following:

If the leg is externally rotated, adducted, flexed This position of the leg is seen in an anterior hip dislocation. This is not a common injury. It may be secondary to the patient sliding from a high place, or getting out of a car and landing on his feet.

If the leg is internally rotated, adducted and flexed Think of a posterior hip dislocation. This may occur in situations where the patient sustains a blow to the knees while in a sitting position (i.e., a fall from a wheel chair). The pain is severe, constant, and located in the inguinal region or thigh. There is a high probability of acetabular rim fractures; avascular necrosis occurs in 20 to 25 percent of patients with a posterior dislocation.

If the leg is externally rotated with shortening Note any trochanter displacement. This leg position can occur in neck and trochanteric fractures. This is a common injury. The closer the fracture is to the head of the femur the greater chance there is for avascular necrosis developing.

If there is no abnormal position, examine and transfer the patient

The leg should be examined following the objective data sheet if there is no abnormal leg position. An abnormal position should preclude a thorough exam. In either case the patient should be transferred and/or referred for a thorough medical evaluation regardless of whether or not a bone injury is suspected; a fall by an elderly person demands a full evaluation in order to correct and/or treat any underlying medical condition, environmental hazard or lack of health teaching.

PART B WORKSHEET

To be used with physician consultation in order to help identify the precipitating factors of the fall.

Chief Complaint: _____

SUBJECTIVE DATA:

Describe events immediately preceding fall, how the patient fell, how he or she landed, and after effects (i.e., pain, limitation of motion, etc.).

Events preceding the fall: This is a concise list of relatively common events that precede falls in the elderly population. If any response is yes, describe completely.

YES   *NO*

_____   _____   Urination: _____

_____   _____   Position change (looking upward, sideways, lying to

sitting or standing): _____

_____ _____ Stumbling: _____

_____ _____ Dizziness, lightheadedness, vertigo: _____

_____ _____ Loss of consciousness or no recall of preceding

events: _____

_____ _____ Pain: _____

_____ _____ Syncopal episode after unusual exercise: _____

_____ _____ Coughing, sneezing, hyperventilating:_____

_____ _____ Climbing or descending stairs: _____

_____ _____ Sudden weakness in legs followed by fall to ground

without loss of consciousness: _____

(Describe positives completely):

PAST MEDICAL HISTORY
YES   NO

_____ _____ Serious illnesses: _____

_____

_____ _____ Hospitalizations:_____

_____ _____ Surgeries: _____

MEDICATIONS:

_____ _____ Antihypertensives _____

_____ _____ Tranquilizers _____

_____ _____ Steroids_____

_____ _____ Others (including over-the-counter medications)____

_____ _____ Anticonvulsants _____

Part B Worksheet

OBJECTIVE DATA:

Blood Pressure: Lying:_____ Pulse for one
  Standing:_____ minute:_____
  Sitting:_____ Temperature:_____

PERFORM COMPLETE PHYSICAL EXAM WITH SPECIAL ATTENTION TO THE
FOLLOWING:
  YES   *NO*

_____ _____ Any abnormalities? (please describe)_____

_____

_____ _____ Cardiovasular system (note heart rate, rhythm, pres-

ence of murmurs, gallops, pulses): _____

_____

_____ _____ Neurologic system (cranial nerves, motor, gait, re-

flexes, cerebellar function, sensation): _____

_____

_____ _____ Musculoskeletal exam:_____

_____ _____ Breast, prostate exam: _____

LAB DATA (Describe All Abnormalities):
  DONE *NOT*
    DONE

_____ _____ CBC:_____

_____ _____ Hemoccult: _____

_____ _____ EKG:_____

_____ _____ Calcium, Phos.: _____

_____ _____ Alk. Phos.: _____

——— ——— Urinalysis (if indicated by history): _____

——— ——— X-rays (as indicated): _____

PART B WORKSHEET RATIONALE

Descriptions of events that occurred around the time of the fall help ascertain whether the fall preceded the injury (as in cardiovascular or neurological problems) or the injury preceded the fall (as in pathological fractures).

SUBJECTIVE DATA:

Events Preceding Fall
Urination

Some falls follow urination, especially in elderly males with prostatic hypertrophy; the delayed bladder emptying may cause a hypotensive episode.

Position changes

Falls may be secondary to 1) orthostatic hypotension from medications, 2) pooling of blood in the extremities, 3) cerebral hypoxia secondary to vertebral artery compression (e.g., looking upward), 4) carotid artery compression (e.g., looking sideways), or 5) vestibular disease.

Stumbling

The patient may have fallen because of environmental factors (e.g., an unattached rug, etc.) or stumbling may be secondary to gait changes seen in neurologic problems (e.g., previous stroke, quadriceps atrophy, foot drop, etc.).

Dizziness,
lightheadedness, vertigo

This is seen in cerebral hypoxia, arrhythmias, and vestibular disease.

Loss of consciousness

Loss of consciousness can be due to 1) arrhythmias (e.g., heart block, Stokes-Adams, sick sinus syndrome), 2) neurologic problems, 3) vestibular disease, 4) cerebral hypoxia or 5) seizures.

Pain

Pain may have occurred prior to the fall because of a pathologic fracture (seen in metastatic disease or osteoporosis). The pain may also have caused the patient to fall from a momentary response to the pain, as in a painful stiff joint.

Unusual exercise

Patients with aortic stenosis may experience syncopal episodes after increased exercise due to a decrease in responsiveness of the heart to meet the increased oxygen demands. Silent myocardial infarctions are another cause of falls after unusual exercise.

Coughing, sneezing, hyperventilating

The patient may experience a vasovagal response and fall as a result.

Climbing or descending stairs

Patients with a weakness of the knee extensors or hip muscles may fall on climbing and descending the stairs; they may also have fallen because they misjudged distances (were unable to see), due to poor lighting or other environmental hazards.

Sudden weakness in legs followed by fall without a loss in consciousness

This is indicative of vertebral basilar artery insufficiency. The paralysis does not affect the upper extremities; it is usually transient, but may last for hours. This is sometimes called drop attacks.

Past Medical History
Hospitalizations
Surgeries

Ask specifically about bilateral oophorectomy because of an increased incidence of osteoporosis in females if they have not received estrogen replacement. Ask about partial gastrectomies, because patients may develop pernicious anemia and then develop B_{12} deficiency neuropathies. Ask about a history of peptic ulcer disease (PUD); the patient with PUD may again have a slow bleed leading to anemia and syncopal episodes. If the patient has a positive history of cancer of the prostate, breast, thyroid, kidney, bladder, or lung, consider a possible bone metastasis with pathological fractures that may have precipitated the fall. Ask about a previous history of cardiovascular or neurological problems (e.g., high blood pressure, heart problems, CVA's or seizures) that could be related to the falls.

Medications

Certain *antihypertensives* can cause postural hypotension, causing the patient to experience lightheadedness on changing positions, and thus fall.

Tranquilizers cause a decreased awareness and confusion leading to falls.

Steroids taken for long periods of time cause an increased incidence of osteoporosis.

Others: Numerous drugs may cause dizziness or lightheadedness. In the elderly population, some patients experience this after taking nitroglycerin, so advise the patient to take the medicine while sitting down.

Anticonvulsants play a role in the abnormal metabolism of vitamin D. Individuals who take anticonvulsants and lack sunlight exposure or vitamin D intake may develop osteomalacia.

OBJECTIVE DATA:
Vital Signs

Look for orthostatic blood pressure changes that may have contributed to dizziness or lightheadedness and thus precipitated a fall. Orthostatic hypotension can occur in alcoholics with neuropathies, those patients taking antihypertensives, anti-Parkinson's drugs and/or tranquilizers. In addition, orthostatic hypotension can occur secondary to a decreased responsiveness of the cardiovascular system because of age-related changes. Falls may be the first manifestation of a systemic illness; for this reason the temperature should be taken. Take the pulse for one complete minute, feeling for a rhythm abnormality that might have precipitated the fall.

COMPLETE EXAM WITH SPECIAL REFERENCE TO:
Cardiovascular exam

Search for any arrhythmia. Aortic stenosis may cause hypoxia to the brain after increased exercise, causing the patient to pass out and fall. Other cardiovascular problems that are responsible for falls include heart block, silent myocardial infarctions, sick sinus syndrome and bradycardia.

Neurologic exam

The complete neurologic exam will evaluate whether a central or peripheral (vestibular) abnormality may have caused the fall. The significance of nystagmus must be considered in light of other signs and symptoms. Look for rotary nystagmus that may be suggestive of labyrinthine disease. A sustained horizontal or vertical nystagmus may be suggestive of brain stem diseases. Look for any muscular weakness, an inequality of reflexes or abnormal cerebellar function that may indicate coordination problems that could have precipitated the fall. Check the gait for its character and quality; Parkinson's, CVA's or other neurological disorders cause gait disturbances that can precipitate falls. Check sensation and proprioception; look for neuropathies secondary to diabetes mellitus, alcoholism and vitamin B_{12} deficiencies that can contribute to a decreased awareness of position sense, causing falls. Check for a cogwheel rigidity on range of motion seen in Parkinson's disease.

Musculoskeletal exam

Look for joint deformities or an instability of structures that may have contributed to falling. Check for foot deformities; foot problems themselves can predispose the elderly to falling.

Breast exam

Examine the lumps that may represent malignant disease with an underlying metastasis to the bone, causing pain or pathological fractures that could precipitate a fall.

Prostate exam

Cancer of the prostate may metastasize to bone, causing either pain or a pathologic fracture.

LAB DATA:

CBC

A CBC is done to rule out anemias seen in nutritional deficiencies, occult bleeding, or anemias associated with an underlying cancer. If bleeding is suspected as being associated with the fall, a baseline CBC should be drawn with a follow-up CBC taken to assess blood loss. Intertrochanteric fractures (not neck fractures) may be associated with a blood loss of 3 to 5 units.

Hemoccult

Hemoccult tests of the stool are done to rule out gastrointestinal bleeding from occult cancer or peptic ulcer disease, etc.; the hypovolemia may cause orthostatic hypotension or anemia both of which can precipitate falls.

EKG

An EKG is done to rule out arrhythmias or silent myocardial infarctions that may have precipitated a fall.

Calcium
Phosphorus

Calcium and phosphorus are tested to rule out hyperparathyroidism as the etiological cause of falls.

Alkaline phosphatase

The alkaline phosphatase may be increased in bone metastasis and/or Paget's disease.

Urinalysis

Examine urine if symptomatology suggests a possible urinary tract infection (UTI) for occasionally falls may be the manifestation of a UTI.

X-rays

X-rays should be taken as indicated by the history and physical. For hip pain, x-rays of the anterior-posterior (AP) and lateral pelvis should be taken; pelvic pain from a fracture can give the same type of pain as a hip fracture.

Osteoporosis or bony metastasis can lead to pathological fractures; these are visible on x-ray. Bony x-ray changes are also seen in Paget's disease (especially the skull, long bones, or vertebrae).

Osteoarthritis of the cervical spine (causing bony spur formation with encroachment and thus causing cerebral hypoxia) can be visualized on x-ray.

The chest x-ray may show evidence of cancer of the lung; this frequently metastasizes to bone.

ASSESSMENT:

This assessment section is designed to increase the practitioner's awareness of conditions that cause falls: 1) Pathologic fractures (the patient sustained an injury, and then fell); 2) Cardiovascular conditions that precipitated a fall from hypoxia; 3) Neurologic problems that cause falls; and 4) Other causes of falls in the elderly.

Conditions That May Cause Pathologic Fractures:

Osteoporosis

Osteoporosis is a condition commonly associated with the elderly population, characterized by a decrease in bone mass. The formation and resorption of bone is a process that takes place continually through our lives, and this process represents a delicate physiological balance. Normal bone formation and resorption depends upon several factors: 1) sufficient dietary intake of calcium and phosphorus, 2) adequate dietary intake of vitamin D or an adequate exposure to the sun (vitamin D is needed for absorption of calcium in the intestine) and 3) the presence of hormones that stimulate bone tissue activity. In order to maintain calcium homeostasis, the skeleton acts as a reservoir. Any condition that causes more bone resorption than formation could result in a decrease in bone density. After the age of 40 to 50, skeletal mass begins to decline. The etiology of this process is not clearly understood, but it is known to occur in women at a faster rate than in men. Some of this increase in bone resorption in postmenopausal women can be attributed to a lack of estrogen (estrogen decreases bone resorption, but has no increased effect on bone formation). This condition is commonly called postmenopausal osteoporosis. There are various other types of osteoporosis. The etiological causes with which osteoporosis can be associated can be divided into five major classifications: 1) disuse (e.g., immobilization, paralysis), 2) drug induced (e.g., steroids, anticonvulsants, anticoagulants, antacids, alcohol, or aspirin), 3) endocrine (e.g., parathyroid hormone, insulin, etc.), 4) nutritional (e.g., calcium or vitamin D deficiency, metals, etc.) and 5) miscellaneous causes (e.g., genetic, trauma, aging, renal, or osteoclast activating factor).

Common osteoporotic etiologic causes include an 1) increased calcium loss via the intestine or kidney, 2) a decreased dietary intake of calcium, or 3) immobility which increases bone reabsorption. The patient may be completely asymptomatic or may present with pain secondary to pathologic fractures. The fractures may occur with any minor trauma or no apparent trauma. The most common sites of fractures are the vertebrae and femur.

Subjective complaints range from no complaints to one of pain (resulting from pathologic fractures). The most common sites of pain are the spine, hips, wrists and humerus. If present, the pain may have occurred prior to the fall or following only minor events such as coughing, sneezing or straining.

There may be no *objective findings* of disease other than found on x-ray (i.e., a decrease in bone density or evidence of pathologic fracture). There may be spinal tenderness and posture changes. In lab tests the calcium, phosphorus and alkaline phosphatase are within normal limits.

Osteomalacia

Osteomalacia is a disorder characterized by abnormal mineralization of bone. It can be secondary to: 1) a lack of vitamin D intake in the diet, 2) inadequate exposure to the sun in addition to a decreased dietary intake, 3) intestinal malabsorption syndromes in which vitamin D and calcium are lost, 4) a renal tubular defect or 5) use of some drugs, particularly Dilantin. Adequate mineralization of bone requires sufficient available calcium and phosphorus concentrations as well as vitamin D to ensure proper absorption of calcium. Demineralization of the bones causes them to be more susceptible to fractures from minor trauma.

The most common symptoms are a generalized skeletal pain sometimes with tenderness; gait changes secondary to pain; and muscular weakness, especially proximal weakness (because of changes in the calcium concentration—calcium is needed for muscle contraction). The patient may present with symptoms only after falling; the fall then leads to identification of the underlying etiology.

Objective findings may include: proximal muscle weakness, bone tenderness, and gait disturbances. The levels of calcium and phosphorus will depend on the underlying etiology of the osteomalacia. For example, osteomalacia secondary to vitamin D deficiency may have a normal or low calcium with a low phosphorus; in renal tubular problems the calcium is normal, there is

a decreased phosphorus and the alkaline phosphatase may be normal
or elevated.

Metastatic cancer

Primary lesions of the thyroid,
breast, prostate, kidney, lung or
bladder may metastasize to the
bone. The subjective symptoms will
be associated with the primary cancer site; there will also be bone pain
present. The patient's underlying
malignancy may be first identified
after the patient has experienced a
pathologic fracture and fall. The objective symptoms will match those
expected in a primary site cancer
(e.g., a breast mass, thyroid mass,
prostate nodule, etc.). If cancer is
suspected, the lab tests should include urinalysis, alkaline phosphatase, calcium, phosphorus, BUN/
creatinine, thyroid panel and scan,
acid phosphatase, chest x-ray and
bone scan. The results of the lab
tests may reflect the site of the metastatic cancer.

Hyperparathyroidism

Hyperparathyroidism may be considered a disease that predisposes
the elderly to pathologic fractures
for the following reason: the increased secretion of parathyroid
hormone may result in a mobiliza-
tion of calcium from the bone into
the extracellular fluid, causing excessive bone resorption and osteoporosis.

Paget's disease

It is not uncommon in the elderly
that Paget's disease may present initially with a pathologic fracture.
The early course of the disease may

be asymptomatic or accompanied by vague bone pain and headaches. The disease is characterized by an increased resorption of bone. The lab findings include normal calcium and phosphorus and an increased alkaline phosphatase.

Postural hypotension

Postural hypotension (secondary to 1) anemias, 2) medications such as tranquilizers and antihypertensive agents or 3) the sluggishness of the cardiovascular system in responding to position changes) can cause a temporary hypoxic episode. During this hypoxic episode the patient experiences dizziness and/or lightheadedness and falls.

Cardiovascular Conditions

It is important to ascertain a history of the events preceding the fall in order to search for cardiovascular conditions that may have precipitated the fall. The cardiovascular conditions may have caused cerebral hypoxia (resulting in dizziness), or arrhythmias associated with syncopal episodes. Some conditions that may be causative are heart block, Stokes-Adams attacks, silent myocardial infarctions, atrial flutter or fibrillation, or ventricular arrhythmias. Aortic stenosis may also be the cause; after unusual exercise the patient may have cerebral hypoxia secondary to an inability of the stenotic valve to meet the increase in oxygen demands. The symptoms may include any of the clinical features associated with the conditions.

Objective findings may include an abnormal cardiovascular exam consistent with the etiology. Electrocardiogram and possible Holter monitoring may be useful in identifying the cardiovascular abnormality.

Neurologic Problems

Neurologic problems may be directly responsible for the fall because of vertigo, lightheadedness, dizziness, etc., or indirectly responsible because of an associated confusion, muscle weakness, incoordination, or gait changes.

Possible neurologic problems include vestibular problems, CVA's with some residual motor dysfunction, Parkinson's disease, diabetic neuropathies, epilepsy or chronic brain syndrome. These conditions can precipitate falls because of 1) gait changes associated with motor dysfunction (e.g., Parkinson's); 2) uncoordination secondary to multiple sclerosis (MS); 3) changes in vibratory sensations and proprioception (as in diabetic neuropathies, vitamin B_{12} neuropathies or alcoholic neuropathies); 4) syncopal episodes with seizures; 5) vertigo, lightheadedness or dizziness secondary to vestibular problems; 6) confusion secondary to chronic brain syndrome; or 7) muscular weaknesses.

The symptomatology and physical findings depend on the neurologic problem. If a neurologic problem is suspected, particular attention should be directed to the neurologic exam: cranial nerves, motor, sensory, reflexes, cerebellar, Romberg, mental status exam, etc.

Others

Asthma

Patients with a history of asthma who have been treated with steroids are at a higher risk for falling because steroids may be associated with an increased incidence of osteoporosis and pathologic fractures.

Arthritis

Arthritis of any type can be a predisposing factor to falls because of joint instability that may result from the disease process. In addition, those patients whose arthritis has been treated with steroids are also at an increased risk for falling (because of the resultant osteoporosis).

Foot problems

Foot problems (i.e., corns, calluses, etc.) are common among the elderly, and may precipitate falls either because of a reaction to pain or because of shoes that fit poorly, causing stumbling.

Immobile patients

Patients who have long periods of immobilization are at an increased risk of falling because of 1) potential episodes of postural hypotension upon arising, 2) increases in the osteoporotic process with periods of prolonged immobilization, or 3) confusion associated with the organic illness that necessitated the immobilization.

Cervical spondylosis

Cervical spondylosis can cause a fall if the patient has osteoarthritis of the neck with encroachment; an upward or sideways neck movement can cause a decrease in cerebral blood flow causing hypoxic episodes.

Pernicious anemia

Pernicious anemia is a condition in which the fundus of the stomach does not secrete enough intrinsic factor to ensure adequate absorption of the vitamin B_{12} (extrinsic factor). In the vitamin B_{12} nutritional deficiencies, there may be a loss of vibratory sensation and proprioception which may lead to falling. Patients with a history of partial gastrectomies secondary to peptic ulcer disease may develop pernicious anemia.

Emotional stress

Patients who have increased emotional stress have a higher risk of falling because of a decreased awareness.

Environmental Hazards
Stairs

Falling on the stairs is a fairly common phenomenon. The elderly person may slip on wet stairs, misjudge the last step, or fall because of decreased visibility secondary to both poor stair lighting or the decreased visual acuity that may accompany aging. Whereas younger people may be able to regain balance when they begin to fall, the aged person's reflex responses are slower, making this a more difficult task. The aged person who is adjusting to new glasses may experience a temporary dizziness and thus fall when looking down to descend the stairs.

Tripping on slippery surfaces, worn out rugs, throw rugs, clutter	Many elderly patients fall because they slip on icy or snowy steps, landings, etc., or they misjudge the distance of curbs or steps. The elderly also frequently fall because throw rugs slide on hardwood floors, linoleum, etc., or they get their foot caught in a worn edge of a carpet.
Mobility aids	Mechanical devices used to aid the elderly in movement, such as braces, crutches, wheelchairs, etc., can malfunction (break, fit wrong, etc.) and cause a fall.

PART C WORKSHEET RATIONALE

This section of the protocol is to be used in two ways: First, Part C is designed to serve as a plan section to Part B. It is assumed that, once a particular organic etiology as a cause of the fall has been determined, the patient's medical regimen will be primarily managed by the physician. The following plan focuses on the part of the management that includes teaching, counseling and preventive health care.

The second purpose of Part C is that of a preventive health screening tool; it is designed to help the health practitioner identify those patients at high risk for falls and to subsequently guide them in appropriate health prevention management. The patient's problem list should be examined; those patients who have a diagnosed illness listed in the left-hand column are at a high risk for a potential fall. Patients, their families, staff in institutions, and others should be made particularly aware of that high risk and institute appropriate preventive health care as per these guidelines.

Organic illnesses causing pathologic fractures (e.g., osteoporosis, osteomalacia, metastatic cancer, hyperparathyroidism and Paget's)

The medical regimen depends on the correction of the underlying etiology (e.g., correction of the condition causing increased calcium loss if possible, with addition of dietary or supplemental calcium and vitamin D). In the treatment of postmenopausal osteoporosis, estrogen replacements may be of some benefit in decreasing bone resorption, but they are not capable of restoring the bone mass lost.

The elderly with osteoporosis should be encouraged to become physically mobile (because immobility enhances bone resorption). The patient should be educated about the disease process and should be taught the importance of proper body mechanics in lifting, etc. The patient should be taught to avoid undue straining and/or sudden jerky movements.

The management of osteomalacia, metastatic cancer, hyperparathyroidism, and Paget's disease should be primarily managed by the patient's physician.

Postural Hypotension

Educate elderly male patients to sit on the commode to urinate when first arising. Some patients experience a vasovagal response with a resultant syncopal episode that can cause a fall. Also see "Immobile Patients."

Cardiovascular Problems

The patient should be taught about the need for compliance to the medical regimen, the side effects of medicines, and how to decrease the risk of falling (i.e., not changing positions rapidly, etc.) If the patient has a pacemaker, she or he can be taught how to take the pulse so as to watch for indications that the battery is failing.

Neurologic Problems

The patient should be made aware of the disease process and associated symptoms. She or he may benefit from physical therapy in hopes of modifying gait alterations. The patient should be taught the importance of decreasing environmental hazards; the side effects of medications should also be taught.

Others
Asthma

The practitioner in collaboration with the physician can ascertain the feasibility of decreasing the steroid dosage to the lowest tolerable dose. If osteoporosis is documented as present, educate the patient to decrease environmental hazards, avoid straining, and utilize proper body mechanics.

Arthritis

The patient may benefit from the use of crutches, walkers, etc., but should be instructed in their proper usage. The patient must be made aware of the role that environmental hazards play in potential falls.

Foot problems

The patient may benefit from referral to a podiatrist. Instruct the patient about the importance of decreasing environmental hazards and wearing good fitting shoes with nonskid surfaces.

Immobile patients

Studies (Rodstein, 1964) and surveys (by author Broderick) have demonstrated that the "risk" hours for falling are from 6 to 10:30 A.M. (the patient is arising, bathing, dressing, etc.) and 5 to 9 P.M. (the patient is busy with dinner-hour and bedtime activities); and in institutions from 2 to 5 P.M. (when shift changes cause lapses in observational periods). Few falls occur at night (those that do are usually due to the patient reaching for something and falling out of bed). The increased risk activities include 1) getting in and out of bed, 2) getting in and out of the bathtub, 3) getting on and off the commode and 4) getting on and off wheelchairs. Practitioners should therefore be particularly skilled in helping the patient understand the risk activities so that together they can problem solve and trouble shoot potential preventable falls.

To prevent falls secondary to postural hypotension episodes, encourage the patient to sit up at the bedside and to ambulate (with help) only when temporary dizziness has passed. Educate the staff to be alert in helping the confused patient to prevent falling.

Cervical spondylosis

If the patient has osteoarthritis of the neck with nerve encroachment, warn of the dangers of looking upward, sideways, or of reaching for things with arms above the head; these activities decrease the cerebral blood flow, causing hypoxic episodes and possibly precipitating falls.

Pernicious anemia

Identification and treatment (with physician collaboration) is necessary. The patient should be made aware of the importance of complying with the medical therapy.

Emotional stress

The patient's health care should include an assessment of his or her coping strategies and problem-solving ability. Psychotherapy may be indicated; if the health team caring for the patient is not skilled in this, the patient should be referred to a mental health therapist. The patient should be taught about the increased risks of falling when particularly preoccupied with stress.

Environmental Hazards
Stairs

The patient's stairwells should be equipped with sturdy handrails which extend to the edge of the last step and are located far enough away from the wall to facilitate easy grabbing. The stairs and stairwells should have good lighting with nonskid strips on the stairs. In institutions, the doors at the top of stairs should be well labeled, preferably with a window in the door that will alert the residents to the stairs.

Slippery surfaces or unstable structures, environmental clutter

The elderly should be strongly encouraged to remain at home on snowy or rainy days. Throw rugs should be discouraged; if used, only those with rubber or nonskid backing should be in the house. Have the patient check for areas of worn carpets and be alert to these present hazards; the edges of the carpet should be tacked down. Rails and bars should be installed in the bathroom around the tub and commode to assist the patient in getting in and out of the tub, etc. Encourage the elderly patient to clean up spills right away and to allow the floor to dry well. Encourage the use of nonskid floor waxes. Warn patients of the hazards of wearing hard rubber sole or leather sole shoes (they provide less gripping surfaces). Have the patient fallproof the house by discouraging extension cords lying on the floor, avoiding chairs on rolling casters, etc. Encourage the use of night lights to illuminate the path to the bathroom at night or keeping a flashlight by the bedside for this purpose. The aged person sometimes accumulates possessions because they provide a sense of security. In the cluttered environment, the patient should be encouraged to discard what she or he deems unnecessary or at least to arrange things in an orderly manner, with wide pathways for walking.

Mobility aids

Mobility aids used by the elderly should be examined for possible malfunctioning parts; correction of any problems should be a top priority.

REFERENCES

1. Brockelhurst, J. C. *Textbook of Geriatric Medicine and Gerontology.* London: Churchill Livingston, 1973, pp. 476–494.
2. DeGowin, Elmer L. *Bedside Diagnostic Examination*, 3rd ed. New York: Macmillan Publishing, pp. 631–632.
3. Freehafer, Alvin A. "Injuries to the Skeletal System of Older Persons." *Working with Older People: Vol. IV Clinical Aspects of Aging.* Washington, D.C.: U.S. Department of Health, Education and Welfare, 1973, Chap. VIII, pp. 180–194.
4. Gilbert, Gordon and Cynthia Vaughn. "The Role of Estrogens in Osteoporosis." *Geriatrics*, Sept. 1977, 42–48.
5. Grimes, W. "Why Some Fractures Don't Heal." *Modern Medicine*, Vol. 45, No. 14, Aug. 15, 1977, 34–37.
6. Neilson, Johannes, Homma, Akira, and Toraen Bjorn. "Geronto-Psychiatric Prevalence Study." *Journal of Gerontology*, Vol. 23, No. 5, Sept. 1977, 556.
7. Rodman, Gerald. *Primer on the Rheumatic Diseases*, 7th ed. Sections 61, 62, 63. New York: The Arthritis Foundation, pp. 120–122.
8. Rodstein, Manuel. "Accidents Among the Aged: Incidence, Causes and Prevention." *Journal of Chronic Disease*, Vol. 17, 1964, 515–526.
9. Rodstein, Manuel, and Alfonso Camus. "Interrelation of Heart Disease and Accidents." *Geriatrics*, Feb. 1973, pp. 87–96.
10. Turek, Samuel L. *Orthopaedics: Principles and Their Applications*, 2nd ed. Philadelphia: J.B. Lippincott Co., 1967, 649–713.

Chapter 3

Hearing Deficit

OVERVIEW

The reduction of hearing sensitivity which occurs with advancing age is termed *presbycusis*. It may be argued that some hearing loss due to presbycusis is present in all geriatric patients, although the extent of this hearing loss may be slight. Certainly, the nurse or physician serving the geriatric population will encounter many patients who present a complaint of hearing loss.

Presbycusis is an irreversible, bilateral, primarily sensorineural loss of hearing sensitivity. It does not present a life-threatening situation, although the communication difficulties frequently encountered by the presbycusic patient may result in serious social or psychological difficulties. Presbycusis is probably the most frequent cause of hearing loss in the geriatric patient, even though other otologic conditions can exist coincidentally.

Hearing loss which has resulted from aging may be expected to differ from patient to patient. Spoor (1967) has examined data from eight separate studies of hearing loss in the elderly and has offered data revealing a relationship between age and hearing loss. These data are presented for men and women respectively in Figures 3-1 and 3-2. Examination of these data reveals that presbycusic hearing loss appears to increase as a function of age, with the higher frequencies (above 1000 Hz) being affected the most. It should also be noted that hearing loss appears to be greater in men than in women for any age group, a finding which may be partially due to factors other than the aging process.

Hearing loss is a symptom which may occur alone or as a manifestation of another disorder. It is the practitioner's responsibility, when encountering a geriatric patient who presents with a complaint of hearing loss, to explore for and rule out all possible conditions which may be medically and/or surgically treatable or which may represent life-

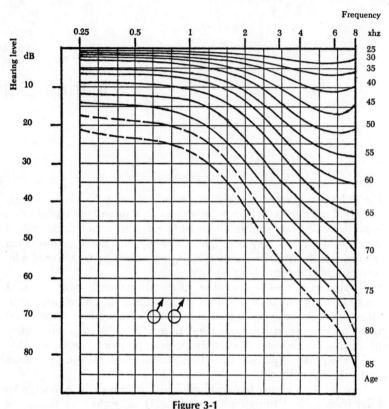

Figure 3-1
Curves giving the relation between hearing level and frequency at different ages for men according to the calculated data.

threatening situations. Only when all other possibilities have been ruled out should a diagnosis of presbycusis be made.

The diagnosis of presbycusis is, therefore, essentially one of diagnosis by exclusion. Therefore, the following protocol is intended to facilitate identification of *conductive pathologies* (external auditory canal, tympanic membrane and middle ear space) as well as nonpresbycusic cochlear pathologies (*sensory*) and retrocochlear pathologies (*neural*). The protocol is intended primarily as a screening device, to be used as a basis for deciding when to refer a patient to a specialist.

It is assumed that the armamentarium of any medical clinic will include an otoscope and tuning forks. Space for recording of audi-

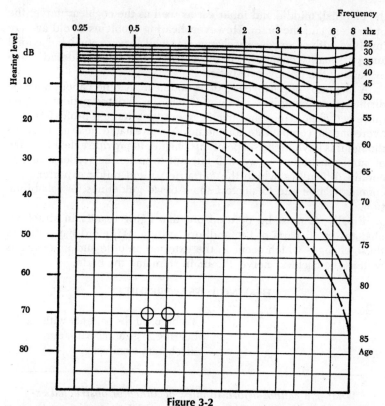

Figure 3-2
Curves giving the relation between hearing level and frequency at different ages for women according to the calculated data. Figures 3-1 and 3-2 from A. Spoor, "Presbycusis Values in Relation to Noise-Induced Hearing Loss," *International Audiology*, 6, 1967, pp. 48–57.

ometric data is provided so that this data may be made part of the patient's record if audiometric evaluation is accessible. Properly performed audiometric testing can provide a significant addition to the information gathered with the otoscope and tuning forks. Comprehensive audiologic evaluation also facilitates the designing of an effective program of aural rehabilitation.

A second purpose of this chapter is to provide an understanding of the social and psychological effects of hearing loss in the geriatric patient. Aging results in structural changes in all parts of the auditory system. Willeford (1971) has outlined these changes which occur in the external, middle and inner ear as well as the cochlear nerve, the brain stem and the brain. However, hearing problems in old age are involved with other sensory changes, as well as perceptual, behavioral and personality changes. These changes must be considered when evaluating the presbycusic patient.

A diagnosis of presbycusis does not mean that the patient must be dismissed as being beyond help. Often, the geriatric patient will require active guidance and management by a trained professional to overcome or compensate for medically untreatable hearing loss. Although it is beyond the scope of this chapter to provide a detailed plan of aural rehabilitation, we will attempt to make the reader aware of certain difficulties which the geriatric patient might experience in communication and to suggest some broad guidelines for rehabilitation.

Finally, it must be pointed out that aging results in structural changes in all parts of the auditory system. Willeford has outlined these changes which occur in the external, middle and inner ear as well as the cochlear nerve, the brain stem and the brain.

HEARING LOSS WORKSHEET

To be used for patients with hearing loss, aural pain, aural discharge, tinnitus.

What you cannot afford to miss: occluded or obstructed external auditory canals, otitis externa, otitis media, perforated tympanic membrane, cholesteatoma, ossicular discontinuity, Meniere's disease, acoustic trauma, presbycusis, acoustic neuroma.

Chief Complaint: _____

SUBJECTIVE DATA:

HEARING LOSS:
YES   NO

_____ _____ Unilateral: R_____ L_____

_____ _____ Bilateral: better ear R_____ L_____

Date of Onset: _____

Patient's estimate of etiology: _____

_____

_____

(Describe All Positive Responses)
YES   NO

_____ _____ Sudden onset: _____

_____ _____ Gradual onset: _____

_____ _____ Fluctuating: _____

ASSOCIATED WITH THE FOLLOWING:

_____ _____ Tinnitus: R_____ L_____ (steady, pulsa-
                 tile, periodic, constant)

_____

_____

_____

_____ _____ Aural pain: _____

_____ _____ Aural discharge: _____

_____ _____ Head cold: _____

_____ _____ Head injury: _____

_____ _____ Feeling of fullness in ears:_____

_____

_____ _____ Nausea: _____

_____ _____ Vertigo: _____

_____

_____ _____ Presence of allergies: _____

_____ _____ Other: _____

DIFFICULT LISTENING SITUATIONS ASSOCIATED WITH THE HEARING LOSS:
(Describe All Positive Responses)
YES   *NO*

_____ _____ Do people's voices sound loud, but not clear, to you?

_____

_____ _____ Do you have difficulty understanding words?_____

_____

_____ _____ Do people's voices sound too soft to you? _____

_____

_____ _____ Do you often find it necessary to ask people to speak

up? _____

_____

_____ _____ Can you understand conversation better when you

are watching the face of the speaker? _____

_____

_____ _____ Do you think that you lipread?_____

_____

_____ _____ Do you hear better in a noisy environment? • _____

_____

_____ _____ Do you have difficulty understanding conversation in a noisy environment? _____

_____

_____ _____ Do you have difficulty using the telephone because you cannot understand the words? _____

_____

_____ _____ Do you have difficulty understanding the speakers on the radio or the television? _____

_____

_____ _____ Do you have difficulty when you are talking to only one person? _____

_____

_____ _____ Do you have difficulty when you are talking with several persons? _____

_____

_____ _____ Do you have difficulty determining from which direction a sound is coming? _____

OTOLOGIC MEDICAL HISTORY:
YES   *NO*

_____ _____ Earaches: _____

_____ _____ Drainage from the ears: _____

_____ _____ Excessive cerumen: _____

Hearing Loss Worksheet

———— ———— Loss of hearing: _____

———— ———— Meniere's disease: _____

———— ———— Otosclerosis: _____

———— ———— Tinnitus: _____

———— ———— Perforated eardrum(s) _____

———— ———— Ear surgery: _____

_____

RELATED MEDICAL HISTORY:
YES   NO

———— ———— Mumps: _____

———— ———— Measles: _____

———— ———— Whooping cough: _____

———— ———— Scarlet fever: _____

———— ———— Viral pneumonia: _____

———— ———— Influenza: _____

———— ———— Viral meningitis: _____

———— ———— Polio: _____

———— ———— Diphtheria: _____

———— ———— Syphilis: _____

———— ———— Tuberculosis: _____

———— ———— Brucellosis: _____

———— ———— Sinusitis: _____

———— ———— Tonsilitis: _____

———— ———— Diabetes: _____

———— ———— Arthritis: _____

———— ———— Malaria: _____

———— ———— Broken nose: _____

———— ———— Skull fracture: _____

———— ———— Concussion: _____

———— ———— Surgery for any reason: _____

———— ———— High blood pressure: _____

DRUG EXPOSURE:

Have you ever taken any of the following drugs?

Group I Acetylsalicylates and Salicylates:

———— ———— Aspirin: _____

———— ———— Quinine: _____

———— ———— Chloroquine phosphate: _____

Group II Diuretics:

———— ———— Ethacrynic acid: _____

———— ———— Furosemide: _____

———— ———— Ethacrynate sodium: _____

———— ———— Fenoprofen calcium: _____

Group III Aminoglycosides:

———— ———— Amikacin sulfate: _____

Hearing Loss Worksheet

_____ _____ Gentamicin (Garamycin): _____

_____ _____ Kanamycin sulfate: _____

_____ _____ Neomycin sulfate: _____

_____ _____ Paromomycin sulfate: _____

_____ _____ Streptomycin: _____

_____ _____ Tobramycin sulfate: _____

_____ _____ Dihydrostreptomycin: _____

Group IV Miscellaneous:

_____ _____ Vancomycin: _____

_____ _____ Polymyxin B: _____

_____ _____ Viomycin: _____

FAMILY HISTORY OF HEARING DISORDERS:
YES   *NO*

_____ _____ Do you know of any member of your family who has

a hearing loss? _____

_____ _____ Has any member of your family ever had treatments

for any problem related to the ears? _____

_____

_____ _____ Has any member of your family ever worn a hearing

aid? _____

_____

NOISE EXPOSURE:
YES　　*NO*

_____ _____ Have you ever been in the military service? If yes,

describe your duties: _____

_____

Have you ever worked around any of the following?

_____ _____ Farm machinery: _____

_____ _____ Trucks: _____

_____ _____ Power tools: _____

_____ _____ Internal combustion engines: _____

_____ _____ Heavy equipment: _____

_____ _____ Airplanes: _____

_____ _____ Air hammers: _____

_____ _____ Locomotives: _____

_____ _____ Stamping equipment: _____

_____ _____ Any machinery which produced loud noises: _____

_____

Do you like to do any of the following?
YES　　*NO*

_____ _____ Shoot guns: _____

_____ _____ Use power tools: _____

_____ _____ Work with noisy machinery: _____

Hearing Loss Worksheet

_____ _____ Work on cars or motorcycles: _____

_____ _____ Ride motorcycles: _____

_____ _____ Ride snowmobiles: _____

_____ _____ Do you now or have you ever had any other exposure

to loud noises? _____

_____

HEARING AID HISTORY:
YES   *NO*

_____ _____ Do you now wear or have you ever worn a hearing

aid?

Make:_____ Model:_____

Date of Acquisition: _____

Serial Number:_____ Type: Behind-the-

ear Body Eyeglasses All-in-the-ear (Circle the

correct type)

Ear in which aid is/was worn? Right Left
Binaural fitting
Earmold Type: Standard Ring Shell Other

Age of present earmold:_____

Apparent fit of earmold: Tight ____ Loose ____

Condition of earmold:_____ Condition

of coupling tubing: _____

Condition of cord (for body aid): _____

Summary statement regarding general condition of

hearing aid and accessories: _____
Place of Acquisition: Hearing Aid Dealer
Audiologist   Speech and Hearing Clinic
Physician's Office

Name of Supplier: _____

Address: _____

Telephone: _____

Why did you obtain a hearing aid? _____

_____

How long have you been wearing/did you wear a hearing aid? _____

_____

How many hours per day do/did you wear a hearing aid? _____

_____

Does/did the hearing aid help you to hear? (yes, sometimes, not much,

not at all—describe) _____

_____

Were you given instructions in the operation of the hearing aid when

you purchased it? Did you understand its operation? _____

AURAL REHABILITATION HISTORY:

Have you ever had instruction in any of the following? (Positive answers to any of these questions should be followed by notation of when, where and by whom the instruction was provided.)

Hearing Loss Worksheet

YES   NO

_____   _____   Speechreading: _____

_____   _____   Auditory training: _____

_____   _____   Speech therapy: _____

OBJECTIVE DATA:

OTOSCOPIC EXAMINATION: (DESCRIBE POSITIVE RESPONSES)
AURICLE
YES   NO

_____   _____   Appearance normal: _____

_____   _____   Microtic: _____

_____   _____   Pre-auricular tags present: _____

_____   _____   Absent: _____

_____   _____   Mutilated: _____

_____   _____   Laceration present: _____

_____   _____   Swelling present: _____

_____   _____   Perichondritis present: _____

_____   _____   Sensitive upon palpation: _____

_____   _____   Furunculosis present: _____

_____   _____   Dermatitis present: _____

_____   _____   Herpes present: _____

MASTOID AREA:
YES   NO

_____   _____   Normal: _____

_____ _____ Swollen: _____

_____ _____ Tender: _____

EXTERNAL AUDITORY CANAL:
YES   *NO*

_____ _____ Inflamed: _____

_____ _____ Swollen: _____

_____ _____ Collapsed: _____

_____ _____ Atretic: _____

_____ _____ Occluded with cerumen: _____

_____ _____ Obstructed with foreign matter: _____

_____ _____ Pustules present: _____

_____ _____ Osteomas present: _____

_____ _____ Excessive hair present: _____

_____ _____ Otitis externa present: _____

_____ _____ Furunculosis present: _____

_____ _____ Keratosis obliterans present: _____

_____ _____ Discharge present: _____

TYMPANIC MEMBRANE:
YES   *NO*

_____ _____ Normal: _____

_____ _____ Perforated (describe): _____

_____ _____ Dull in color: _____

Hearing Loss Worksheet

_____ _____ Inflamed: _____

_____ _____ Injected: _____

_____ _____ Bluish:_____

_____ _____ Positive Swartze's sign: _____

_____ _____ Thickened:_____

_____ _____ Retracted: _____

_____ _____ Extended: _____

_____ _____ Monomeric membrane present (describe): _____

_____

_____ _____ Tympanosclerotic plaques present: _____

_____ _____ Bullous myringitis present: _____

_____ _____ Evidence of growth into the middle ear: _____

_____ _____ Granulation present: _____

_____ _____ Yellowish: _____

EUSTACHIAN TUBE:
YES   NO

_____ _____ Normal in function:_____

_____ _____ Excess tissue around orifice: _____

_____ _____ Valsalva possible: _____

_____ _____ Toynbee maneuver possible: _____

_____ _____ Does Valsalva or Politzer maneuver subjectively im-

prove the patient's hearing? _____

TUNING FORK TESTS:

Schwabach:

Frequency	Better than Examiner's Hearing Sensitivity	Equal to Examiner's Hearing Sensitivity	Poorer than Examiner's Hearing Sensitivity
512 Hz			
1024 Hz			
2048 Hz			

Weber:

	Lateralizes Right	Lateralizes Left	Midline
512 Hz			
1024 Hz			
2048 Hz			

Rinne:

Frequency	Positive	Negative
512 Hz		
1024 Hz		
2048 Hz		

Bing:

	Normal	Conductive
512 Hz		
1024 Hz		
2048 Hz		

Remarks: _____

_____

_____

_____

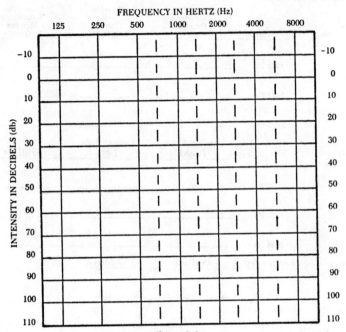

Figure 3-3
Sample audiogram form.

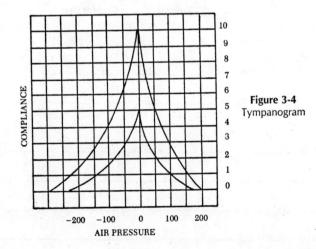

Figure 3-4
Tympanogram

Speech Audiometry
(Speech Results)
Right Ear

SRT: _____ dB HTL

SD: _____% @

_____ dB SL

Left Ear

SRT: _____dB HTL

SD: _____ % @

_____ dB SL

Masking levels: _____

_____

Remarks: _____

_____

Impedance Audiometry
(Acoustic Impedance Measurements)

Reflex Thresholds

	500	1000	2000	4000
R				
L				

Remarks: _____

_____

Summary of site of lesion testing: _____

_____

_____

_____

_____

_____

_____

HEARING LOSS WORKSHEET RATIONALE

SUBJECTIVE DATA:

Unilateral or Bilateral

Presbycusis is virtually always bilateral. If a patient indicates that a hearing problem is primarily unilateral, the examiner can assume with reasonable confidence that some problem other than presbycusis exists. In the case of bilateral impairments, it is useful to determine whether the patient believes that one ear is better than the other ear. If the patient notices some difference between ears, this suggests the possibility of ongoing pathology other than presbycusis.

Onset

Any hearing loss which has been present before the seventh decade of life must be assumed to be due to factors other than the aging process until proven otherwise. The examiner should establish the time of onset of the hearing loss as accurately as possible. Any changes in hearing sensitivity which have occurred since the onset of the loss should be noted along with any accompanying symptoms. General physical condition since the onset of hearing difficulties should be explored. Any factors which might have brought on or contributed to a hearing loss should be noted.

Patient's Estimate of Etiology

The examiner should permit the patient to tell, in his own words with as little guidance as possible, what he or she believes is the cause of the hearing loss. Although such a statement may be erroneous, insight may be gained into the patient's background, the effects the hearing problem has had on the patient's life and his or her expectations for rehabilitation. The patient should be encouraged to provide a complete statement, since some factors to which the patient attaches no significance may be of importance. The examiner should be wary, however, of estimating the severity of the hearing loss from the patient's comments. We have seen patients who have come to us and announced that they were "deaf as a post," but who revealed only moderate hearing losses upon audiologic evaluation. Experience tells us that these patients' subjective assessments of their problems are as important as our audiologic evaluation in determining the extent of the difficulty posed by the hearing loss. It should be noted that we have seen patients who reported no difficulty hearing, but whose audiologic evaluations revealed some impairment. Once again, the patient's subjective estimate must be considered.

Sudden Onset

Hearing loss of sudden onset must be considered to be from factors other than presbycusis, and a problem requiring immediate medical attention.

Gradual Onset

The patient whose hearing loss is principally due to presbycusis will report a gradual, bilateral hearing loss which has occurred over a number of years. However, a patient with active otosclerosis may also report gradual hearing loss. Since otosclerosis usually results in unilateral impairment or asymmetrical bilateral impairment, the examiner should question the patient regarding subjective differences between ears. In addition, the otosclerotic patient may report that he is able to hear better when sounds become louder, or that he may hear better in a noisy environment. The presbycusis patient may report exactly the opposite.

Fluctuating Hearing Loss

Fluctuating hearing loss classically accompanies Meniere's disease. However, the patient whose hearing loss is due to middle ear pathology such as otitis media or negative pressure from eustachian tube dysfunction may report some subjective fluctuation. Subjects in whom allergies or hay fever produce upper respiratory symptoms may also report fluctuation. In addition, the examiner will encounter patients who complain of fluctuating hearing sensitivity whose hearing appears to be within normal limits audiometrically. The complaint of fluctuation of hearing sensitivity may be offered by patients with nonorganic hearing losses.

Associated With:
Tinnitus

Tinnitus is a nonspecific complaint. It may occur in normal hearing sensitivity or in ears having a conductive, cochlear or neural pathology. Low-pitched tinnitus may accompany otitis media, Meniere's disease, glomus jugular tumors or occlusive cartoid artery disease. If the patient reports a continuous, low-pitched tinnitus with a hearing loss, middle ear pathology such as otitis media may be suspected. This tinnitus may become pulsatile when the conductive component becomes advanced. If the tinnitus is pulsatile and low-pitched, but no hearing loss is present, the possibility exists for the presence of a glomus tumor or occlusive carotid artery disease. If the patient reports a high-pitched tinnitus, either constant or intermittent, several etiologies are possible including presbycusis, noise-induced hearing loss, hearing loss from exposure to ototoxic drugs, or retrocochlear involvement.

Aural pain

The patient with this complaint may be referring to a feeling in the pinna, the ear canal, the middle ear or the mastoid. Aural pain is indicative of some problem other than presbycusis. It should be noted that

117

some patients having tempomandibular joint syndrome will also complain of pain in the locality of the ear.

Aural discharge

Aural discharge may result from lesions in the external auditory canal, the tympanic membrane, the mastoid or the cochlea. It requires immediate medical attention.

Head cold

Hearing loss associated with head colds may be the result of middle ear pathology brought on by the upper respiratory infection. This hearing loss will be conductive, but may not be of sufficient severity to be detected by the use of tuning forks. Audiometric evaluation and/or impedance audiometry should detect even a small conductive component in a hearing loss.

Head injury

A severe blow to the head may result in a perforated tympanic membrane, disarticulation of the ossicular chain, or a fracture of the bony labyrinth with resultant escape of cochlear fluids. A perforated tympanic membrane or disarticulated ossicular chain will produce a unilateral conductive hearing loss. Loss of cochlear fluids will produce a sensorineural hearing loss which may be either unilateral or bilateral, depending upon the locus of the fracture. Audiometrically, speech intelligibility may be greatly reduced in proportion to the severity of the hearing loss. A loss of vestibular function may be noted.

Fullness in the ear

Classically, this sensation accompanies Meniere's disease. However, it is also reported by patients who are experiencing some eustachian tube dysfunction and by patients having perforations of the tympanic membrane. Meniere's disease typically produces sensorineural hearing loss, which may be primarily low-frequency in the early stages of the disease but may involve all frequencies as the disease progresses. Eustachian tube dysfunction may or may not produce a low-frequency conductive hearing loss. It will often result in negative pressure in the middle ear which should be revealed by impedance audiometry. Patients having perforations of the tympanic membrane may display a conductive hearing loss, depending upon the location and size of the perforation. Impedance audiometry will demonstrate inordinately large static compliance measurements.

Nausea

Nausea associated with tinnitus, vertigo and hearing loss is highly suggestive of Meniere's disease. The examiner should attempt to determine whether the nausea occurs coincidentally with the hearing loss.

Vertigo

True vertigo is a false sensation of motion. However, many patients who report dizziness are actually experiencing some other sensation. The patient should be asked to describe the sensation in detail, including any action or event which seems to precipitate the attacks.

119

Vertigo may also be spontaneous, however, and this possibility should be explored. The examiner should determine whether the attacks occur with or without nausea and vomiting; vertigo with these symptoms is labyrinthine in origin. It should also be determined whether hearing loss is present. The causes of vertiginous disturbances of the labyrinth include Meniere's disease, effects of ototoxic drugs, paroxysmal positional vertigo, trauma, tumors on the vestibular branch of the VIIIth nerve, vestibular neuronitis and vertebral artery insufficiency. True vertigo can also occur in cerebellar disease, cerebral anoxia and endocrine disease. The geriatric patient who suffers from arteriosclerosis may also demonstrate vertiginous symptoms. When the clinician encounters a patient who presents with true vertigo, he or she may wish to refer this patient for further evaluation, which may include electronystagmography or other techniques employed for evaluation of the vestibular system.

Allergies

Allergies may produce symptoms similar to those presented as a result of upper respiratory infections. Transient middle ear pathologies may occur with the possibility of accompanying conductive hearing loss.

DIFFICULT LISTENING SITUATIONS ASSOCIATED WITH HEARING LOSS

Do voices sound loud, but not clear? Do you have difficulty understanding words?

If the patient complains that speaker's voices sound loud enough but not clear to him, it is an indication that a sensorineural component may be present in the hearing loss. A sensorineural loss often leads to a reduction in speech discrimination ability. Reduced speech discrimination may be responsible for the complaint often voiced by geriatric patients that "people don't speak clearly any more. They just mumble."

If the patient indicates difficulty understanding speech regardless of its intensity, a sensorineural hearing loss is suggested. However, if the patient indicates that an increase in intensity improves his or her ability to understand speech, a conductive or mixed hearing loss must be suspected. It should be noted, however, that some persons with sensorineural hearing losses may benefit from moderate increases in input intensity.

Do voices sound too soft? Do you often ask people to speak up?

This suggests a moderate to severe loss of hearing sensitivity. It may reflect a conductive component, which has the effect of attenuating input intensities. However, a person having a moderate sensorineural loss may also need to ask speakers to speak louder. It is useful to inquire whether an increase in intensity on the part of the speaker greatly increases understanding. A positive answer suggests a conductive component or a mild sensorineural loss.

Is understanding improved by watching the speaker? Do you read lips?

These questions may provide some insight into the patient's assessment of his problem, as well as his willingness to compensate. Some patients claim that they can increase understanding by watching the speaker, and believe that this increase results from lipreading. However, they may demonstrate no ability to lipread when this skill is evaluated formally. When subsequent audiologic evaluation reveals near-normal hearing, we may suspect that the improvement demonstrated by "lipreading" is, in reality, the result of increased attention on the part of the patient. Some patients who profess to lipread or speechread do, in fact, possess some self-taught ability. This may be a favorable indication for future aural rehabilitation success.

Hearing in a noisy environment

Patients having conductive hearing impairments often experience a slight subjective improvement in understanding in the presence of noise, whereas those patients having sensorineural impairments may experience inordinate difficulty understanding speech in the presence of noise.

Difficulty using the telephone

A sensorineural hearing loss with reduced speech discrimination ability may impair the patient's ability to understand telephone conversation. This reduced speech discrimination may be so slight that the patient reports no difficulty in face-to-face conversation. Patients having moderate to severe conductive or sensorineural hearing losses may experience difficulty using telephones. Interestingly, some patients will report less difficulty understanding speech on a telephone than in normal conversation.

Difficulty in listening to the radio or television

As has been noted above, difficulty understanding speech may be due to reduced speech discrimination resulting from a sensorineural loss. However, since reduction in discrimination may often be somewhat compensated for by an increase in volume, it is useful to inquire whether the patient employs inordinate amounts of volume to facilitate understanding.

Difficulty talking to only one person

Patient response to this question may confirm or restate answers to previous questions. The response may be useful for judging the severity of the loss as well as the type of involvement. A positive response suggests either a moderate to severe hearing loss or greatly reduced speech discrimination.

Difficulty talking with several persons

A positive response to this question should prompt the examiner to ask for an example. The patient may indicate he has difficulty in group conversations such as social gatherings, at which several conversations are occurring simultaneously. This may suggest sensorineural involvement. A positive response may also indicate asymmetry in the hearing loss, a condition which might be expected to result in difficulty understanding those speakers located on the side of the poorer ear.

Difficulty determining the direction from which sounds come

Binaural hearing which is symmetrical within a 15 to 20 dB range is necessary to effectively localize sounds. Therefore, the patient who reports consistent inability to localize sound may be suspected of having a unilateral loss of sensitivity or a bilateral loss in which one ear is significantly poorer than the other ear.

Otologic Medical History
Earaches

This refers to the patient's history of earaches prior to the time of the present complaint. A history of earaches may suggest chronic middle ear disease and the presence of a conductive hearing loss due to necrosis of the ossicular chain. Other problems which may be present are chronic otitis media or a perforation of the tympanic membrane. Although middle ear pathology is suggested, the clinician should be alert for the possibility of a sensorineural hearing loss, since middle ear disease may also invade the cochlea.

Drainage from the ears

Drainage suggests a history of middle ear disease (see above) and perforations of the tympanic membrane. Drainage may also result from a cholesteatoma or a lesion in the external auditory meatus. Drainage may also be an initial sign of a malignant ear disease, such as a carcinoma.

Loss of hearing

Determination should be made of when the hearing loss was first noticed and of possible etiologies of the loss. The clinician should not assume that the present complaint is similar or related to the prior complaint.

Meniere's disease

The clinician should determine when and by whom this diagnosis had been made and how the problem has been treated. A patient with Meniere's disease should be referred for otologic evaluation and management. Audiologic evaluation is helpful for assessing the extent of the hearing loss and the need for aural rehabilitation.

Otosclerosis

Otosclerosis has been treated by several surgical procedures. If the patient has had surgery, determine when it was performed as well as the success of the results. Audiologic evaluation will be helpful in the determination of the latter.

Tinnitus

Some practitioners attempt to reduce or eliminate tinnitus by the use of medications such as vasodilators. If treatment has been attempted, determine its success.

Perforated eardrum

Determine what treatment has been used and the extent of its success.

Related Medical History
Past disease

Otologic viral disease may produce sensorineural hearing loss. This loss is usually bilateral, except in the case of mumps, which may produce a unilateral hearing loss. Bacterial diseases, such as bacterial meningitis and encephalitis, may also affect the cochlea and the central auditory pathways.

125

Upper respiratory infections can invade the middle ear, causing conductive deafness. Longstanding conductive pathologies can result in partial or total destruction of the ossicular chain and/or the tympanic membrane. In addition, conductive pathology can invade the cochlea and result in sensorineural hearing loss.

Degenerative diseases, such as diabetes, may result in gradual loss of hearing sensitivity. This loss is usually bilateral and sensorineural, affecting the higher frequencies initially.

Broken nose, skull
fracture, concussion

Traumatic injuries to the head may result in either conductive or sensorineural hearing disorders. Ossicular chain discontinuity may result from a severe blow to the head, producing a conductive hearing loss. A history of a broken nose which has resulted in a deviated septum may also result in a conductive hearing loss. As has been suggested earlier, a skull fracture which affects the cochlea may result in sensorineural hearing loss.

Surgeries

Ototoxic drugs are sometimes used topically as antiseptics after surgery. The effects of ototoxic drugs are discussed later in this chapter.

High blood pressure

The presence of high blood pressure can induce or exacerbate tinnitus. In addition, it may be a factor in sudden ideopathic hearing loss.

Drug Exposure

The medications listed in the four groups in the protocol have the potential to damage the auditory and/or vestibular system. The incidence of damage for any specific drug is not known, although overall incidence is quite low. Bergstrom and Thompson (1976) have suggested the incidence of ototoxicity to be less than 1 percent.

Ototoxic drugs may affect either the cochlea or the vestibular system, or both. These effects may be either unilateral or bilateral. When hearing loss occurs, it is primarily sensorineural, and demonstrates cochlear findings on special auditory site of lesion tests. It may range in severity from mild to profound, and may be progressive after treatment has been terminated. The hearing loss often affects only the high frequencies initially, but may spread to all frequencies tested. It is usually permanent, but may be reversed depending upon the nature of the causative agent.

A definite diagnosis of hearing loss due to ototoxicity is often difficult to make, particularly in the geriatric patient. Audiometrically, drug-induced hearing loss can resemble hearing loss from noise, high fever, illness or presbycusis. Many geriatric patients present a history which includes several of these as possible causes. If drug-related hearing loss is suspected, the examiner should question the patient closely about past medical history, especially regarding the time of onset of the hearing loss and the patient's general physical condition at that time. A general knowledge of the possible effects of ototoxic drugs, coupled with suggestive facts about the history of the patient, may suggest the presence of ototoxic hearing loss.

Acetylsalicylates and salicylates

Perhaps the most frequently used medications which have the potential for causing hearing loss are aspirin and aspirin compounds. Massive doses of aspirin, such as those doses used to relieve the pain caused by arthritis, are generally required to produce a hearing loss. The loss is generally high frequency in nature, reversible upon cessation of medication, and may be preceded by a high frequency tinnitus.

Diuretics

Ethacrynic acid, ethacrynic sodium and furosemide are capable of causing either a transient or a permanent hearing loss when given in massive doses. Vestibular involvement may also be present. Hearing loss due to diuretics may involve all the frequencies tested audiometrically rather than only the high frequencies. Speech discrimination may be inordinately poor.

Aminoglycosides

Aminoglycosides are among the most potent of ototoxic drugs. They may cause permanent sensorineural hearing loss, usually bilaterally. Vestibular symptoms may accompany the hearing loss or may be present with normal hearing. Aminoglycosides may produce a hearing loss during the course of treatment or they may affect hearing sensitivity after all treatment has been terminated. Audiologically, the hearing loss may begin as a high frequency sensorineural loss and progress to involve middle and lower frequencies. The loss may also be progressive in severity, resulting in gradually worsening hearing sensitivity for all frequencies tested. When speech discrimination is affected, it may be inordinately poor compared to the extent of the pure tone involvement.

Miscellaneous

Of the drugs in this category, vancomycin, Polymyxin B and viomycin have been demonstrated to cause possible nephrotoxicity and progressive deafness. Viomycin has been linked to vertiginous episodes.

Family History

Hearing disorders in other family members may suggest the presence of a hereditary hearing loss in the present patient. The clinician should determine whether hearing loss has been present in other family members and/or whether any additional factors may exist which might have contributed to the hearing loss.

Obtaining necessary information may be difficult. The patient may be aware that others in his family suffered from hearing loss, but may not know the reason for the loss. Some patients may be misinformed about the hearing losses of other family members.

An inaccurate conclusion about the presence of hereditary hearing loss can be avoided by obtaining as much information as possible about suspected family members. The clinician should attempt to determine the following regarding hearing loss in other family members: 1) age of the relative at the time of the onset of the hearing loss, 2) possibility of noise exposure which could have contributed to the hearing loss, 3) history of diseases which could have produced the hearing loss, 4) whether the family member was ever treated for hearing loss by a physician, 5) whether the hearing loss was unilateral or bilateral.

Noise Exposure

The noise-producing devices listed here are provided only as examples of potentially damaging noise sources. The examiner will doubtless encounter some patients who will present histories of noise exposure from sources not listed. Furthermore, for any individual patient, even though exposure to potentially damaging noises may be established, it must not be assumed that some loss of hearing will automatically be present.

A differential diagnosis of noise-induced hearing loss is often difficult to make, particularly in the geriatric patient. Presbycusis, exposure to ototoxic drugs, head trauma or longstanding middle ear disease may produce hearing impairments which are indistinguishable audiologically from those impairments resulting from exposure to noise. Classically, hearing loss due to noise exposure is bilateral, sensorineural and high frequency in nature. Maximum involvement is often at 4000 Hz or 6000 Hz, but may be detected at any frequency. Severe noise-induced hearing loss may involve all frequencies, although the loss will generally be more severe at the higher frequencies.

When noise-induced hearing loss is suspected, the examiner should investigate the location of the patient relative to the location of the suspected damaging noise. Persons who have worked many years in the same relative position to a noise-generating source may exhibit a nonsymmetrical hearing loss which is greatest in the ear most directly exposed to the sound. The examiner should also inquire whether the patient has made use of ear protection routinely during his noise exposure. The use of ear defenders such as earplugs or noise-attenuating earmuffs does not rule out the possibility of noise-induced hearing loss, however.

Hearing Aid History

Dissatisfaction with hearing aids may result from one or more of the following: 1) malfunctioning or nonfunctioning hearing aids, 2) improper hearing aid selection, 3) improper hearing aid and/or earmold fit, 4) poor motivation on the part of the hearing aid wearer, 5) ignorance regarding hearing aid use, 6) unrealistic expectations as to the benefits to be obtained, and 7) changing hearing sensitivity. Before questioning the patient regarding general satisfaction with the hearing aid, the clinician should obtain factual information about the instrument. This includes noting the make, model and serial number as well as the particular style (i.e., post-auricle, eyeglasses, body or all-in-the-ear). The clinician should note in which ear the patient is wearing the hearing aid, the type of earmold and its condition. It is sometimes useful to determine the age of the hearing aid, as well as whether the instrument was purchased new.

Why did you obtain a hearing aid?

Patient motivation, or lack thereof, is an important source of dissatisfaction with hearing aids. Hearing aid users may have purchased a hearing aid chiefly to please a spouse or other family member. These patients may be poorly motivated to improve their hearing capabilities, and may be poor candidates for success with a hearing aid. In contrast is the patient who purchases a hearing aid with the expectation that it will completely eliminate all hearing difficulties. This patient may require extensive counseling about the capabilities and limitations of hearing aids.

Many patients may fall between the

above two extremes. We often see patients who express general satisfaction with their instruments but are able to report specific situations in which their hearing aids are less helpful than they would like. Questioning often reveals that these situations include amounts of background noise which serve to mask or "cover up" the speech they wish to hear. These patients also need reassurance and counseling about the limitations of amplification.

How long have you been wearing/did you wear a hearing aid?

Patients who are new hearing aid wearers, i.e., those who have little experience with hearing aids, usually need a period of adjustment and learning before they become successful hearing aid users. These patients often will need counseling and reinstruction in hearing aid use. Additional aural rehabilitative measures such as auditory training may sometimes be helpful.

In contrast, some patients have been successful hearing aid users for some time before becoming dissatisfied with their instruments. This dissatisfaction may stem from a change in the performance of their instruments, a change in hearing sensitivity on the part of the patient, a change in the patient's environment or some combination of these.

How many hours per day do/did you wear a hearing aid?

The length of daily use time may reflect the degree of dissatisfaction with the instrument or the extent to which the hearing aid is needed. What is important is not the *length*

133

of time the hearing aid is worn but *why* the patient chooses to wear or not wear the instrument.

Does/did the hearing aid help you to hear better?

The answer given to this question should reinforce and possibly expand upon information elicited above.

Were you given instructions in the operation of the hearing aid? Do you understand its operation?

This question is perhaps most important for those patients who have recently acquired their first instrument and are still becoming accustomed to hearing aids. Experienced hearing aid users will usually be familiar with the operation of their instruments.

Aural Rehabilitation History

A complete case history for an acoustically impaired individual should include information concerning previous rehabilitative measures. For a patient who has undergone some aural rehabilitation, two categories of information should be available. These categories are patient-initiated information and patient-evaluative information.

Patient-initiated information is all information provided by the patient. This includes his explanation of why the therapy was initiated (i.e., at his request or at the request of others) and of what value the therapy was to him. (Does he feel the therapy increased his communicative abilities, and in what way? Equally important, was the therapy of little or no value and why?) We believe patients who have positive attitudes toward aural rehabilitation are more likely to benefit from therapy than those with negative attitudes.

Patient evaluative information includes results of formal evaluations conducted as part of rehabilitation. Also of importance are summaries, progress notes and therapy plans written by previous therapists. These notes may provide objective information about the patient's success.

In summary, the practitioner should determine what was done for the patient, why the procedures were begun and what the results of the therapy were.

OBJECTIVE DATA

Otoscopic Exam

During this phase of the data-gathering process the clinician will examine the auricle, the external auditory canal and the tympanic membrane looking for any visible signs of an active pathology or the residual effects of previous pathologies. The patient whose hearing loss is due solely to advancing age should yield a normal otoscopic examination. The tympanic membranes may show some deviation in color from the normal pearly white, however, and the examiner must decide for each patient whether the drums are normal for that patient.

Auricle

A microtic or absent auricle may suggest a conductive hearing loss due to the malformation of the ossicular chain. The presence of preauricular tags should alert the practitioner to the possibility of a congenital conductive hearing loss. Perichondritis presents as a red and swollen auricle with a fever. The condition may follow trauma. In furunculosis, the external auditory canal may be reduced in size due to swelling, sometimes with complete closure. Examine lymph nodes in the area of the auricle for enlargement. Herpes affects the auricle and preauricular area and is associated with a facial palsy, vertigo and sensorineural hearing loss.

External auditory canal

The examiner should observe any deviations from normal color and structure. Significant deviations should be investigated further. Examination of the external auditory canal may reveal certain longstanding conditions which do not require referral for treatment. These include the presence of an atretic canal. The practitioner should be aware that although canal atresia will produce a maximum conductive hearing loss, the patient may have normal cochlear hearing sensitivity. In the examination of normal ears, the practitioner should note whether the canal is occluded with cerumen or foreign matter. Complete occlusion produces a conductive hearing loss. The presence of pustules or osteomas (small, hard bony nodules covered with normal skin, usually near the lateral end of the external auditory canal) should be noted. If keratosis obliterans is present, accumulations of desquamated keratin in the bony portions of the external canal will be noted.

Tympanic membrane

As was mentioned above, the tympanic membranes of older patients may often appear dull and retracted. It is sometimes useful to compare the tympanic membranes of patients. In the absence of some active condition or history of a unilateral pathology, both tympanic membranes should be similar in appearance. An inflamed or injected tympanic membrane may signal bacterial otitis when the drum is bluish. A normal-appearing drum with a pinkish hue on the promontory (Swartze's sign) indicates vascular otosclerotic focus. If the drum is bulging and extended, spontaneous perforation is imminent. If the drum appears purple with blisters present on the lateral surface, bullous myringitis is present. Monomeric membranes appear as a single layer of tissue across a perforated eardrum. Tympanosclerotic plaques are deposits of hyalin on the lateral surface of the drum which appear whitish or yellowish. These may sometimes be quite extensive.

Eustachian tube

Eustachian tube dysfunction may be transient, sometimes accompanying symptoms of upper respiratory infections. Excessive tissue growth around the orifice of the eustachian tube may result in a more frequently occurring dysfunction. Eustachian tube function can be assessed by employing either the Valsalva or Toynbee maneuvers while the tympanic membrane is being observed otoscopically. If the eustachian tube is capable of functioning, movement of the tympanic membrane should be noted. Subjectively, eustachian tube dysfunction is suggested by transient feelings of fullness within the ear. This feeling of fullness may or may not be accompanied by a hearing loss. When eustachian tube dysfunction contributes to hearing loss, the Valsalva, Toynbee or Politzer maneuvers may result in a slight subjective improvement in hearing sensitivity. These maneuvers are intended to inflate, or force air into, the middle ear space. In the Valsalva maneuver, the patient attempts to force air out through the nostrils while holding the nostrils tightly closed. The Toynbee maneuver is done with the patient swallowing while holding both nostrils closed. The Politzer technique of inflation introduces air through the nostrils while the nasopharynx is closed by swallowing or by rapidly repeating "K."

Tuning Fork Tests

The practice of using tuning forks as a means of evaluating the auditory system existed long before the advent of modern audiometry. When properly used by a skilled examiner, tuning forks can provide qualitative information about the state of the auditory mechanism and some information about the patient's hearing sensitivity.

It will be noted that the frequencies of 512 Hz, 1024 Hz and 2048 Hz are the only frequencies included. Testing at these frequencies is advised for several reasons. First, inclusion of these frequencies facilitates differentiation between normal and pathological auditory systems and between conductive and sensorineural pathologies. Second, these frequencies constitute the so-called "speech frequencies." Hearing sensitivity from 500 to 2000 Hz has been shown to be important for reception of speech. Therefore, especially with the geriatric patient, useful information can be gained by evaluation at these frequencies. In addition, skillful evaluation at these frequencies may provide information about the severity of the hearing loss for each frequency. This information may be important for diagnostic or rehabilitative purposes.

If, for any reason, the clinician is unable or unwilling to test at the three frequencies mentioned above, the two-frequency evaluation most often performed utilizes the 512 Hz and the 1024 Hz tuning forks. Careful evaluation of these frequencies will be helpful for identification of conductive pathologies, but may miss a sensorineural impairment involving only 2000 Hz and above. Since many geriatric patients may be expected to have a high frequency sensorineural impairment due to presbycusis, the examiner risks overestimating the hearing sensitivity of these patients if only the 512 and 1024 Hz tuning forks are used for examination.

Finally, if only one fork is to be chosen, the 512 Hz fork should be the choice. If a conductive hearing loss is present, it should be most readily detectable at this frequency, since conductive impairments usually involve low frequencies first. The 512 Hz tuning fork is preferable to the 256 Hz fork because of the possibility of tactile stimulation with the latter. Patients may respond to the vibration of a 256 Hz tuning fork without actually hearing it.

Certain precautions must be taken in the use of tuning forks. A tuning fork is manufactured to produce a fundamental frequency, the intensity of which is greater than the intensity of any of its harmonics. To generate this fundamental frequency, the user should strike the fork near the base of the tines. If a tuning fork is activated by striking it near the top of the tines, harmonics of the fundamental frequency may be produced. A patient may then respond to the harmonic rather than the fundamental.

The examiner must also be conscious of the intensity of the tone generated by a tuning fork. Striking the tuning fork with sufficient force to produce the maximum intensity of which a tuning fork is capable may produce inaccurate results. An illustration of this will be provided later, under the discussion of the Weber test.

Another factor which may influence tuning fork test results is the pressure used to apply the stem of the fork to the skull of the patient. The intensity of the bone-conducted signal is partially dependent upon the force used to apply the vibrator to the skull.

In addition to pressure, placement of the tuning fork influences the amount of intensity reaching the cochlea. When performing the Weber test, intensity may be increased by placing the stem of the fork on the nasal bones or teeth rather than on the forehead.

Finally, the examiner must remember that when a vibrating tuning fork is applied to a skull, whether it is on the midline or at the mastoid or the vertex of the skull, both cochlea are being stimulated. Therefore, without the proper use of some means of masking in the nontest ear, it is not possible to know definitely that the patient's response is an indication of the function of the test ear.

The four tuning fork tests described below are perhaps the most commonly used tests.

Schwabach test

This test is useful for comparing the bone-conduction sensitivity of the patient to that of the examiner. It may also be used to compare the air conduction sensitivity of the patient to that of the examiner. The successful use of this test requires that the examiner be aware of the sensitivity of his or her own hearing, i.e., whether it is normal or not. The test is performed by activating the desired tuning fork and placing it on the mastoid of the patient. The patient is instructed to indicate when the tone can no longer be heard. When this is indicated, the examiner immediately applies the tuning fork to his or her own mastoid. If the examiner is still able to hear the tone, it may be concluded that the patient's hearing is poorer than the examiner's at that frequency. However, if the examiner is also unable to hear the tone, his or her hearing may be equal to or poorer than the patient's hearing for that frequency. To resolve this question, the test is repeated, with the examiner applying the tuning fork to his or her own mastoid first, waiting until the tone can no longer be heard and then applying the tuning fork to the mastoid of the patient. If the patient is unable to hear a tone, the hearing sensitivity of the patient and the examiner is approximately equal. However, if the patient is still able to hear a tone, it may be concluded that his or her bone conduction sensitivity is greater in at least one ear than that of the examiner, possibly due to the occlusion effect from a conductive pathology.

Weber test

This test is useful to indicate when the ears of the patients are affected to a different degree, to indicate the presence of a conductive component, or to differentiate between one normal ear and one pathological ear. The test is based on the fact that a tone from a tuning fork applied to a skull will lateralize to an ear having a conductive component. If no conductive component is present, the tone will lateralize to the ear having the best hearing.

The test is performed by striking the chosen tuning fork and placing it on the forehead at the midline. The patient is instructed to indicate the ear in which the tone is heard or the ear in which it is heard the loudest. If the patient indicates that the tone has lateralized to the poorer ear, a conductive component in that ear is indicated. If the patient indicates that the tone lateralizes to the better ear, a sensorineural loss in the poorer ear is indicated.

Patient performance on this test may be affected by several factors. First, patients may become confused when they appear to hear a tone in their poorer ear. They may think this is not possible, and respond (falsely) by indicating that they are hearing the tone in their better ear. This is especially true with geriatric patients. Second, lateralization of a tone to one ear does not eliminate the possibility that a less severe conductive component may exist in the opposite ear.

Even when a conductive component is not present, the test may be affected by artifacts. Remember that in the instance of two sensorineural ears having unequal hearing sensitivity, or of one sensorineural ear and one normal ear, the tone should lateralize to the most sensitive ear. However, if the fork is activated maximally, so that it produces an intensity sufficiently loud to exceed the threshold of the poorer ear, the patient will report hearing a tone in both ears, or in the middle of the head. This response might falsely be interpreted as a normal response. The examiner can guard against this artifact by striking the fork with only enough force to produce an intensity near the patient's best threshold for that frequency.

In summary, a lateralized tuning fork response, in the absence of all other information, indicates only that hearing sensitivity between the two ears is different. Additional information, often from other tuning fork tests, is necessary to clarify the findings.

Rinne test

The Rinne test and the Weber test can provide a clearer clinical picture together than either test can provide alone. The Rinne test compares the intensity of a tone heard at the mastoid with that of an air-conducted tone. The test is performed by placing the stem of the vibrating fork on the mastoid near the posterior-superior edge of the ear canal. The patient is asked to indicate when the tone can no longer be heard. At the patient's signal, the tuning fork is quickly moved opposite the orifice of the external auditory canal. The tuning fork should be held about one inch from the canal, with the tines parallel to a frontal plane of the skull. Air-conducted tones will be heard longer than bone-conducted tones for a normal or a sensorineural ear.

The test artifacts possible in the performance of the Rinne test include the possibility of the patient hearing an air-conducted sound when the tuning fork is on the mastoid. This may occur if the stem of the fork touches the auricle accidentally, producing sound waves in the ear canal. In addition, unless the opposite ear is masked with some noise source, it is not possible to guarantee that the response to the bone-conducted tone was actually from the test ear.

Results of the Rinne are considered positive when air conduction is greater than bone conduction. Results are considered negative, indicating a conductive component, when bone conduction is greater than air conduction. However, this result will occur only when the conductive component is sufficient to provide an air-bone gap of 15 to 20 dB.

Bing test

This test is similar to the Weber in that it also utilizes the occlusion effect. A vibrating fork is placed on the forehead at the midline, just as in performance of the Weber. The patient is asked whether the tone lateralizes to either ear. The external auditory canal is then occluded by gentle pressure with the finger on the tragus. It is important that this pressure occludes the canal without increasing air pressure on the ear drum. The patient is asked to indicate whether this maneuver either causes a lateralization of sound to the occluded ear or an increase in the intensity of sound in the occluded ear. If the patient reports that no change has occurred, the test indicates that a conductive component is present. When hearing is normal or the ear has a sensorineural hearing loss, occluding the canal will result in a perception of intensified sound.

Audiometric Data

The patient should be referred for audiological evaluation in all instances in which the complaint is hearing loss, tinnitus or aural pain whose etiology cannot be detected otoscopically.

Audiogram (pure tone tests)

The most basic audiometric measure routinely obtained is the pure tone air conduction test. This test may be performed either as a *screening* test or as a *threshold* test. The purpose of a screening test is merely to identify persons who may possess a significant hearing loss. No attempt is made to quantify or describe the hearing loss. In contrast, a *threshold* test may be performed to gather information which will either assist in the diagnosis of ear pathology or will be used to guide the development of an appropriate program of aural rehabilitation.

Both the screening test and the threshold test are performed for each ear individually. In the screening test, the earphones are placed on the patient and the examiner sets the intensity level dial (Hearing Threshold Level or HTL) on the audiometer at some preestablished intensity, such as 25 dB HTL. The frequency selector of the audiometer is set to a preestablished frequency, such as 500 Hz. A tone is presented to the patient and the examiner notes whether the patient indicates that a tone has been heard. Several tone presentations may be made at each frequency. The frequency selector is then moved to a different frequency without changing the setting of the HTL dial and another tone is presented. (Note: Some examiners may screen different frequencies at different intensities. For example, the frequencies 500 Hz and 4000 Hz might be screened at 25 dB HTL and the frequencies 1000 Hz and 2000 Hz might be screened at 20 dB HTL.) Each ear is tested for all frequencies to be screened. The results of an audiometric test are recorded as either "pass" or "fail." Since 25 dB HTL is considered to be the limit of normal hearing sensitivity, a screening test at this intensity will establish only whether the patient has hearing sensitivity which is within normal limits for those frequencies tested.

If the examiner desires to quantify the hearing sensitivity of the patient, an air conduction *threshold* test is performed. This test is also performed under earphones and also tests each ear across several frequencies. Most often, the frequencies of 250 Hz, 500 Hz, 1000 Hz, 2000 Hz, 4000 Hz and 8000 Hz are the frequencies tested, although 125 Hz is often included in the test. A threshold hearing test seeks to determine for each frequency the lowest intensity, in decibels, that a subject can detect 50 percent of the time. Results for each ear are plotted on an audiogram, using the symbols shown in Figure 3-5.

The test is administered by instructing the patient regarding the task to be performed and then placing the earphones over his or her ears. Each ear is tested individually, with the choice of initial ear being dictated by which ear the patient believes is the better-hearing ear. A specific frequency, usually 1000 Hz, is selected and a tone is presented briefly. The intensity of the initial presentation is dictated by whether the examiner chooses the ascending or descending method of limits. When the ascending method is selected, the examiner

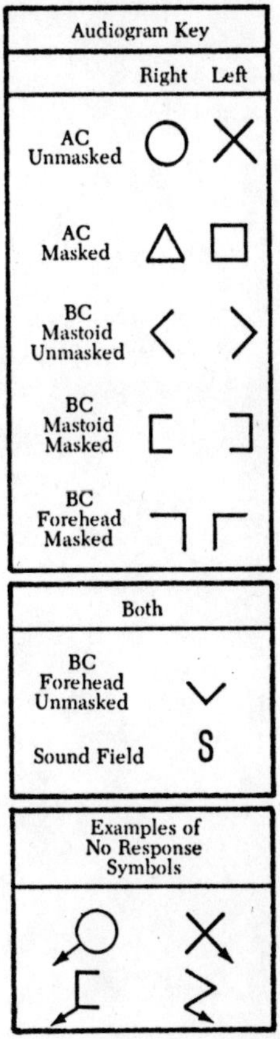

Audiogram Key		
	Right	Left
AC Unmasked	O	X
AC Masked	△	□
BC Mastoid Unmasked	<	>
BC Mastoid Masked	[	]
BC Forehead Masked	˥	ˠ
	Both	
BC Forehead Unmasked	∨	
Sound Field	S	
Examples of No Response Symbols		

Figure 3-5
From Vincent Byers et al. "Guidelines for Manual Pure-Tone Threshold Audiometry." *Journal of the American Speech and Hearing Association*, 20:4, April 1978, pp. 197–301.

begins at a low intensity, presumably below the patient's threshold, and increases the intensity of successive presentations in serial steps of 5 or 10 decibels until the patient indicates that the tone has been heard.

If the examiner selects the descending method of limits, the initial tone presentation is made at an intensity which is presumably above the patient's threshold, i.e., audible to the patient. Successive serial presentations are made at decreasing intensities until the patient no longer indicates he or she has heard the tone. Regardless of which process is employed, several progressions to threshold are made before a different frequency is selected for testing. Both methods yield thresholds which are identical within ± 5 dB when they are properly performed.

After pure air conduction thresholds have been obtained bilaterally, a loss of hearing sensitivity may be observed. When an air conduction loss is noted, it is desirable to obtain thresholds for pure tone bone conducted stimuli at octave intervals from 250 Hz to 4000 Hz. The added information gained by bone conduction testing will reveal whether any hearing loss detected by air conduction is a *conductive* loss, a *sensorineural* loss or a *mixed* loss. When bone conduction thresholds are essentially superimposed upon air conduction thresholds, within ± 10 dB, as in Figure 3-6A, the hearing loss is considered to be sensorineural. However, when the bone conduction thresholds suggest that cochlear hearing sensitivity is better than the sensitivity revealed by air conduction testing, the hearing loss is considered to be either conductive or mixed. A mixed hearing loss is a loss which demonstrates better hearing by bone conduction than by air conduction, but in which bone conduction thresholds are not

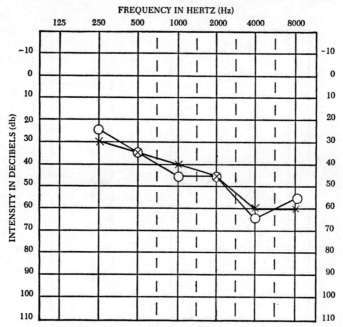

Figure 3-6A
Bilateral Sensorineural Loss

within normal limits. Figures 3-6B and 3-6C illustrate a conductive loss and a mixed loss, respectively.

It will be noted upon examination of Figure 3-5 that different symbols are used for recording *masked* and *unmasked* bone conduction thresholds. If an examiner wishes to determine the bone conduction sensitivity of one ear, it is necessary that responses due to stimulation of the other ear be eliminated. These responses may occur in bone conduction testing because interaural attenuation of stimuli presented through a bone conduction oscilla-

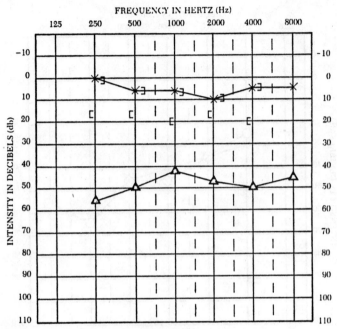

Figure 3-6B
Conduction Hearing Loss, Right Ear

tor is essentially zero. That is, if a bone conduction oscillator is placed upon the left mastoid of a patient and stimulated with a tone, the patient may hear the tone in either ear or in both ears depending upon the intensity of the stimulus and the sensitivity of the patient's ears. Without the use of masking, it is not possible to determine which ear is responsible for the patient's hearing the tone. The proper use of masking will eliminate participation by one ear.

Masking is performed by placing an earphone over the nontest ear and

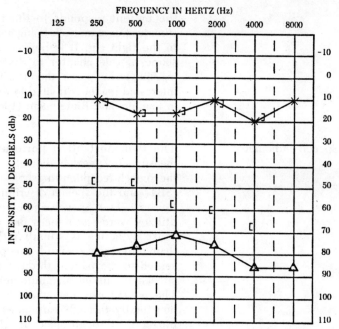

Figure 3-6C
Mixed Hearing Loss, Right Ear

introducing either a broad band or a narrow band noise, depending on the stimulus to be masked. For example, if the examiner wishes to determine the bone conduction sensitivity of the right ear, he or she will place a bone conduction oscillator upon the right mastoid and an earphone over the left ear. Before activating the bone conduction oscillator with a test stimulus, the examiner will introduce noise to the left ear via the earphone. The presence of this noise masks or "covers up" the presence of the bone conducted tone in the left ear. Therefore, the examiner knows that when the patient responds to the test stimulus this stimulus is being heard in the right ear. It is beyond the scope of this chapter to discuss masking techniques or theories. The interested reader is invited to refer to Sanders and Rintelmann (1964).

Speech audiometry

The two most often performed measures in speech audiometry are the speech reception threshold test (SRT) and the speech discrimination test (DS). Speech audiometry utilizes words, sentences or nonsense syllables as stimuli rather than pure tones. Stimuli are presented to the patient through the speech circuit of an audiometer. The patient may hear the stimuli monaurally through earphones or binaurally through speakers. (For certain special types of speech tests, the patient may hear stimuli through both earphones.) The patient is asked to repeat the word heard. An alternative method for eliciting a response is to ask the patient to write down, circle, underline or point to the word heard.

The speech reception threshold (SRT) is defined as the intensity level at which the patient is able to correctly repeat 50 percent of the spondee words he hears. Spondee words are compound words having equal stress on each part, such as *baseball, cowboy, airplane* or *sidewalk.* An SRT equal to or better than 25 dB HTL is considered to be within normal limits.

A speech reception threshold may be obtained separately for each ear under earphones, or binaurally in a sound-field situation. The intensity of the obtained SRT should correspond closely (within ± 6 dB) with the average of the pure tone thresholds (PTA) for 500 Hz, 1000 Hz and 2000 Hz (the speech frequencies). If this agreement does not occur, the SRT may be checked against the best two-frequency averages of the speech frequencies. If an acceptable agreement still does not occur, one or both of the obtained measures (pure tones and SRT) may be suspect. Some geriatric patients may yield SRT's which are higher (poorer) than their pure tone averages by more than the ± 6 dB considered acceptable. Explanation for the lack of SRT/PTA agreement may be found, in these patients, in the fact that some geriatric patients have inordinately poor speech discrimination and, consequently, have great difficulty understanding even the spondaic test words used to determine the SRT. In addition, the test for the speech reception threshold assumes and encourages a certain amount of guessing on the part of the patient. Some older patients are unwilling to guess for fear of making a mistake. The result is a slightly elevated SRT.

The speech reception threshold is a valuable measurement for helping determine the effect hearing loss may have on the communication ability of a patient. For example, if the intensity level of normal conversational speech is considered to be approximately 55 dB HTL, it will be seen that a patient having a hearing loss for speech of 50 dB HTL (as measured by SRT) is hearing conversational speech at a very low sensation level. This patient could be expected to experience a great difficulty understanding speech of normal intensity without a hearing aid.

Speech discrimination score (DS)

Tests for speech discrimination also utilize speech, usually monosyllabic words, as test stimuli. The most frequently utilized test materials are probably the CID W-22 lists developed by Hirsh and his coworkers (1952). These test materials are arranged into 50-word phonetically-balanced (PB) test lists. Phonetic balancing means that speech sounds occur within each test list with approximately the same frequency as they occur in spoken English.

The test is administered by presenting a list of PB words to a patient through the speech circuit of an audiometer. The intensity level for the presentation is usually chosen relative to the SRT. Most often, test words are presented at an intensity of either 26 dB or 40 dB above the intensity of the SRT. Sometimes, it is useful to present the test words at the patient's most comfortable listening level (MCL), or at some intensity level representative of the intensity of normal conversational speech, such as 55 dB HTL.

The test is scored by counting the number of words which the patient repeats correctly and multiplying this figure by two. Score is expressed in percent. Some examiners prefer to present only one-half of a test list, or 25 words, and then multiply the number of correct responses by four. Speech discrimination scores are considered to be within normal limits if they are equal to or better than 94 percent. Patients with normal hearing may be expected to achieve scores within this range. Not all hearing-impaired subjects will demonstrate reduced speech discrimination. Subjects having conductive hearing losses, or mixed hearing loss with near-normal bone conduction sensitivity, will demonstrate normal or near-normal speech discrimination. In contrast, subjects whose hearing impairment is primarily cochlear will usually demonstrate some reduction of speech discrimination. Subjects whose hearing impairment is primarily neural may demonstrate a marked reduction in speech discrimination. Thus, reduced speech discrimination test scores may take on diagnostic significance, especially when considered in relation to other audiometric test results. However, inordinately poor speech discrimination may be noted in the presbycusic patient. For these patients, low speech discrimination scores do not always assume the diagnostic significance of reduced scores in younger patients. Regardless of the age of the patient, speech discrimination testing may be utilized to provide some indication of the effect of a hearing impairment upon communication function, especially when an analysis of the type of errors made is performed. Therefore, speech discrimination testing is often used to assess the effectiveness of a hearing aid, to compare several hearing aids or to determine the effectiveness of a program of aural rehabilitation.

Impedance audiometry

The impedance test battery consists of three tests. These are *tympanometry*, the results of which yield a *tympanogram, static compliance* and measurement of the *acoustic reflex* threshold. The technical aspects and theories of impedance audiometry are explained in Northern (1976).

Tympanometry measures compliance of the eardrum across several conditions of positive, static and negative air pressure in the external auditory canal. The measurements, when plotted on a tympanogram, reveal the point at which maximum compliance of the eardrum occurs. Since an eardrum is known to be most compliant when air pressure is equal in the external auditory canal and the middle ear, a tympanogram indirectly reveals whether air pressure in the middle ear is normal, positive or negative. Different middle ear pathologies yield different tympanometric patterns. A tympanogram which reveals a peak, but with negative pressure, may suggest eustachian tube dysfunction, whereas a "flat" tympanogram is often associated with the presence of otitis media. It should be noted, however, that an absolutely flat tympanogram may be reflective of a test artifact, specifically the presence of the probe tip against the wall of the external auditory canal. The tympanometric patterns associated with different pathologies have been classified by Jerger (1970). Examples of these, along with explanations, may be found in Figures 3-7 and 3-8.

Static compliance, as expressed in cubic centimeters, provides a measure of the mobility of the eardrum and middle ear system. Static compliance expresses equivalent volume of the area between the end of the probe tip and the tympanic membrane. Abnormally stiff middle ear systems are associated with otitis media, eustachian tube dysfunction or otosclerosis. In addition, tympanosclerosis and cholesteatomas may result in reduced compliance. Abnormal flaccidity may be observed in ossicular chain discontinuity and is sometimes noted in the presence of a monomeric membrane. Measurement of equivalent volume is useful for identification of perforations of the tympanic membrane.

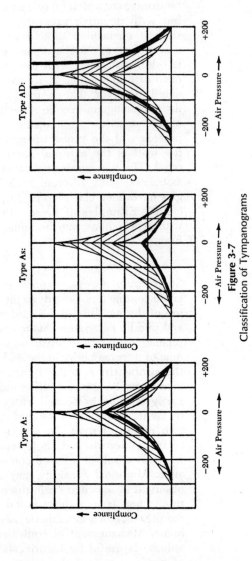

Figure 3-7
Classification of Tympanograms

Type A — Normal

Type As — Indicates slight stiffness of middle ear system (otosclerosis, tympanosclerosis, thickened drums)

Type A_D — Abnormal flaccidity of middle ear system (disarticulated ossicular chain,
monomeric membrane)

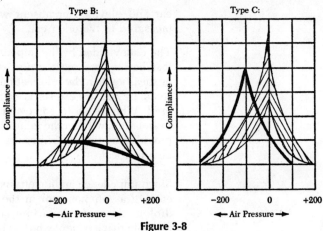

Figure 3-8
Classification of Tympanograms

Type B — Very stiff middle ear system (otitis media, cerumen impaction)

Type C — Negative pressure (eustachian tubal dysfunction, possible middle ear effusion)

The acoustic reflex test measures the changes in compliance which result with the contraction of the stapedial muscle. This contraction can be elicited in a normal ear upon stimulation by sounds of high intensity, usually 70 to 100 dB HTL for pure tones. If the acoustic reflex can be elicited at lower sensation levels, the presence of recruitment, and therefore cochlear involvement is suggested. Absent acoustic reflexes may indicate a mild to severe conductive impairment, a profound sensorineural loss, discontinuity of the ossicular chain or possible retrocochlear involvement. It should be noted that for some pathologies, acoustic reflexes may be normal when measured in one ear and elevated or absent when measured in the other ear.

The data yielded by the impedance test battery are most useful diagnostically when the information derived by all three tests is considered. When each test is evaluated in isolation, without the information provided by the others, results may be equivocal.

Since impedance audiometry is becoming a common tool in the audiologist's armamentarium, it is possible that a patient who has been referred for audiological evaluation will be tested using these techniques. The nurse clinician should, therefore, have some familiarity with the techniques and interpretation of impedance audiometry.

Site of Lesion Testing

In addition to the routine audiometric tests described above, the audiologist often performs special auditory tests intended to identify the locus of a lesion within the auditory system. These tests may be used to confirm or rule out the presence of pathology in the cochlea, on the acoustic branch of the VIII nerve, in the brain stem or in the cortex of the brain. It is beyond the scope of this chapter to describe each of these special tests in detail, or to discuss interpretation of each test. The interested reader is invited to consult Matkin and Olsen (1971).

ASSESSMENT:

External Ear and Ear Canal

Perichondritis

Suspect if there is diffuse red swelling, hot to the touch, or tender. Adenopathy and leukocytosis are commonly present.

Otitis externa; otomycosis

Symptoms will include itching within the canal, pain upon movement of the auricle or pressure on tragus, exudation, swelling, or discharge.

Inspection will show redness and swelling of canal, stenosis, and a normal tympanic membrane.

Hearing will be normal unless canal is blocked, which produces a conductive impairment. Tuning forks will show middle ear involvement.

Keratosis obliterans

Suspect if there is accumulation of deposits of keratin in the external canal and erosion of inferior or posterior canal walls. The patient may report pain and have discharge.

Tumors of the auricle and external canal

Revealed by examination.

Cerumen occlusion

Revealed by examination, audiologic evaluation, or impedance audiometry.

Foreign matter in canal

Usually revealed by examination; may appear as excess cerumen.

Pustules, osteomas

Revealed by examination.

Tympanic Membrane
Bullous myringitis

Yellowish blisters will be seen on the tympanic membrane. There will be a history of recent upper respiratory infection and a feeling of pain and pressure within the ear. Tenderness is noted with pressure on the tragus or with movement of the auricle. Hearing will be normal. Tuning forks will be consistent with slight conductive pathology.

Tympanosclerosis

Deposits of hyalin plaques will be seen on tympanic membrane; these may appear yellowish, covering either a small or large area of the eardrum. Hearing may sometimes be normal or have a slight conductive loss. If the ossicular chain is involved, a severe conductive loss may be present. Tuning forks will be consistent with conductive pathology.

Perforations of tympanic membrane

Revealed by otoscopic examination or by acoustic impedance, which will reveal an abnormally large equivalent volume (greater than 2.5 cc). The patient may report a feeling of fullness and possibly pain at the time of the perforation. Discharge may be present if the perforation is recent. Presence of hearing loss depends upon the size and location of the perforation. If present, hearing loss will be conductive. Tuning forks will be consistent with conductive pathology.

Otitis media
Viral

May follow upper respiratory infection or attack of allergies. Slight pain may be present. Hearing testing may reveal a slight conductive loss. Tuning forks will be consistent with conductive pathology.

Bacterial

Associated with infections of nose and throat. Initial feeling of blocked ear, followed by pain, toxicity and fever. Tympanic membrane appears bluish and injected initially, then thick and red; it may bulge outward. Hearing testing may reveal a slight conductive loss which may progress to a severe conductive loss. Tuning forks will be consistent with conductive pathology.

Cholesteatoma
Congenital

The patient will report a history of slow progressive unilateral hearing loss, but no history of previous infection. Tympanic membrane reveals a whitish bulge, often in the posterior-superior quadrant. Hearing testing will be normal or reveal a mild conductive loss. Tuning forks will be consistent with middle ear pathology.

Primary acquired

Suspect if there is an aural discharge of constant and persistent nature. Otoscopy reveals a perforation of the pars flaccida. Hearing sensitivity is dependent upon the integrity of the ossicular chain. If the cholesteatoma is positioned to conduct sound across the middle ear, hearing may be normal.

Secondary acquired

Suspect if there is a history of chronic ear infection. Otoscopic examination reveals squamous epithelium invading the middle ear. Granulation may be present. Hearing is dependent upon the involvement of the ossicular chain. Tuning forks will be consistent with conductive pathology.

Eustachian tube dysfunction

Suspect if there is a feeling of fullness which may accompany upper respiratory infection or attack of allergies. Subjectively, the patient may note some transient loss of hearing. The hearing is usually normal, although a slight conductive loss may be present. Tympanometry reveals reduced compliance and/or negative pressure. Tuning forks may be consistent with conductive pathology.

Otosclerosis

The patient may have a history of familial hearing disorders. Other family members may have had successful ear surgery. The patient will report a slow, progressive unilateral or asymmetrical bilateral loss of hearing over many years. The onset of hearing loss may have been during the third decade of life. Women may report a rapid progression of the hearing loss during a pregnancy. The patient may report a low frequency tinnitus. Otoscopic examination reveals a normal tympanic membrane. Swartze's sign (pinkish coloration around promontory) may be present. Patient will report a hearing loss, but may report better hearing in noise than in quiet. These patients may also report success with hearing aids. Audiological evaluation will reveal a conductive hearing loss which is usually greatest for the low frequencies. Bone conduction testing may reveal a "Carhart notch," i.e., reduced bone conduction sensitivity at 2000 Hz. Speech discrimination is normal or near-normal. Tympanograms reveal reduced compliance. Tuning forks may be consistent with conductive pathology.

Mastoiditis

Suspect mastoiditis if there is a recent history of acute otitis or discharge from ear. The patient reports pain in the ear or generally over the side of the head. There is a general ill feeling, sometimes with fever; the mastoid area is tender and usually swollen. The skin may be red if an abscess is present. Otoscopic examination may reveal perforated tympanic membrane. Hearing sensitivity is dependent upon the degree of middle ear involvement. Tuning forks may be consistent with conductive pathology.

Cochlear and Retrocochlear Pathologies

Meniere's disease

Expect a sensorineural hearing loss, vertigo, tinnitus and feeling of fullness in the ear. Hearing loss fluctuates early, but progressively deteriorates. The onset may be in the third or fourth decade of life. Initially, Meniere's disease has active stages which occur intermittently; with the onset of the attack, nausea and vomiting occur. Symptom-free periods occur between attacks. Early in the course of the disease, hearing presents a sensorineural loss involving primarily the low frequencies in the affected ear. As the disease progresses, the hearing loss becomes more severe and involves all frequencies. Speech discrimination is reduced in the affected ear. Special auditory site of lesion testing reveals cochlear findings. Tuning forks may be consistent with a sensorineural loss, lateralizing away from the affected ear. In early Meniere's disease, only the low frequency forks may be affected. In a vestibular examination, the affected ear will demonstrate reduced vestibular response to hot and cold stimuli.

Noise-induced hearing loss

In early stages the patient may complain of some hearing difficulty, especially in noisy surroundings. Hearing may be noticeably poorer at the end of the working day (i.e., after extended exposure to a noxious noise). Tinnitus may be present and may be reported as having been the first subjective sign of hearing difficulties. As the hearing loss progresses the patient will report increasing difficulty hearing and understanding speech. These patients will report no history of aural pain, vertigo or nausea. Except in cases where hearing loss can be attributed to acoustic trauma, the loss is progressive over many years. Often, a patient's family will notice the presence of a hearing problem before the patient himself admits its existence. Serial audiograms will reveal early bilateral, high frequency sensorineural hearing loss which becomes progressively worse and begins to involve lower frequencies. Speech discrimination may be reduced if the frequencies of 2000 Hz and below are involved. Site of lesion testing reveals cochlear findings. Tuning forks may be consistent with a sensorineural hearing loss. In severe losses, responses to high frequency forks (2048 Hz and 4096 Hz) may be absent.

Drug-induced hearing loss

Symptoms differ depending upon the drug responsible and the extent of the damage. Hearing loss is usually bilateral and sensorineural, involving the higher frequencies initially. It may be progressive and may not appear until after cessation of medication. Tinnitus may be present and may have preceded any noticeable hearing loss. Vestibular damage may occur. The hearing loss may be reversible depending upon the causative drug. The hearing loss is usually a bilateral, sensorineural loss which may adopt almost any audiometric configuration. Speech discrimination is often poor, even in cases of mild to moderate pure tone losses.

Vascular disorders

Presents as a sudden unilateral sensorineural hearing loss, which may be total or partial. It resembles a hearing loss due to viral labyrinthitis. Case history information concerning any recent illness is important. A positive history of cardiovascular disease may be found in patients with hearing loss due to vascular accidents. Vertigo may also be present.

Viral labyrinthitis

Similar to hearing loss due to a vascular accident. Usually a unilateral, sensorineural loss but may be bilateral. Case history information concerning recent illnesses is important. Extent of loss may be partial or complete, with some recovery often occurring.

Congenital deafness

This is hearing loss that is present at birth, which may be progressive. Some hereditary deafness is not congenital, beginning at some time after birth (see Otosclerosis above). Congenital deafness is usually bilateral, sensorineural and progressive. It may present nearly any audiometric configuration.

Syphilis

Hearing loss due to syphilis may be similar to hearing loss due to Meniere's disease in its early stages. Tinnitus, vertigo and a fluctuating hearing loss may be present. Hearing loss may be either unilateral or bilateral, will be chiefly sensorineural and may present good speech discrimination in its early stages. As the disease progresses, speech discrimination may become poorer with no significant changes occurring in the pure tone sensitivity. Later, sensitivity for pure tones may become poorer.

Retrocochlear Pathology
Acoustic neuroma

Usually insidious in growth, but may be rapid. The patient may first note a unilateral tinnitus with a slow, progressive unilateral hearing loss and vertigo. True vertigo may occur. Later, numbness of the face may occur. In advanced cases, paralysis of the extremities and intracranial pain may be present. Otoscopic examination reveals normal tympanic membranes. Involvement of the Vth, VIIth and VIIIth cranial nerves may be noted. Radiographic examination reveals enlarged internal auditory canal on the involved side. Reduced corneal reflexes and reduced response to tactile stimulation of the posterior wall of the external auditory canal on the affected side may be present. The unilateral sensorineural hearing loss is usually worse in the high frequencies, often with greatly reduced speech discrimination in the affected ear. Abnormal tone decay and acoustic reflex decay are often present. Other auditory site of lesion tests will yield retrocochlear findings. Tuning forks may be consistent with sensorineural loss.

Presbycusis

Suspect presbycusis after all other possibilities have been ruled out. Bilateral sensorineural hearing loss with a negative history of vertigo, pain or nausea. (When any of these symptoms are present, they indicate presence of some pathology other than presbycusis.)

Presbycusis may be grouped into four pathological types: *sensory presbycusis, neural presbycusis, metabolic presbycusis* and *mechanical presbycusis* (Schuknecht, 1964). The physiological changes which occur in each type are of interest because of the resultant effects upon hearing sensitivity and the corresponding effects upon the communicative ability of the patient.

Sensory presbycusis

Sensory presbycusis results from changes near the basal end of the cochlea, specifically from atrophy in the organ of Corti and the auditory nerve. This degenerative change produces a high frequency hearing loss (Figure 3-9A). If the progression of sensory presbycusis is limited to those frequencies above the speech range (i.e., above 2000 Hz), hearing sensitivity for speech will remain relatively unimpaired.

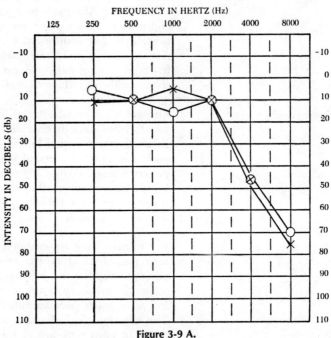

Figure 3-9 A.
Sensory Presbycusis

Neural presbycusis

Neural presbycusis is marked by loss of central nervous system neuron population, particularly in the auditory pathways and cochlea. The result is a reduced processing ability for the neural patterns which have been initiated by incoming acoustic energy. Reduced ability to transmit, integrate and decode these patterns occurs. Audiologically, neural presbycusis manifests itself by a phenomenon termed *phonemic regression*, which may be defined as inordinately poor speech discrimination in relation to the degree of pure tone hearing loss present.

Metabolic presbycusis

Metabolic presbycusis results from changes which occur in the stria vascularis. Audiologically, these patients present a flat audiometric configuration, i.e., a loss which is approximately equal throughout the frequencies tested. Figure 3-9B provides an example of hearing loss due to metabolic presbycusis. The extent of the involvement differs from patient to patient.

Mechanical presbycusis

Mechanical presbycusis is of indeterminant etiology. It appears to be mechanical, perhaps caused by the stiffening of the basilar membrane, rather than chemical in nature. Upon audiometric evaluation, these patients demonstrate a falling audiogram, yielding normal or near-normal hearing thresholds for the lower frequencies with progressively poorer thresholds as tones become higher in frequency. An example of hearing loss due to mechanical

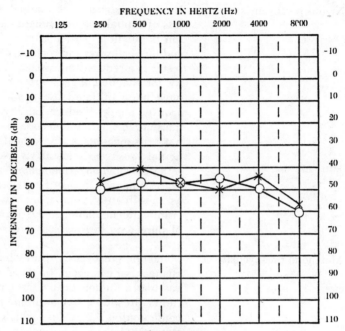

Figure 3-9B.
Metabolic Presbycusis

presbycusis may be seen in Figure 3-9C. Unlike sensory presbycusis, which may demonstrate normal hearing throughout the speech frequencies followed by a precipitous drop in hearing sensitivity, mechanical presbycusis demonstrates a gradually sloping audiogram.

PLAN:

Perichondritis

Refer to a physician.

Otitis Externa

Treatment consists of cleaning and drying the external canal and controlling the pain present. Predisposing causes must be determined and controlled.

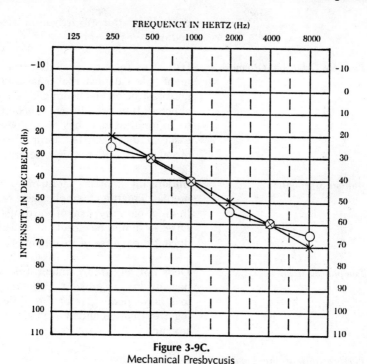

Figure 3-9C.
Mechanical Presbycusis

Keratosis Obliterans	Consultation with and/or referral to a physician is advised. The disease is usually controlled by frequent cleaning with alcohol irrigations.
Tumors of the Auricle and External Ear	Refer to a physician.
Cerumen Occlusion	Removed by irrigation or by use of instruments. Use irrigation only if the tympanic membrane has been examined and found to be intact.
Foreign Matter in the External Auditory Canal	Small foreign bodies may be removed with forceps. Irrigation is sometimes useful. (See above for

contraindications to irrigation procedure.)

Pustules, Osteomas, Otomycosis

Osteomas require no active treatment unless the external canal is totally obstructed and hearing is being affected. If this condition is encountered, referral to a physician is necessary. Otomycosis is a form of external otitis and requires referral.

Bullous Myringitis

Bullous myringitis is a form of otitis media. Treatment emphasizes relieving pain by use of eardrops. Disease should be closely observed during the course of treatment.

Tympanosclerosis

Does not require treatment unless hearing loss is present. If hearing loss is suspected, refer for audiologic evaluation and/or otologic assessment.

Perforations of the Tympanic Membrane

Refer to a physician.

Otitis Media

Otitis media may be treated conservatively with decongestants, or more aggressively with surgical procedure.

Cholesteatoma

Refer to a physician.

Eustachian Tube Dysfunction

This may result in negative pressure within middle ear which may result in a mild hearing loss. Referral for audiologic evaluation, specifically including acoustic impedance measurements, will be helpful in confirming eustachian tube dysfunction. Conservative treatment with decongestants and instructions in the use of the Valsalva maneuver may prevent permanent retraction of the tympanic membranes.

Otosclerosis

Refer to a physician for diagnosis and treatment. If the patient elects not to have medical treatment, referral for audiologic evaluation may be helpful in assessing the extent of the communication problems present. Referral for audiologic evaluation prior to medical referral may provide data which will help confirm otosclerosis.

Mastoiditis

Refer to a physician.

Meniere's Disease

Refer to an otologist or otolaryngologist, perhaps after a referral for audiologic evaluation. Communication difficulties are best managed by instruction in speechreading and auditory training. Hearing aids are sometimes useful. Often, if only one ear is affected, communication difficulties will be negligible.

Noise-induced Hearing Loss

Consultation with a physician may be necessary to establish diagnosis since noise-induced hearing loss resembles other sensorineural hearing losses. When noise-induced hearing loss is confirmed, the patient should be counseled concerning the necessity for use of ear protection if further noise exposure is to occur. Management of communication difficulties begins with assessment of the extent of the problem. Speechreading and auditory training may be helpful and, in cases of mild to moderate hearing losses, may be sufficient to overcome most problems. High frequency emphasis hearing aids are often beneficial. For longstanding, advanced cases of noise-induced hearing loss, speech conservation and speech therapy may be necessary.

Drug-induced Hearing Loss

Audiometric baseline studies are needed to define the extent of the hearing loss. Electronystagmography or other assessments of vestibular dysfunction may be required. The patient should avoid all exposure to ototoxic medications if possible. Since reduced speech discrimination which will lead to communication difficulties may be present, audiologic evaluation is advised. Rehabilitatively, speech-reading, auditory training and, in some instances, use of a hearing aid may be helpful.

Vascular Disorders and Viral Labyrinthitis

Refer to a physician if either disorder is suspected. If the suspected disorder is longstanding and communication difficulties are the primary problem, refer for audiologic testing with emphasis on rehabilitative evaluation.

Congenital Deafness

Consult with the patient's past care source and physician to confirm diagnosis and provide a prediction for course of hearing loss. Refer for audiologic evaluation.

Hearing Loss Due to Syphilis

Refer to a physician.

Acoustic Neuroma

Refer to a physician.

Presbycusis

In *sensory presbycusis* the patient will usually have little difficulty communicating and will have little need for aural rehabilitation. The patient with *neural presbycusis* may present a challenge for successful aural rehabilitation because of poor prognosis for success in using a hearing aid. Although these patients may derive some benefit from the use of amplification, they may also require the development of other channels of communicative input. Patients with *metabolic presbycusis* are usually good candidates for successful hearing aid use because speech discrimination is not greatly affected. Hearing loss from metabolic presbycusis may yield poorer than normal speech reception thresholds due to the loss of sensitivity through the speech frequencies. Once speech is made loud enough to be heard adequately, speech discrimination is good. In *mechanical presbycusis* the steepness of the slope and the extent of high frequency involvement, as well as the presence of loudness recruitment, help determine the need for and the usefulness of a hearing aid.

MANAGEMENT

Management of the patient with presbycusis means attacking the problems caused by the hearing loss rather than the hearing loss itself. Possible problems which may be present as a result of a hearing loss stem, in part, from the reduced communicative input available to hearing-impaired persons. The procedures used to reduce these problems traditionally have been grouped together under the rubric of aural rehabilitation. They include *auditory training, speechreading, speech conservation* and the use of *hearing aids.*

Aural rehabilitation evolves from certain principles and utilizes appropriate techniques of patient management to maintain and/or improve the communication skills of a hearing-impaired person. The type and extent of the communication deficit will dictate the methods employed in therapy. The assessment of a patient's auditory sensitivity is only one aspect of the total evaluation required before effective aural rehabilitation therapy can be developed. As O'Neill and Oyer (1973) have pointed out, evaluation should assess the effects the hearing loss has had upon the patient's speech, his self-image and his social relations.

Ramsdell (1966) has discussed hearing loss from the point of self-image and social relations. He has stated that sound functions at three levels: the background, the warning and the symbolic levels. The primitive background level utilizes hearing to make the person aware of and feel part of the world around him. Loss of hearing at the background level may contribute to feelings of depression. Sounds at the warning level require some overt response on the part of the listener whereas sounds at the symbolic level enable the listener to communicate. Lack of ability to communicate may lead to low self-image, and may result in withdrawal, feelings of uselessness and paranoia.

Aural rehabilitation is best designed and implemented by those professionals, i.e., audiologists and speech pathologists, who have had extensive training in the evaluation and management of the communicative abilities of the acoustically impaired. However, the practitioner who knows something of the fundamental goals of a broad-based aural rehabilitation program will be able to recognize patients for whom therapy might be beneficial, and thereby be better able to initiate appropriate referrals. Furthermore, the practitioner will be able to provide support for the patient who is engaged in what is often long-term therapy.

Therefore, the following discussion is offered as a broad overview of the specific areas cited above. It is suggested that the practitioner who desires a more in-depth discussion consult the references included in the text.

AUDITORY TRAINING

Auditory training may be thought of as a process which seeks to improve an existing input system. The objective of auditory training procedures is to develop a hearing-impaired subject's ability to discriminate sounds. For some severely impaired persons, the goal may be to achieve the ability to make distinctions between widely divergent types of sounds, i.e., gross distinctions. For other patients, the goal may be to distinguish and differentiate between speech and non-speech sounds, while for others the goal may be discrimination of individual speech sounds.

Effective auditory training procedures require an accurate assessment of the abilities and needs of the patient prior to the initiation of therapy. Tasks are then planned which will challenge the patient with increasingly more difficult listening situations.

The extent of a patient's hearing loss will dictate, to some extent, the establishment of goals for an auditory training program. A sensorineural hearing loss often results in distortions of speech sounds which prevent normal speech intelligibility. If the loss is of sufficient magnitude, the person may be totally unable to hear certain spoken sounds. Rehabilitation goals for this person will be different from the goals for the person who merely has occasional difficulty distinguishing among certain speech sounds.

Some persons are unable to hear the high frequency sounds of the language because they have no usable hearing for high frequencies. Others have some residual hearing in the high frequencies but a sufficiently severe loss to prevent their hearing high frequency speech sounds without a hearing aid. It should be noted, however, that the use of a hearing aid may result in reception of the high frequency elements of language but not in their discrimination.

SPEECHREADING

Numerous educators of the hearing-impaired have offered teaching methods and systems intended to teach speechreading. These will not be reviewed here.

Many hearing-impaired patients will report some self-taught ability to speechread, however, and the nurse clinician may offer some suggestions which will facilitate this task. Speechreading is made easier when the speaker has good light directed toward his face. The hearing-impaired person should be advised to move closer to the person with whom he is conversing, since speechreading becomes more difficult as speaker-to-listener distance increases. In addition, reducing this distance will improve the hearing-impaired person's auditory discrimination by improving the signal-to-noise ratio of the speech to which he listens. The hearing-impaired person can make speechreading easier by asking the speaker to talk slower, using natural rather than exaggerated lip movements.

Speechreading is also facilitated by lack of distracting background noises and a minimum of distracting gestures on the part of the speaker. Spoken language is the result, in part, of a rapid succession of movements of the articulators, and the visual perception of these movements requires intense concentration by even the most proficient speechreader. Because of the high degree of concentration required, efficient speechreading is a fatiguing process. Many persons, particularly older persons, are not able or willing to attend sufficiently to the task. In addition, the older person may not possess sufficiently keen eyesight to permit acquisition of proficiency in speechreading.

SPEECH CONSERVATION

Speech conservation is therapy which emphasizes aspects of auditory training, articulation therapy and voice therapy. Its purpose is to prevent deterioration of speech and/or voice patterns, or to improve production of speech if much deterioration has already occurred. These problems may arise from lack of ability on the part of the patient to monitor speech production. Any program of speech conservation must be designed specifically for the patient for whom it is intended. Therefore, referral to a specialist for a thorough audiologic evaluation, as well as for a speech evaluation, is recommended.

HEARING AIDS

The purpose of a hearing aid is to amplify sounds so that a hearing aid wearer can make better use of his residual hearing. A "hearing aid" may be nothing more sophisticated than a hand cupped around the pinna to help gather sound waves and direct them into the ear, or the ear trumpet which Grandpa used long ago.

Today, however, the term "hearing aid" usually refers to a small electronic amplifying device designed, constructed and worn for the purpose of improving the speech reception and discrimination capabilities of the hearing aid wearer. Use of a hearing aid may also improve the hearing-impaired person's ability to localize the source of a sound. These devices are sometimes referred to as personal wearable hearing aids to distinguish them from auditory training units, which also amplify sound electrically. Auditory trainers are usually larger than personal hearing aids and provide a higher quality sound with greater amplification potential. The two types of units differ in other ways which will not be discussed here.

Hearing aids and auditory training units amplify a limited range of frequencies within that range to which the normal human ear is sensitive. Consider the following illustration:

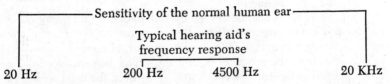

The normal human ear is sensitive to those frequencies from 20 Hz to 20,000 Hz. However, a typical hearing aid may amplify only those frequencies between 200 Hz and 4500 Hz. (Some hearing aids will amplify an even narrower range of frequencies, while some may amplify either above or below this range, or both.) The range of frequencies to which any given hearing aid is sensitive, i.e., those frequencies for which it will provide amplification, is termed its *frequency response*. The frequency response is an important parameter to consider when selecting a hearing aid for a patient.

Another parameter used to describe hearing aid performance is *gain*. Gain may be thought of as the amount of amplification which a hearing aid provides, i.e., the difference between the output intensity and the input intensity. The amount of gain which a given hearing aid will provide is determined by its components. In addition, all hearing aids have an adjustable volume control which permits the wearer to adjust the gain to his personal needs.

Wearable personal hearing aids are available in several styles or types. These are: 1) post-auricle, 2) body, 3) eyeglasses and 4) all-in-the-ear. Within the post-auricle and eyeglasses category are special hearing aids. Examples of these include CROS (Contralateral Routing of Signals) and BICROS (Bilateral Routing of Signals). Figure 3-10 illustates each of the four principal types.

Instruments within each of the categories and subcategories differ in terms of the above-mentioned performance parameters as well as in other performance characteristics, the discussion of which is beyond the scope of this chapter. Selection of a particular instrument for a particular patient should be guided by the specific requirements of that patient. Although hearing aids are not fit by prescription, in the manner of eyeglasses, such factors as type of hearing loss, severity and extent of involvement must be considered. In addition, physical limitations of the patient, social, vocational and preferential requirements should be considered.

It should be remembered that the primary purpose of a hearing aid, i.e., the reason a person elects to wear a hearing aid, is to improve receptive communication abilities. A hearing aid performs this function in one, and possibly two ways. First, a hearing aid may be used to increase the intensity of speech at the ear of the hearing aid wearer. For some persons, making speech louder enables them to better understand what they wish to hear.

Making speech louder to a hearing-impaired patient is of little value, however, unless a concomitant improvement in speech discrimination occurs. Speech discrimination, sometimes referred to as speech intelligibility, may be defined in simple terms as how well a person understands what he hears. It has been shown by numerous investigators that speech discrimination is partially a function of intensity of the speech signal.

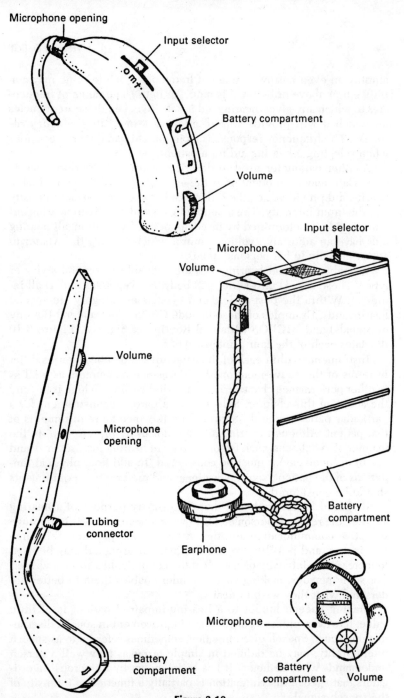

Figure 3-10.
Types of Hearing Aids: (from right to left) Post-auricular, body (top), eyeglass, all-in-the-ear (bottom).

For some hearing-impaired persons, speech discrimination is more than a function of intensity. A person having a sensorineural hearing loss may experience reduced speech discrimination at intensity levels above his or her threshold for speech. For example, at a sensation level of 26 dB (i.e., at 26 decibels above the speech reception threshold), a normal ear or an ear with a pure conductive hearing loss will achieve near-normal speech discrimination. However, at this same sensation level a sensorineural-impaired ear may exhibit reduced speech discrimination. Several investigators have shown that by selectively amplifying those frequencies which demonstrate the greatest loss for pure tones, speech discrimination can often be improved over the unaided condition.

Hearing aids may be used, then, to improve a hearing-impaired listener's reception of speech and, sometimes, his discrimination of speech. For some patients, an improvement in reception capabilities will result in increased discrimination, while for some patients, an increase in discrimination is the main objective.

DETERMINATION OF CANDIDACY FOR AMPLIFICATION

Determination of candidacy for successful use of amplification is best accomplished pragmatically. It is our opinion that any hearing-impaired person who complains of difficulty understanding speech should be considered a candidate for evaluation with a hearing aid. While it is true that some hearing losses are more amenable to amplification than are others, successful hearing aid use is predicated upon many factors other than degree of hearing loss. Furthermore, modern hearing aid technology provides for the possibility of selective amplification which permits the fitting of hearing aids to hearing losses which were considered to be beyond the help of hearing aids 10 years ago.

For example, the use of high-frequency emphasis post-auricle hearing aids has enabled persons with sensorineural losses affecting only the high frequencies to receive some assistance from a hearing aid in many instances. At one time, these patients, who may have normal hearing sensitivity at or below 1000 Hz, were considered poor candidates for amplification. The use of high frequency emphasis hearing aids has permitted the successful fitting of some hearing losses caused by presbycusis or noise exposure.

THE GERIATRIC PATIENT AND HEARING AIDS

The geriatric patient may present special problems for hearing aid fitting and successful hearing aid use. Sometimes these problems may be related to the hearing loss itself. For instance, the mild to moderate loss of some older persons may be accompanied by phonemic regression. For these patients, a hearing aid may make speech louder without greatly improving speech discrimination. Because of the characteristics of a sensorineural hearing loss, however, the presence of loud sounds may cause discomfort to the patient because of the presence of recruitment.

Certain factors not directly related to hearing loss must be considered in deciding whether to fit a presbycusic patient with a hearing aid. Perhaps the most important of these is patient motivation. While the motivational factor is important for a hearing aid wearer of any age, it is sometimes assumed to be present in the younger patient who is self-referred for a hearing aid evaluation. However, many geriatric patients come to the audiology clinic more to please a relative or a friend than to actively seek help for a hearing problem. The nature of a presbycusic hearing loss is a slow development over several years. Therefore, patients having mild to moderate hearing losses may have been able to adjust to decreasing hearing sensitivity without realizing it. These patients then reject suggestions that they have a hearing problem, sometimes preferring to shift the blame for communication difficulties to the speakers to which they listen. They may reject the idea of a hearing aid as being unnecessary. Furthermore, even though some older persons will admit to having a hearing problem, they may prefer to attempt to compensate in other ways, rejecting a hearing aid as being a visible sign of age.

Related to possible poor initial motivation is the question of adjustment to amplification. Contrary to some advertising claims, hearing aids do not necessarily provide normal hearing or natural hearing. If a patient is not properly counseled, he may have unrealistic expectations and may reject a hearing aid when these expectations are not fulfilled. Even those patients who are extensively counseled prior to a hearing aid fitting may have difficulty adjusting to amplification. Older persons who, because of gradual hearing loss, have heard environmental sounds at greatly reduced intensities may be disturbed when these sounds are amplified.

For those patients, then, who initially reject amplification, or for whom reality falls short of expectation, a program of aural rehabilitation may be necessary. It should be noted that some time spent in aural rehabilitation will benefit any inexperienced hearing aid wearer, regardless of their initial degree of acceptance or motivation. We believe strongly that a period of guided adjustment to amplification is desirable for any person who is an inexperienced hearing aid wearer. Older patients especially may need this counseling. We feel that patient progress during the adjustment period should be monitored at regular intervals by professionals who are knowledgeable about hearing aids and their use. Apart from ensuring that the instrument is functioning properly and is being properly worn and maintained, the professional should guide the patient during the adjustment period. Several suggestions can be offered to assist the patient during this time.

First, we believe that the patient must have a clear understanding of what the hearing aid can be expected to do for them. A hearing aid is no panacea. The patient must understand that the instrument will not restore his or her hearing to normal. When the idea is accepted that a hearing aid is a prosthetic device to be used to provide assistance whenever possible, the patient is better able to accept those situations in which the instrument is of reduced value. Given this understanding, he or she is ready to begin exploration of those situations in which the hearing aid will be helpful.

It is advisable that initial experience wearing a hearing aid occur in situations of minimal background noise. The patient may be advised to wear the hearing aid only around the home at first, where the noise levels are somewhat predictable and controllable. It may be necessary to advise the patient to wear the hearing aid only for short periods of time initially, and to remove it if signs of nervousness or fatigue begin to occur. However, the patient should also be advised that adjustment to amplification will be facilitated with increasing exposure to the instrument. For some persons, a concerted effort is needed to adapt to a hearing aid, and the geriatric patient should be given as much encouragement as is necessary to bring about this adjustment.

Finally, depending upon the needs of the patient, encouragement should be given to wear the hearing aid in situations in which background noise levels are greater than the noise levels around the home. The patient should be encouraged to wear the hearing aid "out into the world."

It should be noted that aural rehabilitation for hearing aid wearers may include more than a session or sessions of hearing aid orientation. Extensive auditory training and speechreading instruction may be required to assist the patient in obtaining maximum benefit from the instrument. Some older persons are unwilling to participate in extensive therapy.

One might expect that age and general state of health might have some correlation to success in hearing aid use. In fact, it has been shown by Jerger and Hayes (1976) that expectations for successful hearing aid use decline in patients over 65 years of age. General health

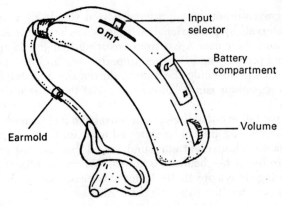

Figure 3-11

may affect patients' ability to physically manipulate a hearing aid, as well as their motivation for using amplification.

Finally, we feel strongly that members of the hearing aid wearer's family be educated as to the expectations and limitations of the hearing aid. They, too, must realize that use of amplification does not restore hearing to normal. Family members should be advised that maximum communication will occur when they speak slowly and naturally. Slight increases in vocal intensity on their part may be beneficial, but shouting will be of little value. Depending upon the general physical health of the hearing aid wearer, it may be advisable to acquaint a member of the family with the basics of operation and maintenance of the hearing aid.

TROUBLESHOOTING FOR THE GERIATRIC HEARING AID WEARER

The clinician who works around geriatric patients will encounter persons who have worn a hearing aid for many years. Generally, these patients will be aware of the benefits and limitations which they may expect from their instruments. Some, however, may complain occasionally about the performance of their aids. The nurse clinician may find it useful to be able to "troubleshoot" malfunctioning hearing aids. She or he need not be an expert regarding hearing aids to determine a few simple facts about a patient's instrument. Figure 3-11 illustrates features of a typical post-auricle hearing aid.

The clinician should look closely at the instrument itself. Is it relatively clean? Are cracks present in its case? Do any of the external switches appear to be broken, nonfunctional or missing? If it is a post-auricle instrument, is the sound tube cracked, broken or occluded with cerumen? The clinician should examine the sound tube, earmold and connecting tubing carefully to determine whether any dust, cerumen or other foreign matter is present which may be preventing passage of sound into the patient's ear.

Next, the examiner should open the battery compartment and check to see if the batteries are properly installed. This may be determined by ensuring that the positive pole of the battery (marked "+") is aligned with the proper contact within the hearing aid. Although it is difficult to incorrectly insert a battery into many modern post-auricle instruments, once an instrument has had its battery compartment sprung slightly, it is by no means impossible. Many geriatric patients may own body-style hearing aids, which are much easier to improperly load with batteries. If the batteries are properly loaded and the hearing aid does not work, the batteries may simply be dead.

If visual examination of the instrument reveals no gross physical defects, the examiner should then attempt to determine if the hearing aid is functional. This may be done by inserting a battery into the instrument, advancing the volume control to the "full-on" position, and attempting to obtain feedback. The hearing aid will feed back (i.e., emit a high-pitched whistle) when it is cupped between the hands with the volume full-on. The whistle is produced when the internal noises of the instrument are emitted by the transducer and picked up by the hearing aid's external microphone. They are then reamplified by the hearing aid and reemitted from the transducer. If the instrument is a body-style hearing aid having an external transducer (earpiece) it is necessary only to move this external earphone into proximity with the hearing aid's external microphone to obtain feedback. Failure to emit feedback suggests that either the instrument itself is nonfunctional or the battery is dead.

If the hearing aid can be made to feed back, the instrument is known to be operating. However, the presence of feedback does not rule out the possibility that the instrument may be distorting the signal which it emits. Gross distortion can be detected by listening to the hearing aid, but requires electroacoustic analysis for quantification.

If the patient complains that the hearing aid "flutters" or seems to go on and off in rapid succession, this may be symptomatic of internal dysfunction within the hearing aid.

Finally, the examiner should determine the condition and fit of the patient's earmold. The earmold should be clean, free from sharp edges or rough spots, and should fit tightly into the patient's ear.

If no obvious physical defects are detected in the hearing aid itself, the clinician must determine whether other factors are contributing to the patient's dissatisfaction. Several questions provided in the protocol will help explore this possibility.

If the clinician concludes that the hearing aid is malfunctioning, referral to outside sources may be necessary. This may be a hearing aid dealer, audiologist or speech and hearing clinic, depending upon which service is readily available. If it is suspected that the patient's dissatisfaction results from improper use of the hearing aid, a brief counseling session may alleviate the patient's problems. For some persons, extensive counseling in conjunction with other rehabilitative measures may be necessary. If it is suspected that the patient has been improperly fitted, referral to a hearing aid dealer or audiologist may be helpful. Most important, if it is suspected that a change in hearing sensitivity has occurred which is partially responsible for the patient's dissatisfaction, referral to a physician is necessary.

REFERENCES

1. Bergstrom, LaVonne. "Congenital Deafness." In *Hearing Disorders*. Jerry L. Northern, ed. Boston: Little, Brown and Co. 1976, pp. 171–177, Chap. 15.
2. _____ and Patricia Thompson. "Ototoxicity." In *Hearing Disorders*. Jerry L. Northern, ed. Boston: Little, Brown and Co., 1976, pp. 136–152, Chap. 12.
3. Byers, Vincent et al. "Guidelines for Manual Pure-Tone Threshold Audiometry." *Journal of the American Speech and Hearing Association*, 20:4, April 1978, pp. 297–301.
4. Hirsh, Ira J. et al. "Development of Materials for Speech Audiometry." *Journal of Speech and Hearing Disorders*, 17, 1952, pp. 321–337.
5. Jerger, James. "Clinical Experience with Impedance Audiometry." *Archives of Otolaryngology*. 92:311, 1970.
6. _____ and Deborah Hayes. "Hearing Aid Evaluation: Clinical Experience with a New Philosophy." *Archives of Otolaryngology*, 102:214, 1976.
7. Matkin, Noel and Wayne Olsen. "Differential Audiology." In *Audiological Assessment*. Darrell E. Rose, ed. Englewood Cliffs, N.J.: Prentice-Hall, 1971, pp. 321–368, Chap. 10.
8. Northern, Jerry L. "Clinical Applications of Impedance Audiometry." In *Hearing Disorders*. Jerry L. Northern, ed. Boston: Little, Brown and Co., 1976, pp. 20–36, Chap. 3.
9. O'Neill, John J. and Herbert J. Oyer. "Aural Rehabilitation." In *Modern Developments in Audiometry*. James Jerger, ed. New York: Academic Press, 1973, pp. 212–252, Chap. 7.

10. Ramsdell, D.A. "The Psychology of Hard-of-Hearing and the Deafened Adult." In *Hearing and Deafness*. Hallowell Davis and S. Richard Silverman, eds. New York: Holt, Rinehart and Winston, 1966, pp. 459–473.
11. Sanders, Jay W. and William F. Rintelmann. "Masking in Audiometry." *Archives of Otolaryngology*, 80, 1964, pp. 541–556.
12. Schuknecht, Harold F. "Further Observations on the Pathology of Presbycusis." *Archives of Otolaryngology*, 80, 1964, pp. 369–382.
13. Spoor, A. "Presbycusis Values in Relation to Noise-Induced Hearing Loss." *International Audiology*, 6, 1967, pp. 48–57.
14. Willeford, Jack A. "The Geriatric Patient." In *Audiological Assessment*. Darrell E. Rose, ed. Englewood Cliffs, N.J.: Prentice-Hall, 1971, pp. 281–320, Chap. 9.

Chapter 4

Urinary
Incontinence

OVERVIEW

In order for the primary health care provider to understand the underlying etiology of incontinence in the elderly female or male, she or he must understand the normal anatomy and physiology of the aging lower genitourinary tract. From an adequate knowledge base the practitioner can utilize the following protocol to determine the etiology and differential diagnosis of urinary incontinence in both the male and female elderly patient.

Urine is formed in the kidneys, where the various processes resulting in its formation are completed (e.g., filtration, reabsorption and secretion). Urine is then transported via the ureters to the bladder. The flow of urine is conducted by the peristaltic contractions of the smooth muscle in the ureters and the hydrostatic pressure in the ureters. The ureters attach to the bladder at an oblique angle thus helping to prevent the reflux of urine.

The bladder is composed of three layers of smooth muscle. The outermost layer (called the detrusor muscle) is the layer which, during contraction, causes micturition. The detrusor muscle also forms the internal urethral sphincter at the insertion of the urethra. Skeletal muscle at the end of the urethra forms the external sphincter. Motor innervation of the bladder is accomplished by both involuntary smooth muscle action and voluntary skeletal muscle action. The involuntary actions include the sympathetic innervation of the bladder and internal sphincter, and the parasympathetic innervation of the detrusor and internal sphincter. The voluntary actions include the somatic innervation of the external sphincter.

When the urine in the bladder stretches the wall to a certain point, stretch receptors in the wall of the bladder transmit impulses via afferent fibers of the parasympathetic nervous system to the brain and spinal cord. These responses bring about the relaxation of perineal muscles and the external sphincter, and the contraction of the detrusor muscle causing micturition. In the absence of an intact bladder innervation, the bladder's smooth muscle will still contract; however, the stretch receptors in this case require a higher degree of stretch (more urine) before causing urination.

The aged genitourinary system characteristically is physiologically changed in ways that can contribute to urinary incontinence. There may be residual urine and a smaller bladder capacity (sometimes half that of younger adults). The onset of the desire to urinate is frequently late, (often at the limit of capacity), whereas younger adults usually have a desire to urinate at about half bladder capacity. In addition, in old age the frequent presence of uninhibited bladder contractions of the detrusor muscle causes an urgent demand to micturate. The declining function of the bladder smooth muscle leads to hypertrophy which largely increases the incidence of the formation of urinary diverticuli.

The elderly male is more prone to incontinence (especially stress) because of two major factors: prostatic pathology and manipulative procedures performed. Prostate pathology (i.e., benign prostatic hypertrophy, cancer of the gland and prostatitis) cause compression on the urethra. This compression gives rise to the symptoms of frequency, nocturia, hesitancy, weakened stream and dribbling.

Incontinence in the elderly female is most frequently the result of a relaxed pelvic musculature (secondary to multiparity and/or estrogen deficiency). Both males and females may have urinary incontinence tendencies exacerbated by diseases that increase intraabdominal pressure (such as obesity, chronic obstructive pulmonary disease [COPD] and ascites).

The three types of incontinence are stress, urgency and overflow. Stress incontinence is defined as an involuntary urine loss as a result of an increase in abdominal pressure such as coughing or straining or poor pelvic muscle tone. Urge incontinence is a urine loss that occurs inappropriately and without patient control. Overflow incontinence is urine loss that occurs independently of stress or patient control.

The following protocol approach divides the causes of incontinence into two types: episodic and continuous. Three types of episodic incontinence are: 1) stress (i.e., caused by multiparity, trauma, increased intraabdominal pressure, etc.); 2) urge (i.e., caused by structural problems or inflammation); 3) overflow (i.e., caused by drugs or psychogenic problems). Three types of continuous incontinence are: 1) stress (i.e., a prolonged uncorrected condition); 2) urge (i.e., prolonged untreated structural problem, inflammation or a declining bladder musculature function); and 3) neurogenic (i.e., diabetes, tabes dorsalis, tumors or trauma).

URINARY INCONTINENCE WORKSHEET

What you cannot afford to miss: bladder tumors, urinary tract infections, urinary tract fistulas, neurological lesions, urethral or bladder obstructions, kidney disease, diabetes, tabes dorsalis, sphincter trauma.
Males: *Prostatitis, benign prostatic hypertrophy, cancer of the prostate, past prostatectomy, sphincter trauma.*
Females: *Pelvic tumors.*

Chief Complaint: _____

SUBJECTIVE DATA: (Describe All Positive Responses)

MALES AND FEMALES:
YES   NO

_____ _____ Onset, duration of incontinence: _____

_____ _____ Dysuria: _____

_____ _____ Hematuria: _____

_____ _____ Nocturia: _____

_____ _____ Frequency: _____

_____ _____ Urgency: _____

_____ _____ Back pain: _____

_____ _____ Dribbling: _____

_____ _____ Diminished size or force of stream: _____

_____ _____ Enuresis (diurnal or nocturnal): _____

_____ _____ Presence of urge to void: _____

_____ _____ Absence of urge to void: _____

_____ _____ Constipation/diarrhea: _____

_____ _____ Retention: _____

_____ _____ Urethral discharge: _____

_____ _____ Nausea/vomiting: _____

_____ _____ Hesitancy: _____

_____ _____ Precipitated by coughing, sneezing, laughing, bending over, etc.: _____

_____ _____ Abnormal characteristics of urine (i.e., color, odor):
_____

_____ _____ Bowel incontinence: _____

_____ _____ Urine leakage from unusual source: _____

_____ _____ History of decreased output: _____

_____ _____ Straining to void: _____

_____ _____ Difficulty initiating a stream: _____

FEMALES:
YES   _NO_

_____ _____ Sensation of sagging of perineal area: _____

_____ _____ Vaginal discharge or irritation: _____

_____ _____ Perineal irritation: _____

Urinary Incontinence Worksheet

MALES:
YES   NO

_____ _____ Vesical or rectal tenesmus:_____

_____ _____ Impotence:_____

_____ _____ Interruption of stream:_____

_____ _____ Urinary retention past/present: _____

FAMILY HISTORY:
YES   NO

_____ _____ Diabetes, syphilis, cancer, TB, hypertension, heart

disease, kidney disease, multiple sclerosis: _____

PAST MEDICAL HISTORY:
YES   NO

_____ _____ Diabetes:_____

_____ _____ Venereal disease, pelvic inflammatory disease:_____

_____ _____ Cancer: _____

_____ _____ Tuberculosis: _____

_____ _____ COPD: _____

_____ _____ Kidney disease and/or frequent urinary tract infec-

tions or stones or history of urethral dilatations for

stenosis:_____

_____

_____ _____ Pernicious anemia: _____

_____ _____ Parkinson's disease: _____

SURGICAL HISTORY:
YES   *NO*

_____ _____ Females: back surgery, bladder repairs, GYN sur-

gery, rectal surgery, spinal surgery: _____

_____ _____ Males: back surgery, prostatic surgeries, rectal or

urethral surgery: _____

FEMALES ONLY:
YES   *NO*

_____ _____ OB history, history of traumatic deliveries,

Gr_____ Para_____ Ab_____

MALES AND FEMALES:
YES   *NO*

_____ _____ Current medications: _____

_____ _____ Use of alcohol: _____

_____ _____ History of recent trauma: _____

OBJECTIVE DATA (Describe all abnormal findings):

Vital Signs: _____BP _____Temp _____Wt. _____Ht.

ABDOMINAL EXAMINATION:
Inspection (exposure from nipple to mid-thigh)
YES   *NO*

_____ _____ Shape of abdomen (scaphoid, obese, distended,

masses, etc.): _____

_____

_____ _____ Asymmetrical: _____

Urinary Incontinence Worksheet

_____ _____ Muscle tone (poor): _____

_____ _____ Ascites: _____

AUSCULTATION:
YES   NO

_____ _____ Bowel sounds abnormal: _____

PERCUSSION:
YES   NO

_____ _____ Liver span abnormal:_____

_____ _____ Spleen abnormal: _____

_____ _____ Bladder palpable: _____

PALPATION:
YES   NO

_____ _____ Masses: _____

_____ _____ Tenderness: _____

_____ _____ Palpable kidneys: _____

_____ _____ Palpable bladder: _____

_____ _____ Inguinal node enlargement: _____

_____ _____ Hernias (umbilical, inguinal, diastasis recti): _____

BACK EXAMINATION:
YES   NO

_____ _____ Spinal, CVA tenderness: _____

_____ _____ Scars from laminectomy, etc.:_____

RECTAL EXAMINATION:
NORMAL ABNORMAL

_____ _____ Check for sphincter tone, perineal sensation, masses,

fecal impactions, fistulas, hemorrhoids, fissures, etc.

_____ _____ Prostate (should be symmetrical, nontender smooth):

_____boggy _____nodular _____tender

PELVIC EXAMINATION: (FEMALES ONLY)

Inspection (Describe All Abnormal Responses)
YES   NO

_____ _____ Bartholin's and Skene's glands abnormal: _____

_____ _____ Reddened, irritated perineum: _____

_____ _____ Vaginal discharge:_____

_____ _____ Atrophic changes: _____

_____ _____ Urethral discharge: _____

_____ _____ Urethra reddened, swollen, caruncle: _____

_____ _____ Cystocele, rectocele, urethrocele: _____

_____ _____ Pelvic musculature relaxation: _____

_____ _____ Fistulas:_____

PELVIC AND RECTOVAGINAL BIMANUAL:
NORMAL   ABNORMAL

_____ _____ Systematically examine vagina, cervix, uterus, ad-

nexa. (Describe all abnormalities.): _____

_____

_____

_____

MALE GENITOURINARY EXAMINATION:
NORMAL   ABNORMAL

_____ _____ Circumcised, uncircumcised: _____

_____ _____ Penis (meatal stenosis, hypospadias, epispadias): ___

_____

_____ _____ Urethral inflammation, discharge, stenosis: _____

_____

_____ _____ Testis: _____

_____ _____ Epididymis: _____

_____ _____ Vas: _____

_____ _____ Hernias: _____

_____ _____ Scrotal exam lying down and upright (check for red-

ness, warmth, hydrocele, varicocele): _____

NEUROLOGIC EXAMINATION: (DESCRIBE ALL ABNORMAL RESPONSES)
NORMAL ABNORMAL

_____ _____ Cranial nerves II through XII: _____

_____ _____ Motor: _____

_____ _____ Sensory: _____

_____ _____ Reflexes: _____

_____ _____ Tremors: _____

_____ _____ Cerebellar function: _____

_____ _____ Proprioception: _____

_____ _____ Mental status: _____

LAB DATA: (DESCRIBE ALL TEST RESULTS)
     NOT
DONE DONE

_____ _____ CBC _____

_____ _____ Blood sugar fasting, 2 hr pc: _____

_____ _____ BUN/creatinine clearance: _____

_____ _____ Urinalysis (micro and macro and C&S): _____

Males:

_____ _____ Three glass urine: _____

_____ _____ Prostatic fluid examination: _____

The following tests should be done in the following situations:

_____ _____ Acid phos/alk phos: (on males if the prostate exam is abnormal): _____

_____ _____ Electrolytes (if patient is confused): _____

_____ _____ Blood serology (VDRL, FTA) if patient has an abnormal neuro (i.e., Argyll Robertson pupils, ataxia, loss of reflexes): _____

_____

_____ _____ Abdominal x-ray (if patient has an abnormal abdominal exam or if you suspect urinary calculi with signs and/or symptoms of hematuria, severe flank pain, etc.) _____

The following tests should be done if the patient's incontinence cannot be explained by inflammation. It is not expected that the nurse will order these tests *without a referral to the patient's urologist; however, a basic review of these procedures has been provided.*

_____ _____ IVP: _____

_____ _____ Cystourethroscopy, cystoscopy:_____

_____ _____ Voiding cystogram: _____

_____ _____ Cystometrogram:_____

_____ _____ Electromyography: _____

URINARY INCONTINENCE WORKSHEET RATIONALE

SUBJECTIVE DATA:

Onset of Difficulties

The determination of the underlying pathology is aided by knowing whether the onset of the problem of urinary incontinence is sudden or gradual. If the problem was sudden, the causative agent could have been derived from trauma, surgery or a recent CVA. Gradual onset of increasing chronicity may be secondary to unsolved structural problems (e.g., worsening pelvic relaxation leading to stress incontinence or neurologic problems).

Duration

Episodic causes of incontinence can be stress incontinence, urge incontinence, or overflow. In females, stress incontinence may be secondary to multiparity or estrogen deficiency. In males, stress incontinence is related to manipulative procedures or prostatic enlargement. In either sex, episodic stress incontinence may be secondary to obesity, COPD or ascites. Urge incontinence that is episodic in either sex may be secondary to inflammatory processes or obstructive pathology. Overflow incontinence that is episodic is related in both sexes to iatrogenic causes. However, continuous overflow incontinence may be the result of underlying neurological disease (e.g., diabetes mellitus, tabes dorsalis, multiple sclerosis), invasive neoplasms, trauma or surgical complications.

Dysuria

Dysuria associated with urinary incontinence, especially urge incontinence, may be the result of inflammatory processes of the bladder or urethra. Dysuria may be due to a primary involvement of the urinary tract infection or it may occur as a secondary process (i.e., in females: cervicitis or contamination from vaginal discharge). In the elderly, infections may be present without dysuria. Dysuria in males may be secondary to urethritis from gonorrhea or prostatitis.

Hematuria

Gross or microscopic hematuria may either be total, initial or terminal. Total hematuria indicates bleeding arising either from the kidney or ureters. Initial hematuria indicates bleeding arising from lesions below the neck of the bladder, and terminal hematuria arises from lesions or inflammation in the trigone area. Painless hematuria associated with incontinence may be secondary to tumors. Painful hematuria with incontinence may arise from inflammatory processes, urinary polyps, diverticuli or bladder stones. In males microscopic hematuria can be secondary to prostatitis.

Nocturia

Nocturia associated with polyuria and incontinence may be indicative of diabetes mellitus. In males, nocturnal frequency associated with hesitancy and dribbling are hallmark symptoms of benign prostatic hypertrophy.

Frequency

Frequency in association with nocturia, polyuria and incontinence without dysuria may be secondary to diabetes mellitus. Frequency with nocturia, incontinence and dysuria may be secondary to inflammatory processes or to structural problems (e.g., polyps, strictures, decreased functioning of the detrusor, etc.). Frequency without associated dysuria but in association with small, frequent involuntary voidings may be caused by neurologic or psychogenic causes. In males, frequency with a difficulty in starting and stopping the stream is usually secondary to prostatic enlargement.

Urgency

Urgency associated with incontinence may be secondary to inflammation (trigonal, urethral or bladder), stones or tumors. In females, frequency and urgency with incontinence may also be the result of radiation injury from cervical cancer treatment. In males, prostate disease may cause urgency.

Back Pain

Back pain may occur in association with a urinary tract infection (as an underlying pathology of incontinence) or as a neurologic cause of incontinence (e.g., disc disease, tumors, trauma). Low back pain may be due to cystitis. High back pain (CVA tenderness) is suggestive of pyelonephritis. In males, back pain may occur from a spinal cancer that has metastasized from a prostatic cancer.

Dribbling

Dribbling associated with incontinence in the female may be secondary to overflow from whatever cause (i.e., neurogenic, obstructive). In males, dribbling may be caused by benign prostatic hypertrophy (BPH), prostatitis, or sphincter trauma. In either sex, dribbling can be due to an autonomous neurogenic bladder secondary to extensive pelvic surgeries, inflammation or tumors.

Diminished Size or Force of Stream

Stream changes accompanied by urge incontinence may be secondary to structural abnormalities (e.g., strictures, polyps, etc.). Diminished force may be seen in neurogenic disease. In males, the stream change may indicate BPH or cancer of the prostate.

Enuresis

In adults, enuresis may be secondary to neurologic causes, bladder neck obstruction or oversedation. Psychogenic incontinence will usually be present during the day (diurnal) but is absent at night. Nocturnal enuresis is usually secondary to a neurologic problem. In males, enuresis may be secondary to trauma from a prostatectomy.

Presence/Absence of Urge to Void

Presence of the urge to void followed by an inability to except with straining is seen in a motor paralytic bladder. Presence of an urge to void prior to incontinence indicates an urge incontinence from inflammatory or structural causes. Presence of an urge to void but with an inability to stop (uninhibited neurogenic bladder) is seen in lesions affecting the motor pathways. Absence of the urge to void associated with incontinence suggests neurogenic incontinence (i.e., secondary to Parkinson's disease, multiple sclerosis, CVA, tumors, trauma).

Constipation/Diarrhea

Constipation may cause incontinence because of pressure that a fecal mass exerts on the bladder. Alternating constipation/diarrhea in association with urinary incontinence may be secondary to a fecal impaction.

Retention

A history of urinary retention in either sex may be secondary to drugs, obstruction, neurogenic causes, psychogenic causes or following administration of general anesthetics. In males, retention is most commonly caused by BPH, although cancer of the prostate and prostatitis can be the underlying etiology.

Urethral Discharge

In either sex, discharge may be indicative of urethritis. In males, prostatitis, gonococcal urethritis, and nongonococcal urethritis may present in this manner.

Nausea and Vomiting

In either sex, nausea and vomiting may be the only objective sign of a distended bladder in the bedridden patient. In this instance, the patient will have overflow incontinence.

Hesitancy

In either sex, this symptom may arise from neurologic disease (especially multiple sclerosis) or from an obstructive pathology. In males, hesitancy most commonly is secondary to BPH.

Precipitated by Coughing, Sneezing, Bending Over, Etc.

Stress incontinence may occur as a result of increased abdominal pressure (e.g., coughing, sneezing, bending over, obesity, COPD, ascites, etc.).

Abnormal Characteristics of Urine (i.e., odor, color)

Incontinence may be an urge incontinence secondary to a urinary tract infection, in which case there may be a foul odor or discoloration of the urine.

Bowel Incontinence

Bowel incontinence in association with urinary incontinence may be secondary to neurologic diseases with neuropathies (e.g., diabetes), tumors or trauma.

Urine Leakage from Unusual Source (i.e., vagina or rectum)

Incontinence may arise from fistulas secondary to surgery, traumatic deliveries, radiation therapy, cystoceles, rectoceles or urethroceles.

History of Decreased Output

Oliguria may be secondary to obstructive pathology, dehydration, renal insufficiency (either acute or chronic), or congestive heart failure.

Straining to Void

In either sex, straining may be indicative of an autonomous neurogenic bladder secondary to neoplasms, inflammatory lesions or following extensive pelvic surgeries. In males, straining is most commonly due to BPH.

Difficulty in Initiating a Stream

Difficulty initiating a stream may be the result of a sensory paralytic bladder caused by pernicious anemia, tabes dorsalis, overdistention or diabetes. In males, the difficulty may be secondary to prostate pathology.

Females
Sagging sensation

A sagging sensation associated with stress incontinence may result from a relaxation of the pelvic musculature.

Vaginal, perineal discharge or irritation

Discharge or irritation associated with incontinence can be caused by urethritis from fecal contamination leading to urge incontinence.

Males
Vesical or rectal tenesmus

In males, the bladder is directly in front of the rectum. Tenesmus may result from a distended bladder pressing on the rectal musculature.

Impotence

In males, impotence may be secondary to diabetic neuropathy, tabes dorsalis, multiple sclerosis, postsurgical complications, psychogenic influences or iatrogenic causes.

Interruption of stream	An interruption of a stream may be indicative of obstructive pathology (e.g., stone at the bladder neck).
Urinary retention	Urinary retention may be secondary to drugs or obstructive pathology (especially BPH in males). Either of these causes may precipitate an overflow incontinence.

Family History
Diabetes mellitus, multiple sclerosis, TBC, syphilis, cancer, stones, kidney disease

A familial history of these diseases should alert the practitioner to potential conditions which can be associated with urinary incontinence.

Past Medical History

Diabetes, MS, or syphilis may be the neurologic causative agent of incontinence. Chronic obstructive pulmonary disease may cause stress incontinence because of a chronic cough which increases intraabdominal pressure. A history of cancer is important because of possible radiation damage. Parkinson's disease may cause an uninhibited neurogenic bladder. Pernicious anemia may cause a motor or sensory paralytic bladder. Frequent urinary tract infections may be secondary to structural abnormalities or poor hygiene, both of which can cause urge incontinence. In males, recurrent UTI's may be indicative of BPH or unresolved prostatitis.

Surgeries

Incontinence may occur as a result of surgical trauma, the development of fistulas secondary to surgery, neurologic damage, or a direct sphincterotomy.

OB History

Multiparity or a history of difficult deliveries may cause stress incontinence due to a relaxation of the pelvic musculature.

Current Medications

Overflow incontinence may be secondary to antihistamines, tricyclic drugs, phenothiazides, sedatives, anticholinergics, quinidine, muscle relaxants or antispasmodics.

Alcohol Usage

Alcohol usage may promote incontinence because alcohol inhibits the antidiuretic hormone (ADH). The anesthetic effect of alcohol may also increase the likelihood of developing urinary retention.

History of Recent Trauma

Disc disease or pelvic fractures may precipitate urinary incontinence.

OBJECTIVE DATA:

Abdominal Examination

Poor abdominal muscle tone is common in the elderly; this factor together with obesity may cause stress incontinence. Palpable masses or the presence of ascites may alert one to the presence of a tumor pressing on the bladder and reducing its ability to retain urine.

Back

Costovertebral angle tenderness may be indicative of an infection. Spinal tenderness may be secondary to disc disease or other neurologic causes. Cancer of the prostate (advanced) frequently metastasizes to bone, particularly the spine causing pain.

Rectal Examination

Check for the character of the sphincter tone. Poor sphincter tone may indicate neurogenic incontinence (secondary to disease, trauma or lesions). The presence of a large fecal mass may indicate a fecal impaction as an underlying cause of incontinence. In males, examine the size, shape and consistency, etc. of the prostate gland. The presence of hemorrhoids may be secondary to the strain of voiding necessary in prostatic disease.

Pelvic Examination

Inflammation in the periurethral glands, perineum, urethra or vagina might indicate urge incontinence. Atrophic changes or muscle relaxation may indicate the source of stress incontinence. The presence of fistulas or palpable pelvic masses can cause incontinence.

Male Genitourinary Examination

It is important to perform a complete genitourinary exam in males. The examiner should be looking for signs of inflammation, stenotic lesions, etc. that may precipitate incontinence. An epididymitis can seed a prostatitis with a resultant incontinence secondary to the inflammation.

Neurologic Exam

Any abnormality in the neurologic exam should alert one to the possibility of neurogenic bladder disease.

Incontinence in association with polyuria, polydipsia, peripheral neuropathies and bowel incontinence may indicate diabetes. Incontinence may be caused by tumors in the central or peripheral nervous system which might produce an abnormal neurologic exam.

Multiple sclerosis may consist of incontinence, loss of proprioception, cerebellar abnormalities and a positive Babinski's sign.

Tabes dorsalis (very rare condition) can present as incontinence in association with areflexia, wide stance gait, paresthesias and Argyll Robertson's pupil.

Laboratory Data

CBC

A complete blood count should be done for routine screening purposes.

In males, anemia may be due to a metastatic cancer of the bone which has metastasized from a primary site in the prostate.

Blood glucose determination

If the subjective data has raised suspicions of diabetes, the tests of fasting blood glucose and postprandial blood sugar should be done.

BUN/creatinine clearance

These are important tests of renal functioning and should be done to determine the patient's kidney status.

Urinalysis

The urine should be examined by dipstick, microscopic exam and culture and sensitivity (if indicated). If the dipstick confirms the presence of sugar and ketones, suspect diabetes. Proteinuria may be indicative of an inflammatory process or secondary to renal complications of diabetes mellitus, and/or renal parenchymal disease. The microscopic urinalysis should be performed with close inspection for WBC's and RBC's (which may indicate an inflammatory process). Casts would indicate an inflammatory and/or renal parenchymal disease. Pyuria without bacteriuria is indicative of tuberculosis. Microscopic hematuria may be secondary to inflammatory processes, glomerulonephritis, cystitis, pyelonephritis, neoplasms, stones, trauma or renal parenchymal diseases. A culture of the urine is done to rule out a urinary tract infection.

Three glass urine (males)

The three glass urine exam (see UTI protocol for further explanation) is done to rule out an inflammation in the prostate, bladder and/or urethra. An inflammation could be the underlying etiology of urge incontinence.

Prostatic fluid exam (males)

A prostatic fluid exam helps rule out the presence of a prostatitis; a prostatitis can cause urge incontinence.

Acid phos/alk phos (males)

An elevation of acid phos is usually indicative of metastatic cancer of the prostate. (Remember that an elevation in acid phos may occur within 24 hours after examination of the normal prostate.) Once the tumor has spread, there may also be an elevation of the alkaline phosphatase.

Electrolytes

An electrolyte imbalance may cause confusion, and as a result the patient may be unaware of the urge to urinate. This condition could lead to overflow incontinence.

Blood serology

If tertiary syphilis is suspected, a VDRL and FTA should be drawn; the FTA is a more sensitive test in screening for latent syphilis and its complications (tabes dorsalis). If the serology is positive suspect neurogenic incontinence.

Abdominal x-ray

The abdominal x-ray will help rule out tumors, bladder or kidney stones as a cause of incontinence.

IVP

An intravenous pyelogram is done to look for stones, filling defects, bladder contour problems, and/or a decreased emptying ability secondary to neurologic causes.

Cystourethroscopy (cystoscopy)

This test will indicate the various types of inflammation, trabeculations and diverticula formation and will also show any occasional unexpected causes of dysuria in the elderly, such as papilloma, stones and carcinoma. This test also shows any increase in common characteristic changes of mild papillary cystitis or trigonitis.

Voiding cystogram

X-raying the bladder after filling it with a radiopaque fluid records bladder morphology and changes in bladder and urethral flow during urination. This test assists in determining neurogenic and nonneurogenic causes of incontinence. Bladder outlet obstruction, whether due to anatomic causes such as the stricture of the urethra, etc. or to functional causes in the uninhibited neurogenic bladder, will be shown by the presence of diverticula.

Cystometrogram

This test is performed by filling the bladder with sterile water, either at a rate of 10 ml./min. or in increments of 50 ml. q. 2 min., or continuously. The changes in bladder pressure are recorded on a graduated paper by means of a cystometer. The examination is completed when micturition occurs, when discomfort becomes severe, or when a large bladder volume has been achieved. Cystometry is of value in determining the bladder function in incontinence.

Electromyography

This is a measurement of the striated muscle contraction or relaxation. An electrode is inserted into the urogenital diaphragm and motor impulses are observed.

ASSESSMENT:

Episodic Incontinence
Stress incontinence

Stress incontinence is involuntary loss or discharge of urine. In the elderly female, it may be the result of multiparity with consequent relaxation of the pelvic musculature, traumatic deliveries that have resulted in the development of fistulas, a loss of the normal urethrovesical angle or estrogen deficiency. In males, stress incontinence usually follows manipulative procedures performed for purposes of diagnosing urinary problems. However, prostatitis and prostatic hypertro-

215

phy can also cause stress incontinence. In either sex, this condition can be secondary to conditions that cause a rise in intraabdominal pressure (e.g., COPD, obesity or ascites).

Subjective data may include:
1. Incontinence on coughing, sneezing, bending over or arising from supine position.
2. Longstanding history of obesity, COPD or ascites.
3. History of recent surgery—males or females.
4. Females—history of multiparity or traumatic deliveries.
5. History of recent or recurrent UTI.
6. Incontinence associated with no warning, no urge and/or no sensation.
7. A history of embarrassment secondary to urine odor.

Objective findings may include:
1. Obesity.
2. Females—weakened pelvic musculature, cystocele, rectocele, vaginal discharge with perineal and urethral irritation.
3. Males—urethral discharge and/or inflammation.

The lab tests (wet prep, urinalysis, etc.) will be negative in primary stress incontinence (i.e., secondary to increased intraabdominal pressure). Stress incontinence, however, may be exacerbated by an infectious process, in which case the lab results will reflect the infection.

Urge incontinence

The patient usually will experience a sudden urge to urinate followed shortly thereafter by incontinence. Urge incontinence in either sex is usually secondary to either structural/obstructive pathology (e.g., strictures, urethral polyps or diverticuli) or inflammatory processes (e.g., cystitis, urethritis, prostatitis or vaginitis).

Subjective data may include:
1. A history of dysuria, hematuria, low grade temperature and/or other urinary symptomatology.
2. A history of a sudden urge to urinate followed by incontinence.
3. Females—vaginal discharge and/or history of radiation therapy for cervical cancer.
4. Males—urethral discharge, pain on defecation (secondary to an underlying prostatitis), hesitancy, dribbling and other symptomatology associated with prostatic hypertrophy and/or infection.

Objective data may include:
1. Females—a urethrocele, cystocele and/or rectocele that is severe enough to produce a residual urine; this residual may lead to an inflammatory process which causes urge incontinence.
2. Females—a vaginal discharge.
3. Costovertebral angle tenderness, temperature (e.g., pyelonephritis), swollen irritated urethra and/or urethral discharge (urethritis or cystitis).
4. Males—tender enlarged prostate

(prostatitis), nontender enlarged prostate (BPH or cancer), urethral discharge, an interruption in the stream of urine indicative of obstructive pathology that may be a predisposition to an infection.

The lab data may show the following causes of inflammation causing incontinence:

1. Microscopic urinalysis with WBC's (more than five to ten per high power field) and/or RBC's (more than five per high power field), indicating a cystitis.
2. Urine culture showing greater than 100,000/ml colony growth, indicating a cystitis.
3. Wet prep result of hemophilus, trichomonas or yeast indicating a vaginitis.
4. A prostatic smear and/or three glass urine test result indicating a prostatitis.

Overflow incontinence

Overflow incontinence that is episodic may be secondary to obstructive lesions or drug therapy (i.e., muscle relaxants, antispasmodics, sedatives, quinidine or phenothiazides). In these cases the bladder continues to fill with urine until the bladder wall itself contracts to decrease the intravesical pressure. A small amount of urine is released and a large residual urine may remain in the bladder. This type of incontinence may also be related to psychogenic causes in which the elderly patient is depressed, confused or has been placed in an environment in which she or he has lost control.

Subjective data may include:
1. Symptoms associated with obstructive pathology (e.g., hesitancy, dysuria, hematuria, etc.).
2. A history of small frequent involuntary voidings.
3. Males—a history associated with prostatic hypertrophy (e.g., difficulty starting a stream, hesitancy, dribbling, frequency, etc.).
4. A history of bereavement or change in environment. Psychogenic incontinence is only present during the day. (If incontinence is due to psychological problems the lab studies will be within normal limits.)
5. Positive history for drugs (listed above).

Objective data may include:
1. Depressive symptomatology.
2. Enlarged prostate (e.g., BPH).
3. Obstructive lesions (e.g., polyps, cysts, etc.) if the etiologic cause of the incontinence would be ascertained only by such lab procedures as an IVP, cystogram, etc.

Continuous Incontinence
Stress incontinence

See episodic stress incontinence; the assessment features are the same except the incontinence is of a longstanding duration.

Urge incontinence

Same as for episodic urge incontinence except the incontinence is of longstanding duration.

Neurogenic incontinence
Uninhibited
neurogenic

The uninhibited neurogenic bladder is secondary to cerebral cortex lesions. In this disorder there is a disruption of the efferent pathways from the higher brain centers. The presence or absence of voluntary control will depend on the extent of the lesion. It may be secondary to Parkinson's disease, CVA, arteriosclerotic changes in the cerebral cortex or multiple sclerosis.

Subjective data may include:
1. A positive history of CVA, Parkinson's disease or multiple sclerosis.
2. The patient will state he or she is aware of a sensation to void, but is unable to inhibit voiding.
3. A history of frequency, urgency and incontinence. Hesitancy may also be the concomitant complaint if the patient has multiple sclerosis.

Objective data may include:
1. Any neurologic abnormality associated with various disease entities (e.g., Parkinson's, multiple sclerosis, myasthenia gravis, etc.).
2. There may be tenderness on compression of the iliac crest from pelvic fractures.
3. A large palpable bladder.
4. Residual urine on catheterization.

Reflex neurogenic
bladder

Lesions or trauma to the cord (about S_2 to S_4) may cause a reflex neurogenic bladder. A tumor, inflammation (meningitis) or trauma that interrupts the afferent and efferent pathways to the brain can be the cause.

Subjective data may include:
1. Involuntary urination.
2. Absence of the sensation to void.
3. Paresthesias or a complete loss of sensation and motor function of the lower extremities.

Objective data may include:
1. Abnormal neurologic signs (e.g., spasticity of lower extremities, muscle atrophy, absent sensation, etc.).
2. Lab studies (e.g., cystometric exam) showing presence of uninhibited bladder contractions.
3. Catheterization reveals residual urine.
4. A functional decreased bladder capacity.

Autonomous neurogenic bladder

The afferent and/or efferent pathways are destroyed secondary to such things as pelvic surgeries, neoplasms, infections, lesions, etc. There may be just a sensory loss as in sensory paralytic bladder (example: tabes dorsalis) or a motor loss as in motor paralytic bladder (example: polio, trauma, tumors). The subjective and objective symptoms of an autonomous neurogenic bladder may include those found in *both* the sensory paralytic and motor paralytic bladder. Diabetic neuropathy can be an example of both sensory and motor pathway dysfunction.

Diabetic neuropathy:

Subjective data may include:
1. Family history of diabetes.
2. History of polyuria, polydipsia, polyphagia, weight loss.
3. A history of straining to void or a sensation of incomplete emptying and dribbling.
4. Females—a history of recurrent vaginitis (especially monilial).
5. Males—a history of impotence.

Objective data may include:
1. Females—may have vaginal discharge and/or vaginal, perineal and urethral irritation secondary to discharge.
2. A decreased sensation of the perineum and/or poor rectal sphincter tone.
3. Signs and symptoms associated with diabetic neuropathy (i.e., paresthesias, decreased or absent reflexes, decreased vibratory sensations, etc.).

Sensory paralytic bladder:

This condition results from any lesion or disease that affects either the sensory fibers to the spinal cord or brain.

Subjective data may include:
1. No feelings of a full bladder and/or a saddle anesthesia.
2. Dribbling.
3. Difficulty initiating a stream and/or a decrease in size or force of urine stream.
4. Complaint of overflow inconti-

nence (small involuntary frequent voidings) or of stress incontinence.
5. With a history of surgery, there may be an onset of symptoms after the procedure.

Objective data may include:
1. A distended palpable bladder.
2. Residual urine on catheterization.
3. Neurologic abnormalities indicative of lesions (if present).

An example of sensory paralytic bladder is tabes dorsalis neurogenic bladder:

Tabes dorsalis is a manifestation of latent syphilis. Regarding urinary incontinence, the problem results from a loss of the sensory portions of the reflex arc. There is usually an overflow incontinence with a resultant residual urine.

Subjective data:
The patient may give a positive past history for syphilis. He or she may also complain of a decreased sensation in the extremities, parethesias and/or a history of stumbling, falling or impotence.

Objective data may include:
1. Neurologic abnormalities (i.e., a loss of reflexes, decreased pain sensation, wide stance gait, decreased proprioception and temperature sensation and/or footslap).
2. Other manifestations of latent

syphilis (i.e., cardiac or musculoskeletal involvements).

Motor paralytic bladder:

This condition results from a destruction of the efferent pathways to the bladder.

Subjective data may include:
1. Inability to initiate a normal micturition; however, the patient can void by taking in a deep breath and straining (diagnostic sign).
2. With a history of trauma and/or surgery, the patient may describe the onset of symptoms beginning after the incident.
3. There may be dribbling present.

Objective data may include:
1. A large palpable bladder.
2. Normal sensory exam but neurologic motor exam consistent with underlying etiology.

PLAN:

Episodic Incontinence

In general, if the incontinence has been short-term the practitioner should rule out the common etiologies and treat if indicated. If the incontinence does not clear after appropriate treatment the patient should be referred to a physician/urologist for a complete work-up.

Stress incontinence (females)

Episodic stress incontinence requires no specific treatment other than the correction of the underlying etiologic cause. If secondary to an inflammatory process in females, treat the cause whether it is a trigonitis, vaginitis, estrogen deficiency or urinary tract infection.

If the incontinence is secondary to pelvic relaxation, attempt to manage by teaching the patient Kegal's exercises to increase muscle tone. Have the patient lose weight; use antispasmodics, double voiding procedures and/or pessaries. If the incontinence is secondary to a cystocele or rectocele, a surgical consultation is advisable. If the incontinence is secondary to increased abdominal pressure (from COPD, ascites, etc.) consult and/or refer the patient for management of underlying disease.

Stress incontinence (males)

Males with a recent history of manipulative procedures should be referred for management. If the incontinence is in the presence of an enlarged nontender prostate, the patient should be referred to his physician/urologist for a work-up of BPH or cancer of the prostate.

Urge incontinence

Treat any underlying inflammatory cause of the incontinence. If the inflammatory process has not responded to treatment or the inflammatory process is not the underlying causative agent of the incontinence, refer the patient to his or her physician. If the IVP or cystogram showed an obstructive pathology, the patient should be referred to a urologist.

Overflow incontinence

The underlying pathology should be treated:

1. If the incontinence (after consultation with the patient's physician) appears secondary to obstructive pathology (indicated from results of IVP, cystogram, urinalysis) refer the patient to a urologist.
2. If the incontinence is secondary to bereavement, the patient needs support, understanding and/or counseling.
3. If the incontinence is suspected to be iatrogenically caused, consult with the patient's physician about changing the drug therapy.

Continuous Incontinence

For continuous chronic incontinence, if the patient has not had a complete urological work-up, she or he should be referred to a specialist/urologist (depending on the suspected etiology of the problem). If the patient's problem has been worked up previously, the practitioner should consult with a physician and follow the plans listed in the attached addendums.

Stress incontinence

See plan listed under episodic. The patient should be provided support, understanding and aids to help the patient deal with odor.

Urge incontinence

See plan listed under episodic.

Neurogenic incontinence

Uninhibited neurogenic

Consult and/or refer; in addition, see attached addendums.

Reflex neurogenic

Consult and/or refer; in addition, see attached addendums.

Autonomic neurogenic

If the incontinence is due to surgery and/or trauma, refer the patient to the appropriate specialist. If the incontinence has never been fully evaluated the patient should be referred to a urologist. If the patient's incontinence has been worked up, consult with the previous health provider and see addendums. In addition, a referral to a rehabilitation center should be considered.

Sensory paralytic bladder:

If of recent onset or chronic with no previous work-up, refer the patient to the appropriate specialist. If the patient's condition has been fully evaluated, see addendum. Also, in addition to referral to a rehabilitation center for treatment of the generalized disease, a regimen of drugs that increase bladder tone may be instituted for rehabilitating atonic bladders.

Motor paralytic bladder:

See Autonomic neurogenic.

ADDENDUM 1
PLAN FOR PATIENTS WITH DIAGNOSED NEUROGENIC BLADDER INCONTINENCE

1. If the patient is conscious/mobile, make every effort to get the patient up to the bathroom or commode every two to three hours.

2. If there is incontinence with an overflow retention, catheterization with a slow decompression of the bladder may be required over a period of 12 to 24 hours. (Object is to restore tone.)

3. Maintain a high fluid intake. (Dehydration leads to mental confusion with an imbalance of electrolytes.)

4. Prevent severe constipation (can cause incontinence by obstruction).

5. Restrict fluids after 6 P.M. (assists in preventing enuresis).

6. Meticulous skin care should be done/taught to prevent decubiti.

7. Anticholinergic drugs (to prevent retention/overflow by decreasing bladder tone) may be indicated.

8. Establish a 24-hour flow chart on the patient to determine the times of incontinence and dry hours. Bedpan/commode should be offered every two to four hours and records kept of whether the patient was wet or dry and whether the patient voided. This technique helps in voiding retraining. Attention may be all that is required; by offering the bedpan/commode and offering assistance at the times of recorded incontinence, the patient's incontinence may be well managed.

9. Drug therapy: After consultation, anticholinergic drugs may be tried. The effect is to reduce the bladder tone and increase the sphincter pressure. Drugs should be given according to the incontinence chart; the incontinence should coincide with the peak action of the drug. Remember it must be a neurogenic bladder for drugs to be effective. Possible side effects of glaucoma may present. Withdraw drugs if hepatic dysfunction is suspected, if jaundice appears or if no effect is noted after several weeks of therapy.

10. A diuretic with a rapid onset of action if taken in the morning may promote daytime diuresis and thus decrease the renal output at night.

11. The decision to use intermittent catheterization will be made on an individual basis; the frequency depends on the amount of residual urine. Intermittent catheterization should be done using as small a catheter as possible.

12. Indwelling catheterization may be necessary; keep in mind that:
    a. a UTI is inevitable if in for more than one week.
    b. possible severe pathologic changes may occur in the kidney from infections.
    c. the catheter should be changed every two weeks. It is imperative that the catheter-to-bag connections not be removed except as a whole unit; otherwise, cross contamination can occur, exposing the patient to pathogens.

d. as a helpful preventive measure against infections, a solution of ¼ percent acetic acid may be used as a constant irrigation system with the Foley catheter. This would seem impractical in a nursing home situation, but manageable in a hospital.

13. High fluid intake is essential (up to 2000 cc.—more may precipitate hyponatremia).

14. Urinary diversion measures have been used for the progressive neurologic disorders (ileal conduits, ileocystoplasties, cutaneous vesicostomies). If the patient and surgeon select one of these methods, appropriate counseling and teaching should be provided to the patient.

15. Drugs that cause urinary retention, such as ephedrine sulfate, are sometimes used at nighttime to combat enuresis.

16. Preventive garments and pads are multiple in style and materials. Good skin care is imperative with the use of lotions and cornstarch. A "gelling pad" has been offered, having the dimensions of a sanitary pad and containing powder which forms a gel when it comes in contact with the urine. This pad can accommodate well over 150 cc of urine. Once the gel is formed there is no further wetting of the skin.

ADDENDUM 2
STAFF EDUCATION GOALS FOR ALL PROFESSIONALS WORKING WITH INCONTINENT PATIENTS

1. Knowledge of the physiology of the bladder.
   a. Bladder capacity
   b. Structures involving control
   c. How aging affects the bladder functions and control

2. Insight, patience and understanding of the patient's incompetence in control of their urinary incontinence.

3. Knowledge of current catheter care whether intermittent or indwelling catheters.

4. Understand the value of promoting maximum activity for patients who are able to be out of bed even for short periods of time.

5. Understand the need for individualized patient care conferences for the problematic patients.

6. Knowledge of the importance of meticulous skin care and protection from the effects of incontinence for bedbound or wheelchair patients; understand the need to position and change the patient every two to three hours to avoid decubiti.

Encouragement by the staff of patient improvement in incontinence control cannot be emphasized too much. The patient is thus made to feel important to everyone and that his or her health is cared about. The staff should be considerate in allowing ample time in the voiding act and ensuring some degree of privacy. The staff should provide emotional support to patients.

ADDENDUM 3
PLANS FOR PATIENT EDUCATION FOR THE PATIENT WITH URINARY INCONTINENCE

1. If the patient is oriented, explain the bladder problem and goals of care and rehabilitation; the patient and the staff should plan these together.

2. Stress the importance of frequent voidings to possibly avoid the embarrassment and associated problems which the incontinent voidings precipitate.

3. For the stress incontinent patients, Kegal's exercises have been helpful and should be initiated and evaluated by the patient and health care staff.

4. Acknowledge support in the understanding of the patients' problems, including willingness to assist with their care.

5. Inform the patient of the need to keep the skin cleansed well and dry (if possible) to avoid complicating skin conditions.

6. Inform patients of the available protective garments used with incontinence.

7. If catheter care is required, education in this task will be required; the patient should be taught about the need for aseptic technique, daily cleansing, catheter change procedures, etc.

8. Emphasize the importance of the need to limit alcohol, tea, coffee, or other caffeine-containing beverages.

REFERENCES

1. Badencoch, Alec. "Urinary Incontinence and Enuresis." In *Manual of Urology*, 2nd ed. Chicago: Year Book Publishers, 1974, pp. 529–540.
2. Boyarsky, Saul. *The Neurogenic Bladder*. Baltimore: Williams and Wilkins Co., 1957.
3. Brockelhurst, J. C. *Textbook of Geriatric Medicine and Gerontology*. Edinburgh and London: Churchill-Livingstone, 1973, pp. 280–320.
4. Caldwell, K. *Urinary Incontinence*. New York and London: Grune and Stratton, 1975.
5. Grimes, John H. et al. "Managing Incontinence in Women." *Patient Care*, Sept. 15, 1977, pp. 120–141.
6. Hudak, Carolyn et al. "Dysuria." In *Clinical Protocols: A Guide for Nurses and Physicians*. Philadelphia: J.B. Lippincott Co., 1976, pp. 165–208.
7. Lapides, Jack. "Neurogenic Bladder." In *Fundamentals of Urology*. Philadelphia: W.B. Saunders Company, 1976, pp. 190–241.
8. Rossman, Isadore. *Clinical Geriatrics*. Philadelphia: J.B. Lippincott Co., 1971, pp. 340–351.
9. Stamey, Thomas. "The Diagnosis of Bacteriuria." In *Urinary Infections*. Baltimore: Williams and Wilkins Co., 1972, pp. 1–30.
10. "The Adult Female Patient—Managing Urinary Incontinence." *Patient Care*, Feb. 1, 1973, pp. 70–86.

Chapter 5

Urinary Tract Infection

OVERVIEW

The definition of a urinary tract infection (UTI) includes only those entities that involve the kidneys and their collecting systems or the bladder. Although various forms of glomerulonephritis present with renal pathology and genitourinary symptomatology, they cannot be considered a urinary tract infection because they are not inflammatory responses, but rather disease entities that occur secondarily to other infections. If this definition is strictly taken, UTI's can be divided into upper and lower urinary tract infections. Pyelonephritis is an example of an upper urinary tract infection, while lower tract infections can be divided into cystitis, urethritis and prostatitis in the male and cystitis and urethritis in the female.

The human body has several defense mechanisms that guard against the development of urinary tract infections. The urine and bladder are normally sterile; there are some bacteria present in the lower urethra particularly in the female, but normally the voiding mechanism cleanses the bacteria from the genitourinary tract. The urethral and bladder mucosa may have some type of antibacterial protective capacity though the exact mechanism is not known.

There are numerous predisposing factors that enhance the likelihood of one developing a urinary tract infection (e.g., age, sex, instrumentation, obstructions causing residual urine, the presence of reflux or neurogenic disease and metabolic diseases). The environment can be another factor since the incidence of UTI's increases among institutionalized patients.

Acute urinary tract infections are frequently second only to upper respiratory infections in causing febrile illnesses in the aged. Chronic urinary tract infections occur secondary to chronic pyelonephritis or recurrent bouts of cystitis, prostatitis or urethritis. The most common organisms causing urinary tract infections are *Escherichia coli*, *proteus* or *pseudomonas*. The latter two are more apt to be the causative agent in hospitalized or institutionalized patients who have indwelling catheters.

Organisms enter the urinary tract by several methods: 1) ascending from perineal contamination in the female, 2) a hematogenous or blood-borne route (such as following an upper respiratory infection or from extraction of infected teeth) or 3) via the lymphatic system (rare).

Utilizing this protocol, the practitioner will be assisted in diagnosing a urinary tract infection and in differentiating the patient's symptoms from other disease entities. The diagnosis of a urinary tract infection can be confirmed by a few lab tests and an adequate history and physical exam.

URINARY TRACT INFECTION (UTI) WORKSHEET

To be used for patients complaining of the constellation of the following symptoms: dysuria, hematuria, nocturia, frequency, urgency, back pain.

What you cannot afford to miss: Obstructive pathology causing UTI's (i.e., stones, tumors, prostatic hypertrophy, diverticula). Neurologic diseases that cause bladder dysfunction and increase the likelihood of the development of UTI's (i.e., diabetes mellitus, multiple sclerosis, etc.). Inflammatory processes (i.e., cystitis, urethritis, prostatitis, pyelonephritis).

Chief Complaint: _____

SUBJECTIVE DATA:

    Age:_____ Gender: _____ Sexually Active:_____
Institutionalized:_____

Describe Positive Responses (include onset, severity, duration, location):

YES   NO

_____ _____ Frequency: _____

_____ _____ Excessive fluid intake: _____

_____ _____ Inadequate fluid intake: _____

_____ _____ Urgency: _____

_____ _____ Dysuria (during or after urination?): _____

_____ _____ Retention: _____

_____ _____ Sensation of fullness: _____

_____ _____ Painless suprapubic swelling: _____

_____ _____ Painful retention: _____

_____ _____ Oliguria: _____

_____ _____ Anuria: _____

_____ _____ History of trauma: _____

_____ _____ Incontinence: _____

_____ _____ Stress incontinence: _____

_____ _____ Nocturia: _____

_____ _____ Discolored, cloudy urine: _____

_____ _____ Hematuria: _____

_____ _____ Malodor: _____

GENITAL:
YES   *NO*

———   ———   Pruritus, burning: _____

———   ———   Urethral discharge (or discharge only after a bowel

movement in males): _____

———   ———   Vaginal discharge, rash (females): _____

———   ———   Dyspareunia: _____

———   ———   Painful ejaculation: _____

———   ———   Perineal pain: _____

SYSTEMIC:
YES   *NO*

———   ———   Fever/chills: _____

———   ———   Confusion: _____

———   ———   Anorexia, nausea, vomiting, weight loss: _____

———   ———   Abdominal pain: _____

———   ———   Back pain: _____

PAST MEDICAL HISTORY:
YES   *NO*

———   ———   Diabetes, multiple sclerosis, syphilis: _____

———   ———   Renal calculi: _____

———   ———   Past urinary tract infections (number and treatment):

_____

Urinary Trace Infection (UTI) Worksheet

_____ _____ Bladder tumors, strictures, diverticuli: _____

_____ _____ History of radiation therapy: _____

_____ _____ History of catheterization, instrumentation: _____

_____ _____ History of benign prostatic hypertrophy (males): __

_____ _____ Allergies: _____

_____ _____ Current medications: _____

_____

_____ _____ Appendicitis (surgery with a normal appendix on pa-

thology report): _____

_____ _____ Diet (large amounts of alcohol, spices): _____

SOCIAL HISTORY:
YES   NO

_____ _____ Alcohol, caffeine use: _____

_____ _____ Excessive use of tea, coffee: _____

OBJECTIVE DATA:
Vital Signs: _____BP _____Temp _____P _____R

_____Wt. _____Wt. 3 Mos. Ago _____Ht.

COMPLETE MALE GENITAL EXAM: (Describe All Positives)
YES   NO

_____ _____ Abnormal penis: _____

_____ _____ Urethral discharge: _____

_____ _____ Strictures: _____

————— ————— Abnormal scrotum: _____

————— ————— Abnormal prostate: _____

COMPLETE FEMALE GENITAL EXAM: (Describe All Positives)
YES   NO

————— ————— Abnormal urethra, Bartholin's or Skene's glands: __

————— ————— Vaginal discharge/irritation: _____

————— ————— Cystocele/rectocele: _____

————— ————— Abnormal uterus, adnexa: _____

ABDOMINAL EXAMINATION: (Describe All Positives)
YES   NO

————— ————— Inguinal tenderness: _____

————— ————— Abnormal masses, tenderness, shape: _____

————— ————— Scars: _____

BACK EXAMINATION: (Describe All Positives)
YES   NO

————— ————— CVA tenderness: _____

————— ————— Spinal tenderness: _____

LAB DATA: (Describe All Results)
        NOT
DONE   DONE

————— ————— Urinalysis—macro examination, dipstick, microanalysis (in males do 3 glass urine): _____
_____

————— ————— Urine culture and sensitivity: _____

The following tests should be done if indicated:

237

_____ _____ CBC (if patient has signs of systemic infection i.e. fever, CVA tenderness or has a history of repeated UTI's):_____

_____ _____ Gram stain/GC culture (if patient has positive history of GC contact or a questionable history in presence of urethral discharge and/or vaginal discharge): ____

_____

_____ _____ Vaginal smear (if female patient has any vaginal discharge): _____

_____ _____ BUN/creatinine (if patient has repeated episodes of UTI and/or if the patient's renal status has not been evaluated within the past year): _____

_____ _____ Biochemical assay (if patient has a history of stones or if patient's calcium , uric acid, phosphorus, etc. has not been evaluated in the past year): _____

_____

_____ _____ Acid phosphatase (if male patient has an abnormal prostate exam): _____

_____ _____ IVP, cysto, cystometrogram (if the patient has repeated UTI's without a urological work-up—consultation with and/or referral to a physician/urologist should be done *before* referring the patient for these tests): _____

URINARY TRACT INFECTION (UTI) WORKSHEET RATIONALE

SUBJECTIVE DATA:
Frequency

Causes of frequency include: inflammation, edema or a loss of elasticity. Frequency is seen in cystitis, benign prostatic hypertrophy, any obstructive pathology, urethritis, central nervous system diseases or diabetes insipidus. The practitioner must differentiate true frequency from that resulting from an increased fluid intake, anxiety, polyuria or the excessive use of tea, coffee or alcohol.

Excessive Fluid Intake

Compulsive water drinkers and the normal thirst in hot weather must be separated from those patients who have true polydipsia. Polydipsia is one of the classic signs of diabetes mellitus.

Inadequate Fluid Intake

This occurs frequently in the aged as individuals elect to drink less due to urgency associated with micturition and decreased ease of mobility.

Urgency

Urgency can be seen in: 1) inflammatory processes (i.e., cystitis, urethritis), 2) obstructive pathology causing a urinary tract infection or 3) a neurologic dysfunction.

Dysuria

The major causes of dysuria include obstruction (such as in stenosis or tumors) and inflammation (such as in prostatitis, urethritis, cystitis). Dysuria may also be present in postradiation trauma or in highly concentrated urine. The absence of dysuria in the aged does not preclude the presence of an infection.

Dysuria during urination may be due to a highly concentrated acid urine, urethral obstruction (such as a caruncle in females), or inflammation (e.g., meatal ulcers, vaginal discharge or urethritis). Dysuria *after* urination suggests cystitis, prostatitis, bladder calculi or vesical tuberculosis.

Retention

Urinary retention is secondary to neurogenic causes, obstructive pathology, and some drugs.

Sensation of Fullness

Sensation of fullness is associated with chronic urinary retention due to BPH, advanced Parkinson's disease, CNS lesions and tricyclic drugs.

Painless Suprapubic Swelling

A painless suprapubic swelling (e.g., distended bladder) may be associated with urinary retention; it can be reduced by catheterization. A suprapubic swelling can also be seen in a sensory paralytic bladder.

Painful Retention

Painful acute urinary retention is often caused by a mechanical obstruction of the urethra such as calculi or an acute prostatitis.

Oliguria

The 24-hour urine output is between 50 ml and 400 ml. Even with dehydration the normal kidney will excrete more than 600 ml per day. Oliguria may be indicative of acute renal failure or a lower urinary tract obstruction.

Anuria

Anuria is defined as a 24-hour urine output less than 50 ml.

History of Trauma

The elderly population is more accident prone due to a decrease in balancing reflexes. A contused or ruptured kidney may result in an increased blood pressure caused by compression of the renal artery; the symptoms include hematuria, ureteral colic and a left or right upper quadrant pain.

Incontinence

Incontinence itself does not cause a urinary tract infection; however, some of the underlying causes of incontinence do (i.e., neurogenic causes or obstructive pathologies).

Stress Incontinence

Stress incontinence is the involuntary loss of urine associated with coughing, sneezing, laughing, etc. It can be associated with poor pelvic muscular support in females (e.g., traumatic childbirth) or after instrumentation procedures in males.

Nocturia

Nocturia can be secondary to inflammation (i.e., cystitis, urethritis, prostatitis), diabetes mellitus or benign prostatic hypertrophy. Nocturia may develop in perhaps 60 to 70 percent of the aged. Other common causes include congestive heart failure, increased fluid intake (especially alcohol, tea, coffee taken late at night) and diuretics.

Discolored, Cloudy Urine

Discolored urine (ranging from colorless to black) is more frequently noticed in males or patients in institutional settings. It may be due to infection, medications, foods, dyes, hemoglobin and/or crystals. Sometimes the abnormal color leads directly to the diagnosis.

Cloudy urine is caused by the presence of abnormal constituents: e.g., pus, bacteria, RBC, casts, epithelial cells or amorphous debris (phosphates are a normal precipitant).

Hematuria

Macroscopic hematuria *with pain* may be indicative of urinary tract infection (e.g., cystitis or prostatitis). *Painless* macroscopic hematuria may be seen in tumors (especially bladder), trauma, prothrombin deficiency, gout, renal tuberculosis, uremia or radiation damage.

Hematuria must be distinguished from hemoglobinuria and myoglobinuria.

Microscopic hematuria with pain is often present in interstitial cystitis or it may arise from another source (e.g., prostatitis and calculi).

Malodor

Malodorous urine may be produced by the presence of bacteria. The incidence of residual urine increases with age; foul-smelling urine may be one of the first signs of a UTI.

Genital
Pruritus or burning

Pruritus is described as a burning, scalding and itching sensation; this may be related to infections in the elderly. Pruritus is often related to a urethral caruncle, monilia vaginitis or a cervicitis.

Urethral discharge

This may appear postdefecation in prostatitis. The nonspecific urethritis and gonococcal conditions may be associated with or without a discharge.

Vaginal discharge, rash	A skin and urethral irritation from a vaginal discharge may result in dysuria due to the close proximity of the urethra. A vaginal rash may be secondary to a monilial irritation (common in diabetes mellitus or postantibiotic therapy). A painful herpetic rash is also sometimes seen in the elderly.
Dyspareunia	The increased friability of the vaginal mucosa in postmenopausal women may result in dyspareunia or postcoital bleeding secondary to atrophic changes or vaginitis. The vaginitis may then cause symptoms that mimic those of a UTI.
Painful ejaculation	Painful ejaculation may be associated with acute prostatitis.
Perineal pain	Perineal pain is associated with acute cystitis and/or prostatitis.

Systemic

Fever/chills	A febrile response to infection is diminished in the elderly. Consider an upper urinary tract infection and other systemic infections as a cause of fever and chills.
Confusion	Confusion is often the first sign of systemic stress in the elderly. Confusion can be secondary to the development of renal failure from chronic pyelonephritis or numerous other causes.
Anorexia, nausea, vomiting, weight loss	The common innervation of the urinary and gastrointestinal tracts and their anatomic proximity are responsible for the frequent occur-

rence of gastrointestinal symptoms in disease of the urinary tract. Nausea and vomiting can be seen in uremia and acute or chronic renal failure. Weight loss can be associated with a cancer of the urinary tract.

Abdominal pain

Abdominal pain can be associated with renal calculi. Suprapubic pain can be associated with a lower urinary tract infection or urinary retention.

Back pain

Back pain especially located at the costovertebral angle can be seen in pyelonephritis. Low back pain may be seen in urinary tract infections or in conditions such as cancer, trauma or prostatitis.

Past Medical History
Diabetes, MS, syphilis

All of these diseases can affect bladder function due to an interruption in the normal innervation. As a result, patients are more prone to the development of residual urine which is a good predisposing factor for the development of UTI's. In addition, diabetic patients are more prone to UTI's and monilial vaginitis which can cause cystitis.

Renal calculi

Ascertain a history of previous stones because of their obstructive pathology which may lead to the development of UTI's.

History of UTI's, number and treatment

If the patient gives a history of chronic UTI's, a complete urologic exam is indicated to ascertain the cause. Treatment and follow-up should be determined because of the likelihood of developing chronic pyelonephritis from unresolved UTI's.

Bladder tumors, strictures, diverticuli

All of these are obstructive pathology which can cause UTI's.

Radiation therapy

Cystitis can occur secondary to radiation therapy.

Catheterization, instrumentation

Catheterization almost always introduces some bacteria into the bladder, which become a common source of UTI's. Instrumentation of any type has the same effect.

BPH

Benign prostatic hypertrophy can cause obstruction with residual urine which predisposes to the development of an infection.

Allergies

It is essential to be aware of any medication allergies *before* prescribing any medications.

Medications

Some medications cause urinary retention which may result in an infection.

Appendectomy with a normal appendix on pathology report

If the patient has a history of a right lower quadrant pain with subsequent surgery for appendicitis, it is important to know the outcome of that surgery; patients who were told after surgery that they had a normal appendix may have had cystitis pain instead.

Diet high in alcohol, spices

Some males experience an exacerbation of a chronic prostatitis when they eat spicy foods (such as Mexican or Italian foods) or when they drink alcohol.

Social History
Alcohol, caffeine

Alcohol and caffeine inhibit antidiuretic hormone (ADH) and thus produce frequency in the absence of other urinary symptoms indicative of an infection.

Excessive use of tea, coffee

Tea and coffee contain diuretic xanthines which can cause urinary frequency.

OBJECTIVE DATA:
Vital Signs (BP, P, Temp, R)

These are objective parameters of the patient's general status. Pyrexia is usually present in pyelonephritis. High blood pressure may occur secondary to chronic pyelonephritis that has resulted in renal parenchymal damage.

Weight Gain/Loss

Weight gain can be secondary to edema from renal parenchymal disease. Weight loss may be secondary to cancer or a chronic disease.

Genital Exam
Abnormal penis

Closely examine the penis for phimósis (obstruction) and the prepuce for any inflammation source. A painful lesion could be chancroid. A painless lesion suggests condylomata accuminata, condylomata lata or a chancre.

Urethral discharge

Urethral discharge is seen in urethritis (GC and nonspecific urethritis [NSU]) or after defecation with prostatitis.

Strictures

Urethral strictures of any type may cause obstruction and thus may become a potential predisposing factor to UTI's.

Scrotum

Examine the scrotum for signs of infection (e.g., redness, warmth, tenderness, etc.). Epididymitis can seed a prostatitis.

Prostate

An enlarged nontender prostate is seen in BPH, which can cause obstruction. An enlarged nodular hard prostate indicates a possible cancer. An enlarged, tender, boggy prostate can indicate prostatitis.

Female Genital Exam
Urethra, Bartholin's/ Skene's

Examine the urethra and glands for inflammation or irritation that cause signs and symptoms of cystitis. Vaginal discharge contamination of the perineal area can cause cystitis.

Cystocele/rectocele

Any size rectocele and/or cystocele could cause residual urine; urinary stasis provides an excellent media for bacterial growth.

Uterus, adnexa

Examine the patient for masses or tenderness. A mass from the uterus or adnexa could be causing symptoms of frequency. Although rarely seen in the female elderly, pelvic inflammatory disease from gonorrhea could cause UTI symptomatology.

Abdominal Exam
Inguinal tenderness

Inguinal tenderness is associated with an infectious process of the legs and pelvic area (e.g., lymphogranuloma venereum [rarely seen] or any infected lesion or vaginal discharge, etc.).

Masses, tenderness, shape

The abdomen should be carefully examined for masses and/or tenderness. Any space occupying lesion could push on the bladder causing symptoms of a UTI. A painless suprapubic mass may be a distended bladder.

Scars

Observation of scars could help the examiner to refresh the patient's memory about his or her past medical history (e.g., surgeries including nephrectomies, appendectomies, or surgery for stone removal from the ureters).

Back Examination
CVA, spinal tenderness

Costovertebral angle tenderness may indicate pyelonephritis. Spinal tenderness may indicate a metastatic prostate cancer. Also, injuries causing a fracture or a radiculitis can cause bladder dysfunction; this dysfunction can lead to residual urine.

Lab Data
Urinalysis

A clean catch specimen is vital to an accurate diagnosis. The patient should be instructed as follows:

Female: The perineum should be cleansed thoroughly (using a front to back wiping motion) with several cotton pad/balls. The labia should be spread wide throughout the entire procedure. The area should be rinsed copiously with water. If there is any vaginal discharge this should be "plugged" with a tampon, cotton pad, etc. The female should begin urinating; midway through the urination a sterile container should catch the free-flowing urine (the specimen should not touch the labia, leg, toilet seat, etc.).

Male: A three glass urine collection should be obtained on *all* males as follows:

Retract the foreskin fully. Cleanse the glans with a detergent soap and remove all the soap with a wet sponge.

The first voided specimen (about 10cc) should be collected in a sterile culture tube.

The second voided specimen should be collected midstream in a sterile culture tube (about 10 cc); then stop voiding.

The prostate is then massaged and the secretions are expressed by the clinician into a sterile container. If the prostate is tender, omit this step.

The third voided specimen is then collected immediately postmassage as in the first step.

Macro exam
Color

Color differences may indicate the following: a deep yellow to green color may indicate bilirubin in the urine (the urine froths when shaken). A red to black color may be due to blood, hemoglobin or myoglobin.

Odor

A sweet odor could be due to a large amount of ketone bodies from diabetic ketoacidosis.

An ammonia odor may be due to urine infected with urea splitting organisms such as proteus. A malodor in the urine may indicate an infected urine (most commonly *E. coli*).

Appearance

A cloudy appearance may be due to the presence of WBC's, crystals, and bacteria or from allowing the urine to sit for over an hour.

Specific gravity

Specific gravity is a test of the concentrating ability of the kidneys. Low values occur in diseases that affect the concentrating ability of the kidneys (e.g., chronic pyelonephritis, diabetes insipidus, gout, prolonged potassium deficiency or compulsive water drinking). High values occur in acute glomerulonephritis, diabetes mellitus and/or dehydration.

Dipstick
Protein

Sixty to 80 percent of the urinary protein is albumin. False albuminuria may occur due to exudates from infection of the urinary tract, pus cells, prostatic secretion, exercise or fever. Proteinuria is seen in the kidney involvement of diabetes mellitus, acute or chronic glomerulonephritis, rapid progressive glomerulonephritis, nephrotic syndrome, polycystic kidney disease, septic emboli, and pyelonephritis. Persistent proteinuria of 1+ or greater should be quantitated by a 24-hour collection and analysis. A significant amount of Bence-Jones protein in the urine may indicate the presence of a multiple myeloma.

Glucose

If the glomerular filtration rate is decreased as from diabetic neuropathy or nephrosclerosis, the renal threshold for glucose will rise, but if the renal tubules show an impaired ability to absorb glucose as in acute tubular necrosis, the renal threshold will fall. Glycosuria may be present in those patients who have a decreased renal threshold. Significant elevations are indicative of diabetes mellitus; if diabetes mellitus is suspect, a two-hour pc blood sugar and a fasting blood sugar should be done.

Ketones

The testing is presently limited to detecting acetoacetic aciduria. Excess lipolysis is classic in diabetic ketoacidosis and starvation ketosis.

pH

Urine is usually acid (low pH). If urine is allowed to stand it becomes alkaline due to urea breakdown. Calculi are readily formed in acid urine. If urine is kept alkaline and of low density, stone formation can be prevented.

Urobilinogen

Increased amounts may occur in infections of the liver or obstruction of the extrahepatic biliary system.

Blood

Blood may occur in the urine from a variety of causes including urethrotrigonitis, congestive prostatitis, renal calculi, glomerulonephritis, renal tuberculosis, hemorrhagic cystitis, pyelonephritis, renal vein thrombosis, sickle cell anemia and/or hemophelia.

A three glass urine in males is helpful in isolating the source of bleeding. In initial hematuria (blood in the first glass only) the site of the hemorrhage is the urethra. Terminal hematuria (blood in the third glass) indicates a small hemorrhage from the trigone region of the bladder or prostate. Total hematuria (blood in all the glasses) indicates a bleeding from the kidney or ureter.

Microanalysis

All urine should be refrigerated within three minutes of collection and cultures sent within one to three hours.

Microscopic examination should be done immediately for white blood cells, red blood cells, bacteria, crystals and casts.

Microanalysis will aid in the diagnosis. In pyelonephritis the urine will contain WBC's, bacteria, WBC casts (and sometimes proteinuria). Urethritis in males will show WBC's and bacteria in the first voided specimen only. There will be no casts or RBC's. In prostatitis the third voided specimen may contain WBC's and bacteria. In cystitis the urine sample (or second voided specimen in males) will contain some RBC's, WBC's and bacteria; there will be no casts.

WBC

There are normally fewer than 10 WBC's per high power field (HPF) in spun urine sediment. A greater value may indicate an infection.

RBC

There are normally fewer than 5 RBC's per high power field (HPF) in spun urine. Two to three RBC's in a freshly voided spun urine per HPF is a normal shed. A greater value may be caused by a vaginal contamination, fever, infection, cancer, silent renal calculi, subacute bacterial endocarditis and/or trauma to the kidney.

Bacteria

The urine is normally sterile. One bacterium seen in a drop of unspun urine implies a colony count of 100,000 or more. The presence of bacteria indicates a uropathology. The most common organism in women is *E. coli*. The most common organism in males is *Bacillus proteus*.

Casts

Hyaline casts are composed solely of protein and may be considered normal in small numbers; they are commonly seen in febrile illnesses. They may contain one to two WBC's or RBC's. Epithelial casts are composed of degenerating tubular epithelial cells and are sufficiently obliterated so that they are referred to as fine or coarse granular casts. They may imply nephrosis or glomerulonephritis.

Refer the patient if there are any other types of casts seen in the urine (i.e., red blood cell casts, white blood cell casts, etc.).

Crystals

Crystalluria is more a result of extremes of urine pH than an increased excretion of a substance. Crystal formation is temperature dependent. (Consider the heavy crystal sediment that appears normally in refrigerated urine.) Clinical implications can be drawn only· on freshly voided urine at body temperature.

Cells

The presence of more than a few vaginal epithelial cells indicates a contaminated specimen.

Urine culture and sensitivity

The urine culture is needed to determine the colony count of bacteria. The sensitivity is needed to determine the appropriate therapy.

Complete blood count (CBC)

There may be an increase in the white blood count in acute prostatitis and pyelonephritis. Anemia may be seen in chronic renal disease or any chronic disease. The WBC is usually not elevated in cystitis or urethritis.

GC culture gram stain

The gram stain is positive for gonorrhea if there are gram-negative intracellular diplococci. The gram stain is more accurate on males than females because the presence of mixed vaginal flora reduces the likelihood of positively identifying the gonococcal organism. The incidence of GC is less likely in the elderly because of the usual pattern of a single long-term partner. With a positive or suspicious history, however, a culture should be taken for GC in the following areas: females (cervical, rectal), males (urethra) and in homosexuals or in a history of oral or rectal intercourse (pharyngeal and rectal).

Vaginal smear

The wet prep is performed to evaluate the causative agent of a vaginal discharge. Search for trichomonas, yeast or nonspecific (hemophilus) organisms that could have ascended from the perineum causing a cystitis or urethritis.

BUN/creatinine

The BUN and creatinine should be drawn in order to ascertain the state of the renal function in the elderly. An abnormal result could indicate a chronic pyelonephritis or other renal pathology.

Biochemical assay

The biochemical assay should be performed as a routine screening in order to pick up abnormalities that could adversely affect the urinary tract system. For example, an increase in serum calcium or uric acid could increase the likelihood of stone formation; the stone could have been the obstruction that resulted in a chronic urinary tract infection.

Acid phosphatase

An exam on a male that reveals a hard stony prostate in a patient with recurrent cystitis could indicate a prostate cancer causing obstruction. An acid phosphatase should be drawn on all patients with abnormal prostate exams to rule out prostatic cancer.

IVP, cysto, cystometrogram

These tests should be performed (after physician consultation/referral) on patients with recurrent infections. The results may reveal the cause of the chronic UTI's (i.e., obstruction, bladder dysfunction, etc.).

ASSESSMENT:

Males: Lower UTI's (urethritis, cystitis, prostatitis)

Acute urethritis

Urethritis in males may be acute or chronic. There are several types of urethritis (i.e., GC, nonspecific, chemical). Urethritis usually arises from an ascending infection from the urethra. At times it can be secondary to a descending infection from the prostate.

Subjective data from acute urethritis may include frequency, dysuria and/or a constant itching or burning sensation in the urethra. In GC or NSU symptoms may appear several days after intercourse. In NSU there is usually a history of alcohol consumption. In addition, the patient may give a history of his partner being treated for vaginitis (e.g., trichomonas). Chemical urethritis may arise from such things as spermicidal jellies or perfumed soaps. On physical examination the urethra may be reddened or irritated. The exudate/discharge may range from none to heavy; the character may range from clear to purulent.

The lab tests should include a gram stain. Look for gram-negative intracellular diplococci; even if the gram stain is negative do a GC culture. If the culture is negative the patient probably has nonspecific urethritis. If there is no discharge present have the patient obtain a three glass urinalysis. If the patient has urethritis the first specimen should contain organisms. Trichomonas, if the cause of the urethritis, is difficult to confirm in males. In any type of urethritis the midstream specimen will be clear; this helps determine that the infection is not arising from the bladder. However, if prostatitis is the underlying cause of the urethritis, the third specimen will contain WBC's and bacteria. (See prostatitis.)

Chronic urethritis

Chronic urethritis may be secondary to an unresolved acute urethritis or a chronic prostatitis. The symptomatology is the same as for acute urethritis.

If the chronic urethritis is secondary to a chronic prostatitis, the prostate may be boggy, firm or fibrotic. In chronic prostatitis the massage will reveal discharge with pus and bacteria, and the third specimen of urine will contain pus and bacteria. If secondary to unresolved urethritis, the first specimen will contain organisms and the second and third should be clear.

Acute cystitis

Cystitis in males may be acute or chronic. Cystitis in males is always secondary to 1) a kidney infection that is seeding the bladder with bacteria, 2) an acute or chronic prostatitis or 3) a residual urine as from neurogenic dysfunction or obstruction.

Subjective symptoms may include dysuria, frequency, urgency (that may cause incontinence), nocturia and hematuria (usually terminal). If cystitis is secondary to acute prostatitis or pyelonephritis the patient may complain of fever or low back pain. Cystitis may follow instrumentation or catheterization. The patient may give a history of obstruction (e.g., BPH or strictures) or neurogenic diseases. The abdominal exam may reveal a bladder tenderness or enlargement. A CVA tenderness may indicate an underlying pyelonephritis. If there is a neurogenic disease present there may be poor sphincter tone on rectal exam.

In acute prostatitis there will be a boggy, tender prostate. If the cystitis is secondary to a chronic prostatitis, the prostate may be boggy, firm, and fibrotic. If secondary to BPH the prostate may be firm and nontender.

Chronic cystitis

Chronic cystitis usually occurs as a result of a chronic kidney infection, reflux, residual urine, stenosis or prostatitis. It is the most common cause of chronic bacteriuria and pyuria.

Symptomatology may be the same as in acute cystitis or there may be no symptoms. If secondary to neurogenic disease or obstructive pathology, the bladder may be distended and painful to palpation.

If prostatitis is the underlying etiology, the findings will be consistent with acute or chronic prostatitis. Chronic cystitis secondary to neurogenic disease may show poor sphincter tone on rectal exam.

Acute prostatitis

Acute prostatitis may occur as the result of: 1) an ascending infection from the urethra, 2) the spread of infection by the hematogenous route, or 3) an acute congestive prostatitis secondary to lack of intercourse.

Subjectively, the patient may complain of dysuria, frequency, nocturia, urgency, purulent penile discharge after defecation, painful defecation, bloody ejaculate, initial or terminal hematuria, fever, cloudy urine, perineal aching and/or low back pain. If the gland is severely edematous, urinary retention may be the presenting symptom.

Objectively, fever is usually present and is associated with urethral discharge containing pyuria and bacteriuria. On the rectal exam the prostate may be exquisitely tender and boggy; do *not* massage. The CBC may show an elevation of the WBC. On the three glass urine test the first (if associated with a concomitant urethritis) and third urine specimens may contain pyuria and bacteriuria.

Chronic prostatitis

There may be no subjective complaints at all; however, the patient may complain of a mild discomfort on ejaculation, a mild low back pain or perineal aching, or symptoms of acute epididymitis (e.g., scrotal pain, redness, warmth, etc.). There is no history of fever. The prostate exam will reveal a firm, fibrotic mild to nontender prostate. Massage will produce a purulent discharge with leukocytes and bacteria.

The urine usually contains WBC's and bacteria. The WBC is usually not elevated except when acute epididymitis is present, in which case the scrotum would be tender, reddened and warm.

Females: *Lower UTI's (cystitis, urethritis)*

Acute and chronic cystitis

Cystitis is much more common in females than in males. It may arise from vaginal infections that have contaminated the urethra and ascension of the infection to the bladder, or it may result from chemical reactions (e.g., bubble baths, feminine hygiene sprays, etc.).

The subjective data is the same as for males. In addition, there will frequently be vaginal discharge, perineal pain or itching.

Objective findings may include a reddened or swollen urethra, inflammed Bartholin's and/or Skene's glands; if urethral diverticulum is the underlying etiology, palpation of the urethra will be painful and a purulent exudate may be expressed.

Chronic cystitis

See Males: Lower UTI's.

Urethritis

Females may have urethritis. Symptoms will include complaints of dysuria, frequency and urgency. Objectively the urethra may be reddened, irritated and/or tender. The pelvic exam may show a redness of the genitalia and/or a vaginal discharge. The vaginal wet prep may show a trichomonas, yeast or hemophilus infection. The urinalysis may show some bacteriuria and/or pyuria. The culture may be positive for GC. In females, one of the most common causes of urethritis is a chemical irritant (e.g., bubble bath, feminine hygiene sprays, perfumed soaps, etc.).

Upper Urinary Tract Infections
Acute pyelonephritis
(males and females)

Acute pyelonephritis is the result of a bacterial infection. A cystitis which has been treated inadequately can be the source. Conversely, a pyelo that is continually seeding the bladder with bacteria can perpetuate a cystitis.

Acute pyelonephritis is most common in females. The aged patient may present with confusion or hypothermia and/or may subjectively complain of frequency, dysuria, back

261

pain, fever, chills, nausea and/or vomiting. Hematuria may be present if there is a concomitant cystitis.

Objectively there may be fever (sometimes as high as 103° F or above), CVA tenderness, and an elevated serum WBC count. There will also be bacteriuria, pyuria, occasional RBC's and WBC casts in the urine.

Chronic pyelonephritis (males and females)

Chronic pyelonephritis can prove to be fatal, for it (like chronic glomerulonephritis) may produce progressive scarring and atrophy of the kidney with a resultant development of renal failure. Chronic pyelonephritis can be secondary to both bacterial and nonbacterial etiologies. Thus, the discussion of chronic pyelonephritis can be made on the basis of *chronic obstructive* and *chronic nonobstructive*. *Chronic obstructive pyelonephritis* occurs as a result of an unresolved acute infection or repeated acute infections that occur because of a urinary tract obstruction. It has an insidious onset and may or may not present as acute pyelonephritis.

In *chronic nonobstructive pyelonephritis*, the past medical history may be uneventful. There may or may not be a past history of UTI's. In almost all cases, vesicoureteral reflux is present. The diagnosis is made by x-ray. The onset is always insidious and its presence may be discovered accidentally or on a routine physical exam. Chronic nonobstructive affects both sexes equally. Its incidence may be increased in the aged because of the higher incidence of obstructive pathology.

Subjective findings of chronic pyelonephritis may include acute symptomatology or the patient may be asymptomatic. Loss of the tubular function causes a decreased concentrating ability with a resultant polyuria and nocturia.

Objectively, the physical exam may be normal. The microscopic urinalysis may be sterile or it may show clumps of WBC's, WBC casts, and bacteria; there are usually no RBC casts or RBC's. The dipstick urinalysis may show a mild proteinuria and a decreased specific gravity due to a decreased concentrating ability. The diagnosis is made by x-ray. The IVP has the following characteristics: 1) calyceal blunting, 2) narrowing of the parenchyma over the calyx and 3) the kidney poles are the most common site.

PLAN:

Males: Lower UTI's
Acute urethritis

See *Overall Management Plan* section. In all cases of urethritis, have the patient refrain from alcohol consumption and intercourse for several days.

GC urethritis

If the GC culture and/or gram stain is positive, treat with the appropriate antibiotic therapy. The patient should be recultured in two weeks.

Nonspecific urethritis	Obtain a GC culture to rule out gonorrhea. Treat with appropriate antimicrobials and have the patient return in two weeks for follow-up.
Chemical urethritis	Discontinue the causative agent.
Trichomonas urethritis	Treat both partners with the appropriate medication.
Urethritis secondary to prostatitis	See treatment for prostatitis and have the patient return for follow-up.
Chronic urethritis	Consult with and/or refer to a urologist.
Acute cystitis	See *Overall Management Plan* section. Consult with and/or refer to a physician if obstructive pathology, BPH or neurogenic bladder disease are suspected to be the underlying cause of the cystitis. If this is the patient's first episode of cystitis: 1) obtain a urine culture and sensitivity, 2) treat with appropriate antimicrobials and 3) reculture the patient's urine in two weeks. If this is a recurrent episode (within the past year) consult with a physician.
Chronic cystitis	Consult with and/or refer to a physician; the underlying etiology of the infection must be ascertained. Appropriate tests include an IVP, cystogram, CBC, urinalysis and culture. Treatment includes appropriate antimicrobials, sitz baths, and bladder antispasmodics.
Acute prostatitis	See *Overall Management Plan* sec-

tion. Do not catheterize or manipulate the prostate in any way; if urinary retention is present refer the patient immediately. Treatment includes antimicrobials, hot sitz baths, analgesics if indicated, bed rest, antispasmodics and force fluids. The patient should be scheduled for physician follow-up.

Chronic prostatitis

Consultation and/or referral to the patient's physician is indicated. Management includes CBC, urinalysis, gram stain/culture of the patient's discharge and antimicrobials.

Females: Lower UTI's
Acute cystitis

If the cystitis is secondary to vaginal discharge, both the vaginitis and cystitis should be treated. If the cystitis is secondary to a chemical irritation, the patient should avoid use of the irritant. Treatment may include appropriate antimicrobials, antispasmodics, sitz baths. A follow-up urine culture should be done in two weeks. See *Overall Management Plan* section of this protocol.

Chronic cystitis

If the patient has had no recent IVP and cystogram, these tests should be ordered and the patient referred to a urologist (to determine the underlying cause of the cystitis).

Urethritis

See *Overall Management Plan* section. The patient should avoid the irritant if identified. Treat any underlying vaginitis.

Upper Urinary Tract Infections

Acute and chronic pyelonephritis (males and females)	Consultation with or referral to the patient's physician is indicated. The patient will probably need to be hospitalized for acute pyelonephritis.

ADDENDUM 1
OVERALL MANAGEMENT PLAN FOR THE ELDERLY PATIENT

A. Medication Instructions

Precise instructions should be given. Verbalization of the patient's understanding of directions should be required, for the elderly often mask a hearing deficit and leave without clearly comprehending the regimen. Emphasize the need for compliance, especially in taking all of the medication as directed. Care should be made to instruct the patient regarding disposal of the remainder of previous medication. The elderly frequently take medication only until their acute symptoms are relieved, saving the rest for a future time. It is important to have the patient return for follow-up after completing treatment; ask the patient to bring his or her medicine bottle to the appointment.

To avoid drug induced complications, the patient needs to know what symptoms to watch for. Explanation of side effects/adverse reactions should be simple and direct. Instruct the patient to stop the medication and call the health provider if side effects/adverse reactions appear.

B. Compliance Instructions

Return in two days if symptoms persist. By this time the results of the urine culture and sensitivity should be available and the medication being taken should match the sensitivity.

Return in one week after finishing the antibiotic. (The patient should return earlier if the symptoms have not improved.) At this time the subjective findings should be reviewed. A repeat urinalysis should be done with a culture and sensitivity (if indicated by presence of bacteriuria). The presence of a sterile urine indicating a cure or the presence of asymptomatic bacteriuria needs to be determined. If bacteriuria persists the patient should be referred.

Discuss the signs and symptoms of the recurrence of an infection with the patient to aid in establishing expectancies and discuss the need to seek early treatment. Ideally, urine should be recultured in three months even if the three-week culture was negative. This documents the effectiveness of treatment, patient education and compliance.

ADDENDUM 2
PATIENT EDUCATION HANDOUT

A. For patients with *nonspecific urethritis* and/or *cystitis* instructions include:

1. Increase fluid intake to 2500 to 3000 cc/day.

2. Avoid *milk products* (when tetracycline is prescribed), citrus juices and oxalate foods such as spinach and rhubarb.

3. Include hippuric acid foods such as cranberry juice in the diet daily.

4. If available, use a shower, not tub. If a bath is necessary, use a low water level and be brief.

5. Avoid bubble bath, perfumed soaps, hygiene spray and hexachlorophene soaps. Rinse the perineum well.

6. Use cotton underwear.

7. Avoid harsh laundry soaps, bleaches, etc. Rinse clothing well.

8. Avoid panty hose and/or tight slacks.

9. Avoid prolonged car rides without established frequent stops for voiding purposes (to prevent urinary stasis).

10. In nonspecific urethritis, a relapse is often associated with sexual intercourse. If it occurs, both partners may need to be treated.

11. Void frequently to reduce the bacterial growth in pooled urine.

12. Void pre- and postcoitus.

13. In men prostatitis is often a secondary complication of bladder infection. Watch for signs and symptoms of pelvic aching, discharge, etc.

14. Women should void with their knees well spread to avoid vaginal involvement.

15. Women should wipe the perineal area from the front to back with a single swipe to avoid carrying organisms from rectum to the vaginal-urethral area.

16. Women should cleanse the anal area after each BM with a wet disposable towel.

17. Feminine hygiene sprays are contraindicated and should not be used.

18. Prompt attention should be given to abnormal or excessive vaginal discharge.

19. If the vaginal mucosa is dry/painful during intercourse, a water soluble lubricant such as KY Jelly should be used.

20. Avoid overuse of douching because it disrupts the normal bacterial protection of the vagina. If douching is desired (unless instructed otherwise) plain water should be used.

B. For patients with *prostatitis* instructions include:

1. Prostatitis may be a long-term condition. For this reason increased attention to compliance is necessary.

2. Increase daily intake of fluids to 2500 to 3000 cc.

3. Void frequently.

4. Void before exercise.

5. Take sitz baths for perineal comfort.

6. Foods that have been consistently connected to prostatitis flare-ups should be avoided. They may be precipitating foods for that patient. Avoid alcohol and spices (because some men experience a worsening of their prostatitis with these foods).

7. Avoid strenuous exercise. In some instances, prostatitis may follow strenuous exercise.

REFERENCES

1. Badenoch, Alex W. *Manual of Urology.* Chicago: William Heinemann Medical Books Publications, 1974.

2. Bors, Ernest and A. Estin Comarr. *Neurological Urology*. Baltimore: University Park Press, 1971.
3. DeGowin, Elmer L. and Richard L. DeGowin. *Bedside Diagnostic Examination*, 3rd ed. New York: Macmillan Publishing, 1976.
4. Everett, Houston S. and John H. Ridley. *Female Urology*. New York: Hoeber Medical Division, Harper and Row, 1968.
5. Krupp, Marcus A. and Milton J. Chatton. *Current Medical Diagnosis and Treatment*. Los Altos: Lange Medical Publications, 1977.
6. Lapides, Jack. *Fundamentals of Urology*. Philadelphia: W.B. Saunders Company, 1976.
7. _____. *Quick Reference Laboratory Manual*. Phoenix: Medical Services of Arizona, 1976.
8. Rossman, Isadore. *Clinical Geriatrics*. Philadelphia: J.B. Lippincott Co., 1971.
9. Stamey, Thomas A. *Urinary Infections*. Baltimore: Williams and Wilkins Co., 1972.
10. Taylor, Robert B. *A Primer of Clinical Symptoms*. New York: Harper and Row, 1973.
11. Walker, H. Kenneth, W. Dallas Hall, J. Willis Hurst. *Clinical Methods*, Vols. I and II. Woburn, Me.: Butterworth, Inc., 1976.

Chapter 6

Peripheral Edema

OVERVIEW

Edema is defined as an abnormal accumulation of fluid in the interstitial spaces. Under normal circumstances, a fluid balance is maintained by two factors: 1) pressure gradients and 2) permeability of the capillary membranes. The movement of fluids and solutes is such that a state of osmotic equilibrium must exist between two compartments separated by a membrane. In this instance, the compartments are the vascular system and the interstitial spaces. The forces that control the movement of fluid from the vascular system into the interstitial spaces are: 1) the hydrostatic pressure within the vasculature and 2) the oncotic pressure in the interstitial fluid. Conversely, the movement of fluids from the interstitial spaces into the vascular compartment is controlled by: 1) the oncotic pressure of the vasculature (secondary to the presence of plasma proteins) and 2) the hydrostatic pressure (tissue tension) within the interstitial fluid.

In normal circumstances, these forces will result in a net movement of fluids from the vasculature (at the arteriolar end of the capillary) into the interstitial spaces, and at the venous end of the capillary (the fluid moves from the interstitial spaces into the venous and lymphatic system).

If all of the above normal conditions exist, a balance in the exchange of fluid between the vasculature and the interstitial spaces will be maintained. However, if any one of the above conditions is altered, there will be an imbalance in the exchange of fluid; if the imbalance is not corrected, edema will develop.

The mechanisms involved in bilateral peripheral edema are: 1) conditions that result in an *increased hydrostatic pressure* of the blood, 2) *decreased oncotic pressure* of the blood or 3) *increased oncotic pressure* of the interstitial spaces. The most common cause of bilateral peripheral edema that occurs as a result of an increase in *hydrostatic pressure* of the blood is seen in congestive heart failure.

When either ventricle begins to fail, there is a decrease in the amount of blood ejected from the ventricle during systole which causes an increase in volume of blood contained in the ventricle resulting in a build-up of pressure in the vessels behind that ventricle. This pressure build-up results in an increase in the venous pressure (hydrostatic pressure of the blood) which can exceed the oncotic pressure in the interstitial spaces so that fluids exude from the venous system into the interstitial spaces. In addition, the decreased cardiac output seen in congestive failure results in a decrease of circulating blood volume in the arterial system, which causes a decrease in the perfusion of the kidneys, which activates the renin angiotensinogen system. The salt and water that are retained not only increase the circulating blood volume, but also increase the hydrostatic pressure at the arterial end of the capillary, so that fluid moves from the vasculature into the interstitial spaces further aggravating the formation of edema.

Bilateral edema that occurs secondary to a *decrease in the oncotic pressure* of the blood is seen in conditions in which there is hypoalbuminemia (e.g., renal diseases, liver disease, cirrhosis, and malnutrition). The low serum albumin content results in an alteration of the colloid oncotic pressure of the vasculature so fluid moves from the vasculature into the interstitial spaces.

The third cause of bilateral peripheral edema is an increased oncotic pressure of the interstitial spaces. Conditions that result in an alteration of the permeability of the capillary membrane (allowing proteins to escape from the vasculature into the interstitial spaces) cause an increased oncotic pressure of the interstitial spaces, resulting in edema formation. Examples of this are exposure to chemicals and/or certain bacterial toxins.

Unilateral or localized edema involves three mechanisms: 1) *increased hydrostatic pressure* of the blood, 2) *increased oncotic pressure* of the interstitial spaces (altered capillary permeability) and 3) *lymph obstruction*. Unilateral edema can also be a systemic problem that appears unilateral only because the patient is positioned to make one extremity more dependent than the other.

An increased hydrostatic pressure of the blood in unilateral edema can occur secondary to tumors, varicosities, thrombophlebitis or tight garments. The mechanism involved is the same as for bilateral edema. Localized edema secondary to an increased oncotic pressure of interstitial spaces is seen in allergic reactions, burns, and injuries.

Unilateral edema secondary to obstruction of the lymphatics occurs as a result of increased hydrostatic pressure in the capillary bed. The fluid is forced into the interstitial spaces because of this change in pressure. Ultimately, this obstruction will also result in a decreased circulating blood volume; the sequence of events (described under the edema of congestive heart failure) aggravates the edematous state. Edema secondary to lymph obstruction may occur secondary to inflammation, trauma, surgery or irradiation.

Understanding the pathophysiology of edema helps the practitioner determine the etiology of the condition and then begin a therapeutic regimen to correct the edematous state.

PERIPHERAL EDEMA IN THE ELDERLY WORKSHEET

To be used for elderly patients
with peripheral edema.

What you cannot afford to miss: congestive heart failure from any origin, renal disease, including nephrotic syndrome, hepatic disease, neoplasm causing obstruction to lymphatics.

Chief Complaint: _____

SUBJECTIVE DATA:

Date of Onset: _____Sudden/Gradual: _____

Duration/course: _____

Relieved by: _____

YES   NO

_____ _____ Is the edema unilateral and/or localized (affecting

one limb causing tight ring, tight shoe, etc.)? _____

If *localized, is it associated* with: (If not localized, move to the next section.)

(Describe Positive Responses)
YES   NO

_____ _____ Recent sunburn, burns, injuries, allergies: _____

_____ _____ Standing or sitting long hours: _____

_____ _____ Worse at the end of the day: _____

_____ _____ Wearing tight clothes, especially garters, girdles,

knee-high stockings: _____

_____ _____ Pain: _____

_____ _____ Hot weather: _____

_____ _____ Is edema generalized (or present in bilateral extrem-

ities)? _____

If *generalized edema or present bilaterally, is it associated* with:
(If not generalized, move to Past Medical History.)

(Describe Positive Responses)
YES   NO

_____ _____ Unexplained weight gain: _____

_____ _____ Symptom constellation of shortness of breath, cough,
chest pain, paroxysmal nocturnal dyspnea, orthop-

nea, hemoptysis: _____

_____

_____ _____ Decreased urine output: _____

Peripheral Edema in the Elderly Worksheet

_____ _____ Hematuria:_____

_____ _____ Polyuria/nocturia/increased thirst: _____

_____ _____ Fatigue/weakness:_____

_____ _____ Anorexia/nausea/vomiting: _____

_____

_____ _____ Abdominal pain: _____

_____ _____ Periorbital edema: _____

_____ _____ Increased abdominal girth:_____

_____ _____ Confusion/mental changes:_____

_____ _____ Itching: _____

_____ _____ Weight loss: _____

_____ _____ Jaundice: _____

_____ _____ Alopecia: _____

_____ _____ Rashes: _____

_____ _____ Fever/chills:_____

_____ _____ Facial changes:_____

_____ _____ Changes in urine/stool: _____

_____ _____ Excessive water intake: _____

PAST MEDICAL HISTORY:
YES   NO

_____ _____ Diabetes mellitus:_____

_____ _____ Repeated urinary tract infections/renal disease: ____

———— ———— Renal calculi: _____

———— ———— Collagen vascular disease: _____

———— ———— Alcoholism/jaundice: _____

———— ———— Hepatitis/liver disease: _____

———— ———— Hypertension/cardiac disease: _____

———— ———— Cardiac medicines/special low sodium diet: _____

———— ———— Surgery with removal of lymph nodes: _____

———— ———— Cancer: _____

———— ———— Thrombophlebitis/limb paralysis: _____

———— ———— Medications (please list old and new):_____

_____

———— ———— Operations/hospitalizations: _____

_____

_____

———— ———— Allergies (food, medicine): _____

_____

OBJECTIVE DATA:

Vital Signs: _____BP lying _____BP sitting

_____BP standing _____Pulse × 1 full min.

_____Resp. _____Temp. _____Wt.

Peripheral Edema in the Elderly Worksheet

(Describe Positive Responses)

YES   NO

_____ _____ Unilateral or localized edema: _____

_____ _____ Bilateral or generalized edema: _____

_____ _____ Associated with heat or erythema:_____

_____ _____ Pitting edema: _____

_____ _____ Brawny edema:_____

_____ _____ Abnormal thyroid:_____

_____ _____ Neck veins distended:_____

CHEST:

YES   NO

_____ _____ Dullness:_____

_____ _____ Abnormal breath sounds: _____

_____ _____ Decreased fremitus: _____

HEART:

YES   NO

_____ _____ Displaced PMI: _____

_____ _____ Heaves, lifts, thrills: _____

_____ _____ Irregular rate and/or rhythm: _____

_____ _____ Murmurs:_____

_____ _____ S^3/S^4 gallop: _____

ABDOMEN:

YES   NO

_____ _____ Distention:_____

YES   *NO*

_____ _____ Distended veins: _____

_____ _____ Spider angiomas/ascites: _____

_____ _____ Masses/tenderness: _____

_____ _____ Hepatomegaly: _____

_____ _____ Splenomegaly: _____

_____ _____ Palpable lymph nodes: _____

_____ _____ Palmar erythema: _____

_____ _____ Abnormal temperature of extremities: _____

_____ _____ Jaundice: _____

_____ _____ Hemiplegia or paralysis: _____

_____ _____ Calf tenderness, redness, pain/+Homan's sign:_____

_____ _____ Abnormal reflexes: _____

_____ _____ Abnormal mental status exam: _____

_____ _____ Abnormal pulses: _____

_____ _____ Varicosities: _____

LAB DATA: (DESCRIBE ALL TEST RESULTS)

The following tests should be performed on all patients with undiagnosed peripheral edema.

DONE   *NOT*
       DONE

_____ _____ Urinalysis (microanalysis and macroanalysis):_____

_____

_____ _____ Electrolytes: _____

_____

_____ _____ BUN/creatinine: _____

_____

_____ _____ SMA-12 (total protein, albumin, cholesterol, calcium,

phosphorus): _____

The following tests should be performed on patients
in the following conditions.

_____ _____ CBC (if the patient has not had this test performed

recently): _____

_____ _____ Liver function tests (if the patient has a past history

of ETOH abuse or liver problems): _____

_____ _____ Chest x-ray (if the patient is suspected of having

CHF): _____

_____

_____ _____ EKG (if the patient is suspected of having CHF): ___

_____

_____ _____ Protime, platelet count (if the patient has petechiae,

liver disease, or history of abnormal bleeding):_____

_____

_____ _____ ESR (if the patient is suspected of having serum sick-

ness or glomerulonephritis): _____

_____ _____ ASO titer (if the patient has a history of onset of
edema after a recent untreated pharyngitis where

glomerulonephritis is suspect): _____

_____ _____ Thyroid tests (if the patient has a history or physical

suggestive of hypo- or hyperthyroidism): _____

_____ _____ Flat plate of abdomen (if indicated after physician

consultation): _____

_____ _____ 24-hour urine for protein/creatinine clearance (if the
patient is suspected of having acute or chronic renal

disease, nephrotic syndrome, or liver disease): _____

EDEMA WORKSHEET RATIONALE

SUBJECTIVE DATA:

Onset of Difficulties

Edema from allergies (e.g., insect
bites, foods, etc.) usually develops
rapidly. It may be localized and associated with erythema and warmth,
or it may be generalized and associated with such symptoms as SOB,
wheezes, respiratory stridor, facial
puffiness, etc.

A gradual onset of edema may be
associated with congestive heart
failure, nephrotic syndrome, acute
or chronic renal failure and glomerulonephritis.

Duration

It is important to note the time relationship and duration of the
edema. Edema seen late in the day
and decreasing at night may be due

to a volume redistribution (e.g., idiopathic or secondary to tight clothes). Early morning edema associated with facial puffiness may persist all day and, perhaps, worsen (e.g., edema secondary to the nephrotic syndrome).

Actual disappearance of edema can occur as a result of the shifting of fluids to other areas, such as the sacrum or lungs during the night. Paroxysmal nocturnal dyspnea (PND) occurs as the result of hypervolemia produced by the redistribution of peripheral edema when the body is changed from a vertical to a horizontal position.

Relieved By

Bilateral edema secondary to varicosities, wearing tight fitting clothes or dependent edema may be relieved by lying down or elevating a dependent extremity. Generalized and severe edema may decrease by lying down, but the patient may then complain of paroxysmal nocturnal dyspnea due to a shifting of fluid volume by the reclining position. Paroxysmal nocturnal dyspnea is seen with the edema of CHF.

Localized Edema

Edema affecting one extremity only is considered local. If both hands or feet are swollen, or there is swelling around the periorbital areas, generalized edema is probably present. Unilateral (localized) edema may result from lymph stasis, varicosities, injury, insect bites, thrombophlebitis, cellulitis or pelvic tumor.

Associated with:

Recent sunburn, burns, injuries, allergies	Increased fragility of the capillaries from these conditions can result in a colloidal leak.
Standing or sitting long hours, worse at end of day	Orthostatic edema results from an impairment of circulation by inactivity. It is a problem of gravity and disappears when the dependent areas are elevated.
Wearing tight clothes, especially circular garters, girdles, knee-high stockings	Wearing tight clothing causes stasis edema by constriction of the circulation; it will disappear when the constriction is removed.
Pain	Pain may accompany edema when caused by varicose veins or thrombophlebitis. The pain is increased in the dependent position. In thrombophlebitis there may be a dull ache or frank pain in the calf; in more extensive cases, there is a pain in the whole leg that is accentuated with walking.
Hot weather	"Summer edema," so common to women, is probably caused by increased hydrostatic pressure, although the exact cause is unknown.

Generalized Edema
Associated with:

Weight gain	An unexplained weight gain may gradually increase to nearly 10 percent of the patient's weight before pitting edema becomes evident in generalized edema. Weight gain may be the chief complaint for the patient with generalized edema.

SOB, cough, chest pain, PND, orthopnea, hemoptysis

As a symptom constellation shortness of breath, cough, chest pain, paroxysmal nocturnal dyspnea, orthopnea and hemoptysis is indicative of congestive heart failure. Breathlessness is usually the first complaint; the other symptoms occur as the untreated etiology continues.

Decreased urine output

A history of decreased urinary output may be secondary to acute renal failure, acute glomerulonephritis, etc. However, in the elderly, one must also consider a decreased fluid intake as a cause of low urine output.

Hematuria

Hematuria (either macroscopic or microscopic) may be indicative of numerous conditions (e.g., acute renal failure, acute glomerulonephritis, urinary tract infections, renal calculi, serum sickness, collagen vascular diseases, and chronic glomerulonephritis). This symptom's significance is increased in the presence of other symptoms/signs of renal disease.

Polyuria/nocturia/ increased thirst

Polyuria and polydipsia together can be early signs of progressing renal insufficiency. In chronic renal failure, more and more nephrons are destroyed, and fewer nephrons are called upon to increase their workload. As a result, the glomerular filtration rate decreases, and the blood urea nitrogen level increases. The increased solute load of the serum contributes to an increased glomerulo filtration rate and a rise in the plasma concentration of urea. This results in a decreased concentrating ability of the kidneys and a loss of the excretion of salt-free urine.

As salt is lost in the urine, the serum concentration decreases, the thirst center in the hypothalamus is stimulated, and the patient drinks more and urinates more. The patient with chronic renal failure must not only drink more water, but must excrete more water to handle the load of urinary solutes.

Nocturia is secondary to a redistribution of fluid volume when the patient assumes a recumbent position. This reclining position plus a decreased workload results in an increased perfusion of the kidney. Nocturia may be seen in CHF, chronic renal failure or uncontrolled diabetes mellitus.

Fatigue, weakness

These are very nonspecific symptoms that may be indicative of numerous conditions (e.g., an acute renal failure, chronic renal failure, acute glomerulonephritis, cirrhosis, congestive failure, nephrotic syndrome and/or myxedema). The fatigue and weakness may be secondary to anemia seen in most of the above conditions or an increased fluid load.

Anorexia, nausea, vomiting

These may be GI manifestations of congestive heart failure, liver disease, or hyponatremia seen in acute or chronic renal failure or nephrotic syndrome.

Abdominal pain

Abdominal pain may be secondary to a congested liver from cirrhosis or right-sided failure from whatever cause. Abdominal pain and other GI symptoms listed above may be seen in nephrotic syndrome and/or acute glomerulonephritis or may be secondary to discomfort caused by ascites.

Periorbital edema

Periorbital edema is associated with generalized edema from such things as severe allergic reactions, edema of nephrotic syndrome, myxedema or acute glomerulonephritis.

Increased abdominal girth

Increased abdominal girth is seen in generalized edema of cirrhosis, CHF, nephrotic syndrome, carcinoma or secondary to ascites. It may be due to systemic causes such as impaired water excretion, hypoalbuminemia or increased sodium retention. Local causes of ascites are liver disease with associated portal hypertension or obstruction of the hepatic blood flow from congestion.

Confusion or mental changes

Confusion or mental changes may be secondary to hypoxia associated with CHF, azotemia of acute or chronic renal failure or myxedema.

Itching

Pruritus may be seen in liver disease or chronic renal disease.

Weight loss

Weight loss may be secondary to the anorexia of liver disease, etc.; however, weight loss may not be apparent because of edema. Weight loss may also be secondary to nutritional deficiencies, etc.

Jaundice

Seen in liver disease of whatever origin.

Alopecia

Alopecia may be seen in myxedema, and/or liver disease.

Rashes

Purpuric rashes may be seen in liver disease and/or immune complex diseases (e.g., serum sickness).

Fever/chills

Fever may be indicative of an infectious process, cirrhosis or acute glomerulonephritis.

Facial changes

Periorbital edema may be present. A parotid gland enlargement may be seen in chronic alcoholism. A dull facial expression may be seen in myxedema.

Changes in urine/stools

Light stools and dark urine are seen in alcoholic hepatitis.

Excessive water intake

Psychogenic water drinkers may develop edema secondary to overhydration. Water excess results from an intake in excess of the capacity for excretion. It may occur following too large a water ration during parenteral administration, or as the result of excessive oral intake of water.

Past Medical History
Diabetes mellitus

The renal parenchymal disease associated with diabetes mellitus may be the underlying etiology for the picture of chronic renal failure.

Repeated UTI's/renal disease

Repeated UTI's may have contributed to impairment of the renal functioning thus contributing to the development of chronic renal failure.

It is important to ascertain a previous history of renal disease that may have damaged the parenchyma; that damage may now be contributing to the development of chronic renal failure as an etiology of edema.

Renal calculi

Renal calculi and the obstruction associated with them may give rise to renal parenchymal damage, thus contributing to the development of chronic renal failure.

Collagen vascular disease

This is important historical data to elicit because of the renal pathology associated with such conditions as scleroderma, lupus, etc.

Alcoholism/jaundice

A history of alcoholism is important historical data because of the liver disease associated with longstanding alcohol abuse. Chronic alcoholism may lead to acute alcoholic hepatitis or chronic cirrhosis. Ascites are more likely to occur in the chronic conditions. A history of jaundice may also lead to evidence of a past hepatic disease resulting in liver damage.

Hepatitis/liver disease

In a patient with a past history of hepatitis, the current problem of peripheral edema may be secondary to liver damage from chronic persistent hepatitis (resulting in portal hypertension and other clinical manifestations and complications of the disease).

Hypertension, cardiac disease, cardiac medicines, low sodium diet

A positive past medical history of conditions like cardiac disease, rheumatic heart disease, etc. alert the practitioner that the patient's edema may be secondary to congestive heart failure. Right-sided heart failure causes liver enlargement which may result in liver damage. Sometimes it is difficult to know whether the hypertensive disease came first with subsequent renal damage or vice versa; however, in the presence of longstanding hypertension, the present condition of edema may be secondary to either renal failure or CHF. The elderly patient with cardiac or renal disease may be on a low sodium diet. Therefore, in the presence of edema assess the compliance to the special dietary regimen.

Surgery with removal of lymph nodes

The circulation of the lymph is impaired when there is damage to lymph nodes. Because the small amount of protein which leaks into the interstitial fluid is returned to the blood via the lymph system, lymph stasis edema is rich in protein and very difficult to remove.

Cancer

If the edema is localized, a history of cancer would tend to make one think of some metastasis causing obstruction to the flow of lymph— either as a result of an invasive lesion or as a result of surgical procedure or irradiation.

Thrombophlebitis/limb paralysis

If the edema is localized and associated with redness, warmth, pain, etc., a new thrombophlebitis may be the underlying etiology. If the history is positive for past episodes and currently there are no signs of inflammation, the edema or accumulation of fluid may be the result of some vascular insufficiency that has occurred from a previous episode of thrombophlebitis. Edema from limb paralysis may be caused by the effect of vasoconstriction (from autonomic nerve control) complicated by a decreased lymphatic and venous flow from muscular inactivity.

Medications

It is important to ascertain the kinds, amount of medications, and compliance to medicines. Some medications (e.g., steroids and certain nonsteroid anti-inflammatory agents) may cause fluid retention. Some medications are known for their nephrotoxicity which would precipitate acute renal failure.

Operations/Hospitalizations

The practitioner may obtain important data of the patient's past health which may provide clues for the present edema.

Allergies

Allergic reactions to foods or medications may range from a mild to severe reaction in which there is generalized edema, respiratory stridor, etc. Ask about food and medication intake for the days preceding the edema. Common food allergies are chocolate, nuts, citrus fruits, shellfish, etc. Medication allergies may range from mild pruritic rash to serum sickness or anaphylaxis.

OBJECTIVE DATA:

Vital Signs
  Blood pressure, pulse rate, weight

Obtain these parameters on all patients. Untreated or inadequately treated high blood pressure and renal parenchymal disease are closely interrelated. An elevated BP may be associated with poor compliance to the therapeutic regimen that is now responsible for the development of CHF; it may also be indicative of acute glomerulonephritis, acute or chronic renal failure or liver disease with liver congestion and right-sided heart failure.

It is important to check the pulse for one full minute in order to ascertain any irregularity in the rhythm that may be the underlying cause of congestive heart failure. Digitalis toxicity with its arrhythmias also is an important entity to consider as the underlying cause of edema from CHF.

The weight is an essential objective parameter to obtain so that recent changes (i.e., weight gain or weight loss) can be documented; weight is an important baseline data to ascertain the course of treatment for edema.

Unilateral/Localized Edema

If the edema is both unilateral and localized, one must consider the following etiologies: 1) obstruction of lymph and vascular supply secondary to thrombus, surgical complications, allergic reactions, varicosities, pelvic tumors or tight fitting clothing; 2) in paralyzed limbs secondary to vasomotor impairment; or 3) unilateral may also be present in inflammatory processes (e.g., cellulitis, boils, burns, exposure to irritants or corrosives).

Bilateral Edema

Bilateral or generalized edema can be associated with renal disease, liver disease, CHF, myxedema, or psychogenic overhydration.

Associated with Heat, Erythema

Heat and erythema associated with localized or unilateral edema may be indicative of an inflammatory process. If no trauma is apparent, inspect the area for evidence of an insect bite or sting.

Pitting Edema

Soft pitting edema may be seen in renal disease, CHF, liver disease, myxedema, or the edema associated with injuries and allergies. Pitting may not become evident until the body weight has increased by nearly 10 percent.

Brawny Edema

Edema of longstanding duration may eventually become brawny. (The surrounding tissues become hardened and thickened.) Brawny edema may be seen in peripheral vascular disease and in vascular insufficiency with longstanding stasis.

Thyroid

It is important to examine the thyroid gland for enlargement because hypothyroidism may be unnoticed in the elderly until they present in a myxedematous state with secondary CHF. Once this condition is identified, it can be easily treated.

Neck Veins

When assessing distended neck veins, do so in light of other symptoms. Distention of the neck veins is seen in right-sided heart failure from longstanding high BP, cardiac disease, or liver disease. Distention of the neck veins may occur later in CHF. If right-sided heart failure is suspect, test for the hepatojugular reflex. Pressure on the liver will displace some of the blood from the liver to cause much neck vein distention. This sign occurs before distended neck veins and denotes congestion and constriction of liver circulation. Distention may also be secondary to local causes (e.g., obstruction from neoplasms, large thyroid, etc.).

Chest

It is important to inspect, auscultate and percuss the chest to search for evidence of effusion, pneumonia, etc. Pneumonia may precipitate CHF. Pleural effusions may be the result of: 1) CHF (from cardiac, renal or liver disease) or 2) longstanding COPD (its complications may be responsible for pneumonia). Inspect for lesions, structural deformities, the quality of respirations, etc. Lesions and deformities may be the source of respiratory compromise that may have been previously compensated for, but in the presence of other factors may now be responsible for decompensation. Tactile fremitus is increased in pneumonia (consolidation) and in fibrosis from old inflammatory processes, or may decrease in pleural effusions and pneumothorax. Dullness may be secondary to pleural effusion, pneumonia, neoplasms or atelectasis. Adventitious sounds may be secondary to acute inflammatory processes, CHF, longstanding COPD, etc.

Heart

The location of the PMI (if displaced laterally or medially) is important information which helps denote cardiomegaly (i.e., LVH, RVH). Cardiomegaly may also be secondary to acute processes or chronic process (e.g., HBP, rheumatic heart disease, etc.).

Abnormalities in rate and rhythm secondary to drug toxicity, conduction defects, etc., may precipitate congestive failure. Bradycardia of whatever origin, in itself may precipitate CHF because of a decreased cardiac output; it is also associated with myxedema.

If murmurs are present, note their location, quality, duration, radiation, etc. and whether they have been present previously. In a negative past history for murmurs, current murmurs may be the result of some new dynamic process (e.g., subacute bacterial endocarditis (SBE), anemia, congestive failure, fever, etc.). Systolic murmurs *may* be functional or flow murmurs and may disappear when the anemia or any other underlying etiology is corrected. Diastolic murmurs are also indicative of organic disease, and a search for their etiology must be made. An S³ gallop is indicative of congestive failure. The S⁴ or atrial gallop sound is related to atrial contraction and may occur with or without any clinical evidence of cardiac problems. Patients with primary myocardial disease, coronary artery disease, hypertension and severe forms of aortic and pulmonic stenosis may have an S⁴.

Rubs may be heard in pericarditis secondary to acute SBE. Subacute bacterial endocarditis may occur as a result of seeding from instrumentation or other causes. Subacute bacterial endocarditis may also cause acute or chronic glomerulonephritis. Rubs may be heard in pericarditis after myocardial infarctions or acute renal failure. Remember, the elderly may have silent myocardial infarctions with the atypical presentation of increased SOB without a history of chest pain.

Abdomen

Distention in early stages may be more difficult to ascertain in the elderly because of their flaccid abdominal musculature; it may be secondary to bloating, or to more serious conditions (e.g., ascites associated with liver disease, CHF, neoplasms, etc.).

Distended abdominal veins are seen in liver disease and/or right-sided failure (occurring secondary to congestion, distention and obstruction of either the lymph or blood flow).

Spider angiomata are fiery red, branching lesions seen on the abdomen, trunk, face and neck. They are arterial in nature, blanch when pressure is applied and return to a red color with pulsating spurts. Spiders are seen frequently in liver disease and may be associated with palmar erythema.

Ascites (the presence of fluid in the abdominal cavity) may be secondary to CHF (right-sided failure), myxedema, renal disease, liver disease, neoplasms, etc. If abdominal distention is present, look for bulging flanks and/or the presence or absence of fluid waves.

Masses may be detectable by inspection on thin, cachectic, elderly people; however, the majority of masses are discovered on palpation. Tenderness of the liver may be seen in right-sided heart failure with the primary etiology being liver disease (obstruction of portal circulation). There are many other causes of liver tenderness.

Hepatomegaly

Hepatic and visceral engorgement secondary to an elevated venous pressure are common in right-sided failure. This manifestation of cardiac failure is reflected by anorexia, bloating and right upper abdominal pain. Numerous hepatic diseases must also be considered in hepatomegaly with edema. Portal hypertension results from the scarring of hepatic cells and the constriction of venous channels in intrinsic hepatic disease. Either enlargement or contraction of the liver may partially constrict the inferior vena cava. Ascites and dependent edema associated with chronic hepatic disease is the result of increased capillary pressure and decreased oncotic pressure.

The finding of hepatomegaly is supported not only by palpation of the liver edge, but also by an increased expansion of the liver denoted by percussion.

Splenomegaly

In the normal adult, the spleen should not be palpable. In reference to the symptom of edema, splenomegaly may be seen in subacute bacterial endocarditis with the complication of acute glomerulonephritis, and in anemias (that are presenting as CHF), collagen vascular disease or liver diseases.

Palpable Lymph Nodes

If present with unilateral or localized edema and in the presence of erythema and warmth, consider edema secondary to some inflammatory process (e.g., cellulitis, boils, etc.). Where obstructions of lymphatic vessels occur, the result is the nonpitting brawny edema of lymph stasis. The skin becomes coarse and rough and recurrent infection may be a problem.

Palmar Erythema

Palmar erythema (a diffuse redness over the hypothenar and thenar areas) is closely associated with the presence of spider angiomata. These are attributed to liver disease.

Temperature of Extremities

Warmth in the presence of edema may denote an inflammatory process (e.g., cellulitis, thrombophlebitis, boils, allergic reactions, or the edema secondary to trauma).

Coolness may denote vascular insufficiency.

Jaundice

Jaundice or icterus are terms used to designate the stain in body tissues and blood that occurs as a result of an excess of bile pigment. They must not be confused with yellow skin caused by carotene, quinacrine, etc. If jaundice is present with edema, hepatic disease must be considered. Jaundice is usually indicative of a serum bilirubin concentration of 2 to 4 mgm/100 ml. It is usually more evident in the sclera, trunk or face. A yellowish discoloration of the skin may also be seen in myxedema. Jaundice may be the first presentation of carcinoma of the pancreas. The importance and etiology of this symptom must be evaluated with the presence or absence of other clinical symptomatology.

Hemiplegia or Paralysis

Edema seen in hemiplegia is said to be caused by the effect of autonomic nervous control of vasoconstriction, complicated by a decreased lymphatic and venous flow from muscular inactivity. In the elderly, consider CVA as a cause of paralysis.

Calf Tenderness, Redness, Pain, + Homan's Sign	These findings may be indicative of thrombophlebitis. Measure both calves for their circumference. Evaluate on the basis of history and physical findings.
Abnormal Reflexes	A decreased return phase of the reflex may be indicative of hypothyroidism. In myxedema, this is usually seen with a dull facial expression, mental dullness, generalized edema (including periorbital edema) and signs of CHF. Reflex changes may be seen after a CVA or secondary to various neuropathies (e.g., diabetic or nutritional as seen in alcoholism or vitamin deficiencies).
Abnormal Mental Status Exams	A change in mental status may occur as a result of an acute brain syndrome from hypoxia, etc., or a chronic brain syndrome secondary to longstanding alcohol abuse.
Abnormal Pulses	Note the presence, absence, quality, etc. of the pulses. They may be decreased or absent in vascular problems (e.g., thrombus, embolus, vascular insufficiency, etc.).
Varicosities	Varicosities may be the sole etiology of unilateral or bilateral dependent edema. However, other etiologies should be excluded before attributing the cause of edema solely to varicosities.

LAB DATA:

Urinalysis	The urinalysis should include both the macroscopic and microscopic exams. The urine color may be bloody in acute glomerulonephritis

or acute renal failure; or dark secondary to increased bile pigments in liver disease.

Proteinuria may be seen in varying amounts in nephrotic syndrome. Proteinuria may also be present in acute renal failure, chronic renal failure, acute/chronic glomerulonephritis, congestive failure and liver disease.

Presence of bile in urine can be indicative of inflammation or obstructive liver disease. The presence of RBCs or RBC casts usually denotes glomerulonephritis. In this instance, WBC casts may also be present which denotes the inflammatory response of this disease. RBC casts may also be seen in renal disease secondary to collagen vascular problems or serum sickness. Granular and epithelial casts may be seen in nephrotic syndrome along with massive proteinuria and fat bodies. Fat bodies may be seen in nephrotic syndrome.

In the aged, one must also consider trauma to the kidney secondary to a fall that might present as hematuria. In addition trauma that causes hypovolemia may precipitate acute renal failure.

Electrolytes

Electrolyte disturbances are commonly associated with both renal and cardiac disease. Hyponatremia may be seen in acute renal failure, chronic renal failure, liver disease, and dehydration. Hyponatremia may also occur as a result of the patient drinking more water than the kidneys can excrete. Hyponatremia may present with muscle twitchings and convulsions. Hyperkalemia may be seen in acute or chronic renal failure and have the danger of inducing a cardiac standstill.

BUN/Creatinine

Azotemia is defined as an elevation in the serum BUN/creatinine. This elevation may be a reflection of impaired renal functioning that causes nitrogenous wastes to be retained or it may occur as a result of many factors (e.g., urinary obstruction, decreased perfusion of the kidney, liver disease, or renal disease).

SMA-12

The number and types of tests included in the group may vary in each institution. Common inclusions are total protein, serum albumin, calcium, phosphorus and cholesterol.

Hypoalbuminemia is seen in nephrotic syndrome, liver disease, acute and chronic glomerulonephritis and chronic renal failure. It may occur secondarily to loss of albumin in the urine, malnutrition or malabsorption. Serum calcium may be decreased in acute or chronic renal failure and nephrotic syndrome. Phosphorus may be increased in acute or chronic renal failure. Cholesterol is increased in nephrotic syndrome and arteriosclerotic heart disease. Triglycerides may be increased in the nephrotic syndrome.

CBC

Normocytic normochromic anemias may be present as a result of chronic disease, and can be attributed either to increased destruction of RBC's or a decreased production. Anemia in itself may precipitate CHF. Anemias may be seen in late, acute renal failure; chronic renal failure; acute or chronic glomerulonephritis; cirrhosis or liver disease; nephrotic syndrome or anemia associated with neoplasms. Leukocytosis may be seen in early, acute renal failure or inflammatory processes. Leukopenia may be seen in liver disease, viral infections or overwhelming bacterial infections.

Liver Function Tests

Liver function tests are usually elevated in liver disease. Transaminases are nonspecific and must be evaluated in light of other clinical symptomatology.

Chest X-ray

The chest x-ray is obtained to ascertain the cardiac silhouette, appearance of the lung fields, and to ascertain the presence of pneumonia, neoplasms, effusions, etc.

EKG

The EKG is done to denote abnormalities in the rate, rhythm, or conduction system, and to identify ischemic changes, etc.

Protime

Clotting abnormalities may be seen in anemias and in liver disease.

Platelets

Thrombocytopenia may be seen in liver disease, and (late) in acute renal failure and serum sickness.

Bleeding disorders may arise from a low platelet count.

ESR

The sedimentation rate is a nonspecific test that is elevated in any inflammatory process. With reference to the complaint of edema, the ESR is increased in collagen vascular disease, acute glomerulonephritis, and subacute bacterial endocarditis as a cause of CHF. It is also increased in the nephrotic syndrome.

ASO Titer (Anti-streptolysin Titer)

If acute glomerulonephritis is suspect on the basis of a history of recent URI and physical findings, then draw an ASO titer. An elevation of the ASO titer may or may not be indicative of strep nephritis.

Thyroid Tests

Hyperthyroidism may precipitate CHF on the basis of an increased cardiac output. Hypothyroidism may precipitate CHF on the basis of decreased cardiac output, arrhythmias, etc. Myxedema may be diagnosed on the basis of a low T^3-T^4 and historical and physical findings.

Flat Plate of Abdomen

Look for hepatosplenomegaly, size of kidneys, presence of renal calculi that may cause urinary obstruction or neoplasms.

24-Hour Urine for Protein/Creatinine Clearance

In patients who present with proteinuria, it is helpful to ascertain quantitatively the amount being excreted in the urine over 24 hours. Protein excretion in excess of .50 mg/day is considered abnormal. Albumin is normally too large to be filtered by the glomerulus; thus, documented proteinuria is suggestive of an altered permeability of the glomerular membrane. Excessive proteinuria occurs in acute and chronic glomerulonephritis, nephrotic syndrome, acute and chronic renal failure, and malignant hypertension.

An index of glomerular functioning can be made by the measurement of creatinine clearance in a 24-hour urine sample, while a serum creatinine is drawn at the same time. Remember that the amount of creatinine that is excreted and formed is dependent upon the amount of muscle mass present. It is not usually affected by dietary protein intake or breakdown. The measurement of creatinine clearance may also be used to ascertain the excretion rate of other substances (e.g., phosphorus).

ASSESSMENT:

Localized Edema
Lymph stasis edema

The underlying mechanism is the impairment of the flow of lymph resulting from a mechanical or an inflammatory obstruction (e.g., trauma, node resection or irradiation, or malignant disease).

Subjectively, the patient complains of painless edema of one or both extremities. There may be a history of episodes of lymphangitis, cellulitis, node resection or irradiation. Malignant disease may be suspected by historical data (e.g., weight loss, anorexia, etc.) or by such objective data as masses, etc. Initially, the edema is pitting, then becomes brawny with time. Palpable nodes may be found in the area draining the affected limb. Look for surgical scars, irradiation burns or skin changes.

Colloidal leak edema

The causes of colloidal leak edema result from capillary fragility. These include trauma, burns, hypersensitivity reactions or insect bites. The patient presents with a history of one of the above. The edematous area frequently is painful. Erythema and usually heat accompany the edema. The edema is usually pitting.

Edema due to increased plasma, increased hydrostatic pressure or decreased tissue pressure

Summer edema is a common complaint of women in hot weather. Subjectively, the review of systems is negative. There are complaints of swelling of ankles on hot days which is worse at night after standing or sitting. The edema disappears on cool days and usually decreases overnight to reappear the next day. There is soft, pitting edema of the feet and ankles. The chest and cardiac exams are normal. The CBC and urinalysis are within normal limits.

Edema of old age or weight loss

Weight-loss edema may accompany convalescence and cachexia. It is probably due to decreased tissue pressure, increased capillary pressure and/or decreased oncotic pressure.

Subjectively, the patient may describe a recent dieting or illness resulting in loss of weight or loss of muscle tissue, especially in the elderly. If weight loss was not intentional, organic or functional causes should be searched for.

Objectively there may be loose, sagging skin and soft edema, especially in the periorbital and dependent areas.

Edema due to interference with venous return

Thrombophlebitis

Subjectively, the patient gives a history of sitting for a long period of time with little activity; later, the patient may complain of a dull ache, tight feeling or frank pain in the calf. The pain increases when the limb is in dependent position and in walking. A feeling of anxiety is common. There is also frequently a history of previous thrombophlebitis.

Swelling is slight (measure both calves) accompanied by tenderness, induration, and rubor. It is rarely bilateral. Pain and spasm of the calf muscles is produced by dorsiflexion of the foot; warmth of the affected leg, slight fever and tachycardia may occur.

Chronic venous insufficiency

Chronic venous insufficiency may be the result of damage caused by deep vein thrombophlebitis. It may also occur as the result of neoplastic obstruction of the pelvic veins.

There is often a history of leg injury or phlebitis. It is characterized by progressive edema of the leg, but ankle edema may be the first sign. Itching and dull discomfort made worse by periods of standing are common complaints. Pain occurs if ulceration is present.

Thin, shiny, atrophic, cyanotic skin is followed by a brownish pigmentation. Eczema and superficial areas of weeping dermatitis often develop. Subcutaneous tissues are thick and fibrous and subject to recurrent ulceration.

Varicose veins

Subjectively, the patient complains of a dull, aching heaviness and feeling of fatigue brought on by periods of standing. This may be accompanied by cramping.

Objectively, dilated, tortuous, elongated veins are visible when standing. Brownish pigmentation and thinning of the skin above the ankles is common in varicosities of longstanding duration. Edema is usually worse at the end of the day.

Edema due to paralysis or stroke

Edema develops in the affected limb because of neurologic problems combined with a decreased lymph and venous flow associated with muscular inactivity.

The patient has a history of stroke

or injury leading to paralysis; there are no signs or symptoms of conditions that cause edema (e.g., cardiac, renal or liver problems). There is pitting edema of the paralyzed limb only; this may become brawny in time.

Orthostatic and stasis edema

Normal venous return against gravity is accomplished by the milking of the veins by muscular activity. Muscular relaxation of dependent parts, therefore, favors venous stasis. In the elderly, there is often added venous constriction caused by hours of sitting or by circular garters which many elderly women prefer to wear. Though underlying causes for edema must be ruled out, this is a common cause of peripheral edema in the institutionalized elderly.

There is little or no edema in the A.M.; pitting edema increases as the day progresses, especially after standing long hours.

The remainder of the physical exam is normal or noncontributory. Underlying cardiac or renal disease may be ruled out by physical exam, CBC and urinalysis.

Generalized Edema

The three most common causes of generalized edema (congestive circulatory failure, renal disease and hepatic disease) are included in this group. The purpose of this protocol is to rule them out as the cause of edema; for this reason, the management is not covered in detail.

Congestive heart failure

Subjectively, the patient may complain of chest pain, abdominal pain, nausea and vomiting. Weakness and fatigue are common. Dyspnea on exertion, orthopnea, paroxysmal nocturnal dyspnea about 1½ hours after retiring, nonproductive cough indicate pulmonary congestion of this disease. There is a history of rapid gain of weight (five to ten pounds) for no apparent reason. Oliguria is characteristic of right-sided failure. History may include longstanding cardiac disease, high blood pressure, renal disease, liver disease, anemia, etc.

Objectively, if a pleural effusion is present the chest exam may include dullness, decreased fremitus and rales and rhonchi. Pneumonia and signs of consolidation may also be present. The heart exam may show a displaced PMI (due to LVH, etc.). Arrhythmias may or may not be present. Pitting edema of lower extremities will be worse at the end of the day, almost disappearing by morning, but may be transferred to a sacral area in bedridden patients. Pulse may be rapid with alternating degrees of forcefulness. An S^3 gallop or murmur may be present. Blood pressure is frequently elevated, neck veins distented when sitting, and cardiomegaly may be found. Hepatomegaly with hepatojugular reflux and ascites may also be found. Chest x-ray may show cardiomegaly, pulmonary congestion. EKG—cardiac changes (see CHF protocol) and arrhythmias may be found. Urine may show 2 + to 3 + protein without RBC's or casts in uncomplicated circulatory failure. There may also be casts and RBC's from longstanding renal parenchymal disease. If congestive heart failure is suspected to be the etiology of the edema, the cause of the congestive heart failure should be sought. For a more complete discussion of CHF, refer to the CHF protocol.

Renal Disease

Renal disease may be primary cause of edema, or it may be the contributing cause such as seen in longstanding high BP with renal parenchymal damage that occurs secondarily. Other secondary causes are renal disease associated with collagen vascular diseases or diabetes mellitus.

Acute renal failure

Acute renal failure may occur as a result of: 1) acute glomerulonephritis, 2) acute pyelonephritis, 3) entities that cause acute tubular necrosis (e.g., sudden illness or injury that may be associated with shock, hypovolemia, etc.), 4) severe vasoconstriction that causes decreased renal perfusion, 5) the ingestion of toxic chemicals (e.g., accidental or intentional overdoses) or 6) rapid hemolysis (e.g., after extensive burns or hemorrhage).

Subjectively, the patient may explain a history of any of the above and/or the symptomatology for acute renal failure (e.g., oliguria, hematuria, weakness and fatigue, and the nausea, vomiting and anorexia that occur secondary to hyponatremia).

Objectively, high blood pressure may be present. Fever may or may not be present. The patient may be alert; however, mental status changes secondary to hyponatremia are not uncommon.

Lab data includes:
Urine—the total output is scanty and most often bloody. The dipstick may be positive for blood and protein. The pH may be high due to the presence of RBC's.
CBC—Leukocytosis and anemia may be present.
Serum calcium—may be low.
BUN/creatinine clearance are elevated.
Electrolytes may show a hyponatremia and hyperkalemia.
A *flat plate of the abdomen* is done to ascertain the size of the kidneys and the presence of stones.
The *EKG* may show signs of hyperkalemia (e.g., high peaked T waves, absence of a P wave, arrhythmias, and/or bradycardia).

Chronic renal failure

Chronic renal failure may occur as a result of a longstanding renal parenchymal disease. The onset of chronic renal failure occurs more slowly. The early signs and symptoms may include only the complaints of polyuria and nocturia. Later symptoms may include anorexia, nausea and vomiting secondary to hyponatremia or GI manifestations of CHF. Other symptoms that occur late are signs of CHF (e.g., breathlessness, insomnia and pallor secondary to the anemia associated with renal parenchymal disease).

Objectively, high blood pressure is usually present. There may be a yellowish coloration of the skin (not to be confused with icterus). The cardiac exam may be consistent with that of CHF. Edema is usually generalized and pitting. The neurologic exam may reveal mental status changes and muscle twitchings may be secondary to a decreased serum calcium or hyponatremia. If these imbalances and chronic renal failure are untreated, the patient may progress to convulsions and/or coma.

The lab data may include:
CBC—reveals a normocytic normochromic anemia of chronic disease. The anemia may be secondary to an increased destruction of RBC's or decreased production.
Calcium—the serum calcium is low.
Electrolytes—hyponatremia and hyperkalemia may be present.
BUN/creatinine clearance—the BUN and creatinine are usually elevated.
Serum albumin—usually decreased due to a loss of protein in the urine.
The EKG may show signs of electrolyte imbalance, (e.g., hyperkalemia, arrhythmias, bradycardia, etc.).
The chest x-ray may reveal an enlarged cardiac silhouette or other signs of CHF.

Acute Glomerulonephritis

Acute glomerulonephritis is most commonly associated with a post-streptococcal infection. However, it may be a complication of subacute bacterial endocarditis or (in a younger population) a complication of any of the collagen vascular diseases.

Subjective data may include a history of a recent URI, hematuria, fever, weakness, fatigue, generalized edema or weight gain. The generalized edema may be a facial edema. However, in older patients peripheral edema may be a more common presentation.

Objectively, the patient is usually hypertensive and the chest and cardiac exams may reveal signs of failure. The abdominal exam may reveal pain and hepatomegaly secondary to CHF. If the patient has SBE, splenomegaly may be present.

The lab data may include:
Urine—the urine is a dark bloody color. The dipstick is positive for blood and protein. The specific gravity may be increased. The microscopic urinalysis shows RBC, RBC casts, WBC casts and granular casts.
BUN/creatinine clearance elevated.
Electrolytes show decreased sodium and elevated potassium.
CBC shows anemia.
ASO titer is elevated.

Chronic Glomerulonephritis

Chronic glomerulonephritis may occur as a result of a renal parenchymal disease of longstanding duration.

The subjective data may include evidence of repeated UTIs and repeated bouts of pyelonephritis. A history of obstructive uropathy or other urologic problems *may* be completely negative.

The objective data are the same as for acute glomerulonephritis.

Nephrotic Syndrome

Nephrotic syndrome is a clinical syndrome that is composed of generalized edema, massive proteinuria, and hypoalbuminemia. It occurs when there has been dramatic glomerular damage.

Subjective data may include a previous history of glomerulonephritis, etc. The onset of the nephrotic syndrome is usually insidious with a gradual progression of the edematous state. Signs and symptoms may be associated with the hypoalbuminemia or signs of CHF.

Objectively, the patient may appear pale, lethargic, with facial edema and/or generalized edema. The edema is characteristically soft and pitting. Hepatomegaly may be present secondary to CHF. The chest and cardiac exams may also have findings consistent with CHF. The BP may be within normal limits.

The lab data may include:
CBC showing anemia.
Urinalysis may show a massive pro-

teinuria with microscopic granular epithelial casts, lipid bodies and RBC's on the microscopic exam.
BUN/creatinine clearance elevated.
24-hour urine protein shows massive proteinuria.
Serum albumin low.
Serum calcium low.
Cholesterol and triglycerides elevated.
Chest x-ray, EKG, and electrolytes may show signs of CHF.

Liver Disease

There are a number of clinical entities categorized under the heading of liver disease. It is not the purpose of this protocol to discuss each, but some general signs and symptoms and objective findings are presented.

Subjectively, the historical data may include a wide variety of etiologies for the current problem of proteinuria. General symptomatology of hepatic disease includes a history of nausea, vomiting, fatigue, weakness, anorexia, weight loss, jaundice, dark urine, clay-colored stools, alopecia, ascites, intermittent ankle edema, purpuric rashes, itching and a low-grade temperature. There may be a history of alcohol abuse.

Objective findings may include scleral icterus, spider angiomata (on the face, neck, chest), increased jugular venous pressure, signs of CHF on the chest and cardiac exams, abdominal distention and/or ascites, large abdominal dilated veins, hepatomegaly, and/or tenderness over the liver, splenomegaly, muscular wasting, ankle edema, palmar erythema and jaundice.

The lab data may include:
CBC may show anemia or leukopenia.
Platelets may reveal thrombocytopenia.
Liver function tests may be abnormally elevated.
Protime may be normal or prolonged.
Serum albumin may be low.
Electrolytes may reveal hyponatremia and hypokalemia.
Urine may show protein and/or bilirubin.

Myxedema

Myxedema is a severe form of hypothyroidism. If the hypothyroidism is of longstanding duration and remains untreated, the clinical presentation may be that of peripheral edema and signs of CHF. It is important to recognize this because the CHF can be easily treated and alleviated by treatment of the underlying disease.

Subjective data may include a history of cold intolerance, weight gain, fatigue, skin and hair changes (increased dryness and coarseness of the hair and/or alopecia), constipation, fatigue, confusion, signs of CHF, dysphagia, and/or a history of thyroid surgery.

Objective data may include a yellowish discoloration of the skin (be careful not to confuse it with jaundice) dry skin, coarse hair, hoarseness, facial edema, dull affect, thick tongue, mental status changes, signs of CHF, slowed return phase of the deep tendon reflexes, and/or enlarged thyroid.

The lab data may include:
CBC may show either a normocytic or macrocytic anemia.
T^3-T^4 may be depressed.
Chest x-ray may reveal cardiomegaly or other signs of CHF.
EKG may reveal arrhythmias, a prolonged P-R interval, low voltage or T-wave inversions.
Serum cholesterol may be elevated.

Iatrogenic Edema

Several medications predispose to fluid retention. This protocol delineates specifically those that are frequently given to the elderly.

Subjectively, the patient complains of an onset of edema shortly after initiating therapy with one of the steroids (e.g., corticosteroids, estrogens, androgen, anabolic agents and progesteronal compounds), or some nonsteroidal antiinflammatory agents (e.g., phenylbutazone, oxyphenbutazone, and occasionally indomethacin). The fluorinated corticosteroids are less likely to cause edema.

The iatrogenic edema is a generalized, pitting edema due to sodium retention. Leukocytosis may be present in the patient taking steroids.

315

Protein Deficiency of Poor Nutrition

Edema due to protein deficiency may be found in the poor and elderly due to inadequate nutrition or following bowel surgery.

The patient reports a high carbohydrate, low protein diet (over an extended period) or a history of bowel surgery. She or he may also complain of apathy, irritability, and/or anorexia.

Objectively, there may be skin changes (rash, desquamation, hyperpigmentation or depigmentation), cheilosis, stomatitis, muscular wasting, conjunctivitis, and/or pitting edema. Anemia, hypoalbuminuria, and hyperglobulinemia may also be found.

Sodium Intake Exceeding Capacity of Kidney to Excrete

Sodium intake that exceeds the capacity of the kidney to excrete it is usually due to underlying kidney disease; it may also be due to a poor diet or poor patient education.

The patient subjectively gives a history of renal disease. The patient has been asked to adhere to a low sodium diet but frequently the patient is not complying or family or friends may be bringing foods high in sodium to the patient.

Objectively, the patient has a wide daily variation in weight and edema plus symptoms of an underlying disease.

OVERALL PLAN

Diuretics

Before initiating any diuretic therapy, the patient should be carefully assessed, the cause of the edema determined and treatment of that disease initiated. Treatment of the underlying disorder may or may not include a diuretic. It is to be noted that mild edema is not harmful and, conversely, too vigorous a diuresis can cause serious problems. The elderly have an increased sensitivity to any drug and it is important to keep this in mind when giving diuretics. A target weight loss should be no more than two to three pounds a day.

Whenever diuretic therapy is being used in the elderly, care must be taken to prevent dehydration resulting in reduction of blood volume and circulatory collapse; the possibility of thrombosis and embolism, dilutional hyponatremia and hypokalemia should be also watched for. The patient should be carefully monitored both clinically and by periodic determination of serum electrolytes to detect possible electrolyte imbalance. Other problems commonly found in the institutionalized elderly, which can be traced to diuretics, are constipation and orthostatic hypotension.

In view of the problems connected with diuretic therapy in the elderly, their use cannot be justified for long-term therapy of benign and nonprogressive conditions.

Staff Education

Education is the most effective way to gain staff cooperation in management of peripheral edema in the elderly. Points to include are as follows:

1. Some basics in physiology of edema with differentiation of the causes, and emphasis on those which commonly affect the institutionalized elderly.
2. Nursing management of edema, considering measures which can be implemented to avoid the use of diuretics.
   a. Avoidance of constricting clothing.
   b. Decreased sodium intake.
   c. Frequent changes in position; walking whenever possible.
   d. Elevation of the affected extremity.
3. Common problems encountered in the prolonged use of diuretics because of alteration in fluid and electrolyte balance.
   a. Symptoms of hypokalemia, hyponatremia, hypochloremia.

    b. Constipation, oliguria or dehydration.

    c. Orthostatic hypotension.

Patient Teaching

Many of the elderly are capable of cooperating in management of their edema. Patient teaching should include:

1. The value of active exercise in avoiding and treating peripheral edema.
2. The need to avoid excessive ingestion of salty foods. It will often be necessary to discuss which foods and OTC medications have a high sodium content, so that the patient can avoid them.
3. The advantage of periodically elevating the feet.
4. Problems associated with circular garters, tight clothing.

Flow Sheet

The following flow sheet for peripheral edema is an example of a tool that can be used to monitor the patient's progress. The sheet can be inserted directly into the patient's chart, maintained by the patient and public health nurse, etc. The actual frequency of monitoring each item must be a joint decision by the practitioners managing the patient's care. This decision needs to be based on the patient, his or her diagnosis for the cause of the edema, present health status, etc.

FLOW SHEET FOR PERIPHERAL EDEMA	PATIENT'S DIAGNOSED CAUSE OF EDEMA							
	FREQUENCY TO MONITOR	DATES:						
BP								
Weight								
Intake (ml/day)								
Output (ml/day)								
Frequency of Extremity Elevation/Day								
Daily Exercise (describe)								
Elastic Stocking Use								

Diet (calories/day)								
Medication (List #'s corresponding to key)								
Edema (describe)								
CBC								
Urinalysis								
Na$^+$								
K$^+$								

Key to Medications

1. _____
2. _____
3. _____
4. _____
5. _____
6. _____

SPECIFIC PLAN:

Localized Edema
Lymph stasis edema

Do CBC and urinalysis to rule out systemic disease.
Overall therapy:
1. To aid flow to lymph out of extremities:
   a. Intermittent elevation of extremity. For the lower extremities, elevate the foot of the bed 15 to 20 degrees at two-hour intervals (if practical, during sleeping hours) and one to three hours during the day.
   b. Constant use of elastic bandages or well-fitting elastic stockings; the patient should be taught the correct use of these stockings.

c. Massage toward the trunk either by hand or by pneumatic pressure device.
2. Good hygiene to avoid cellulitis. Any infection should be treated with adequate rest, elevation and antibiotics.
3. Intermittent courses of diuretics in times of exacerbation or in uncontrolled lymphedema to prevent a grotesque deformity.

Colloidal leak edema

The treatment approach would depend on the underlying etiology. Consult and/or refer to the patient's physician in managing the underlying cause of the edema.

Edema due to increased plasma, increased hydrostatic pressure or decreased tissue pressure

Do a CBC and urinalysis if it has not been done recently. Observe the pattern of swelling for one week.

Overall therapy:
1. Elevate feet whenever possible during the day.
2. Avoid tight clothes, especially circular garters, hose with elastic tops, tight panties, and panty girdles.
3. Avoid salty food. Diuretics are not indicated.
4. Elastic stockings or support stockings may help.

Edema of old age or weight loss

Do a CBC, urinalysis and complete physical exam to rule out underlying disease.
Overall therapy:
1. Diuretics are not indicated.
2. Frequent changes in position are helpful to move the edema.
3. Exercise may help increase tis-

sue pressure over a period of time.

4. Avoid excessive salt intake.

5. A good high protein diet may help to increase oncotic pressure.

Edema due to interference with venous return

Thrombophlebitis   Refer patient to the physician.

Chronic venous insufficiency

To rule out systemic disease, do a complete physical exam, CBC, and urinalysis. Diuretics are not indicated.

Overall therapy:

1. Intermittent elevation of legs during the day and elevation at night.

2. Avoidance of long periods of standing.

3. Use of well-fitting, heavy-duty elastic stocking from midfoot to just below the knee.

4. Instruction on the proper hygiene of the skin in order to prevent infection.

Varicose veins

Overall therapy:

1. Use of elastic stockings, from the proximal foot up to but not including the knee, while standing or sitting.

2. Elevation of legs (preferably on bed) from one to two hours during the day.

3. Being alert for common complications: thrombophlebitis and stasis ulcers.

Edema due to paralysis or stroke	The patient should be on physical therapy. Any return of mobility will help alleviate the edema. The physical therapy and leg care should include passive ROM, massage toward the trunk, and elevation (to assist return flow of lymph and venous blood). Diuretics are not indicated.
Orthostatic or stasis edema	If patient is able to walk, it is essential that she or he do so. The distance and number of times will depend on ability. Diuretics are not indicated.
	Elevate the feet on the bed at least an hour during the day (two to three times a day if unable to walk). Sitting, even with feet elevated, will cause constriction especially in the thin patient. Avoid tight clothes. Tight belts, undershorts or panties, girdles (especially circular garters), rolled and tied stockings, or socks with elastic tops should be avoided.

Generalized Edema

Congestive heart failure	Order CBC, electrolytes, SMA, urinalysis, BUN/creatinine, chest x-ray, and EKG. If preliminary findings indicate CHF, refer to CHF protocol.

Renal disease

Acute renal failure	If acute renal failure is suspected, refer to a physician.
Chronic renal failure	If an assessment of chronic renal failure is suspected, the patient must be evaluated by a physician.

Acute glomerulonephritis	If an assessment of acute glomerulonephritis is suspected, refer the patient to a physician.
Chronic glomerulonephritis	If an assessment of chronic glomerulonephritis is suspected, refer the patient to a physician.
Nephrotic syndrome	Refer the patient with suspected nephrotic syndrome to a physician.
Liver disease	If an assessment of liver disease is suspect, refer the patient to a physician.
Myxedema	If the patient shows signs of myxedematous hypothyroidism, refer to a physician.
Iatrogenic edema	Consult with the patient's physician regarding the selection of a medication which retains the same desired therapeutic properties with less sodium retention. Decrease salt intake; this will decrease water retention and also result in a potassium saving.
	Use of diuretic may be necessary if the edema is not controlled by the above means (i.e., if the causative agent is essential therapy).
Protein deficiency of poor nutrition	Consult with a physician if the etiology of the edema is suspected of being caused by protein deficiency. Nutritional counseling (including the use of a dietician) is essential.

Overall Plan

Sodium intake exceeding kidney capacity to excrete	Redo a complete dietary history to ascertain the foods the patient is eating and has eaten. Patient education as to the importance of sodium intake restriction is essential. Depending on the severity of the edema, the patient should be referred to his or her physician if there is no improvement with the above approach.

REFERENCES

1. Chinn, A. *Clinical Aspects of Aging, Working with Older People*, Vol. 4. Rockville, Md.: Department of Health, Education and Welfare, 1971.
2. "Clinical Concepts of Edema." *Patient Care*, December 1969.
3. DeGowin, E. and R. DeGowin. *Bedside Diagnostic Examination*. New York: Macmillan Publishing, 1976.
4. Friedman, H. *Problem-Oriented Medical Diagnosis*. Boston: Little, Brown and Co., 1975.
5. Hudak, C. *Clinical Protocols*. Philadelphia: J.B. Lippincott Co., 1976.
6. Krupp, M. and M. Chatton. *Current Diagnosis and Therapy*. Canada: Lange Medical Publications, 1977.
7. MacBryde, C. M. and R. S. Blacklow. *Signs and Symptoms*. Philadelphia: J.B. Lippincott Co., 1970.
8. Moyer, J. and M. Juchs. *Edema, Mechanics and Management*. Philadelphia: W.B. Saunders Company, 1960.
9. Smith, D. and L. Gipps. *Care of the Adult Patient*. Philadelphia: J.B. Lippincott Co., 1966.
10. Walker, H., W. Hall, and J. Hurst. *Clinical Methods*. Wolburn, Mass.: Butterworth, Inc., 1976.
11. Wollach, J. *Interpretation of Diagnostic Tests*. Boston: Little, Brown and Co., 1974.

Chapter 7

Skin Diseases

OVERVIEW

Appraisal of the skin in the aging person requires a vigilant practitioner. Since 86 percent of the elderly have one or more chronic conditions (Brotman, 1974) the practitioner is often faced with multisystem complaints and there is a tendency to overlook the seemingly less dramatic skin changes or conditions. Often these lesions are discovered during a routine examination or reported as an incidental complaint by the patient. An ability to recognize the significance of these lesions' pathological implications requires knowledge of the clinical picture of the common skin lesions, their incidence and expected course. With this information the practitioner can discriminate anticipated skin changes from more abnormal conditions, establish a diagnosis and initiate the appropriate plan of action.

Recognition of skin lesions in man's largest, most visible organ requires an appreciation that the aging skin has borne witness to the passage of time. In the geriatric patient, the skin evidences the cumulative effects of heredity, environment, health habits and preexisting pathology. The interplay of these forces results in a number of anticipated involutional changes.

Anticipated involutional skin changes found routinely during an exam involve the skin's general appearance. Notably, it appears lax, primarily because of the loss of subcutaneous fat, elastic tissue, and the effects of gravitational pull. On palpation the skin is generally less elastic, lacks turgor and is thin; it may exhibit marked thickening in some localized areas. A generalized dehydration also appears as a result of decreased sebaceous and sweat gland activity and reduced water content. Patches of rough fishlike scales may be evident due to the hypertrophy of the horny layers.

The nails also become more keratinized, resulting in thick, brittle appendages with a tendency to peel and become distorted. On the scalp, the hair grays or lightens in color, thins out and becomes less wavy; in the nose and ears, hair becomes thicker.

Characteristic changes in the face and neck occur with age. A generalized decrease in melanin production gives the face and neck a more uniform color of opaque or white. Spotting or clustering of pigmented areas result as melanocytes lose their ability to spread out in a uniform pattern. Lines of facial expression around the mouth, eyes and nose are exaggerated by drying and the loss of elastic tissue. In addition, the mucous membrane in the mouth becomes (thin) like parchment. Atrophy of the salivary glands contributes to the dry mouth sensation and to halitosis. Small facial vessels become more prominent and hormonal changes contribute to chin whiskers in women.

The genitalia also show age-related changes. The external genitalia undergo involutional changes such as sparse pubic hair and a reduction in the size of the genitals; the vaginal outlet decreases. Hormonal changes contribute to a smooth, dry, glistening appearance of rugae and mucosa with increased friability. The cervix may be difficult to identify secondary to multiple deliveries or vaginal repairs.

A major concern for the practitioner is to discover lesions in the elderly skin that may be a cutaneous cancer. Some areas of skin in the elderly are more prone to this than others. Neoplastic changes can arise in exposed areas chronically irritated by sun, chemicals or friction. Outdoor laborers, tar pitch workers and pipe smokers have a higher incidence of precancerous and cancerous conditions. Especially susceptible are blue-eyed, fair complexioned individuals, who have a limited number of protective melanocytes. The risk of excessive sunlight exposure is evidenced in the United States by the greater mortality rate from skin cancer in the southeast and south central states than in northern states.

The commonality of skin changes and skin conditions in the elderly make it necessary for the practitioner to develop some skill and expertise in managing these problems. Although some plans of action may require the specialized skills of a dermatologist, most are within the realm of the primary care practitioner.

SKIN CHANGES—SKIN CONDITIONS WORKSHEET

To be used in patients with
pruritus, skin changes, lesions,
growths and skin problems.

What you cannot afford to miss: Cutaneous cancers.

Chief Complaint: _____

SUBJECTIVE DATA:

Date Commenced: _____
Describe All Positives

ONSET—DURATION:
YES   NO

_____ _____ Acute (< 3 weeks): _____

_____ _____ Subacute: _____

_____ _____ Chronic (> 3 months): _____

LOCATION—DISTRIBUTION:
YES   NO

_____ _____ Local: _____

_____ _____ Regional: _____

_____ _____ Generalized: _____

_____ _____ Universal (total involvement): ____

_____ _____ Symmetrical: _____

_____ _____ Asymmetrical: _____

Skin Changes—Skin Conditions Worksheet

TYPE AND CHARACTER OF LESION:

YES　　*NO*

_____　_____　Primary:_____

_____　_____　Secondary: _____

COURSE:

YES　　*NO*

_____　_____　Continuous: _____

_____　_____　Progressive: _____

_____　_____　Intermittent:_____

_____　_____　Cyclic:_____

_____　_____　Stable:_____

_____　_____　Subsiding: _____

ASSOCIATED WITH:

YES　　*NO*

_____　_____　Occupation: _____

_____　_____　Leisure activities: _____

_____　_____　Habits: _____

_____　_____　Season: _____

_____　_____　Immediate environment: _____

_____　_____　Food: _____

_____　_____　Drugs:_____

_____　_____　Relocation and travel: _____

——— ——— Mechanical factors: _____

——— ——— Previous trauma (Koebner's phenomenon): _____

ANY ASSOCIATED MANIFESTATIONS:

Local

YES *NO*

——— ——— Pruritus: _____

——— ——— Pain: _____

——— ——— Burning: _____

——— ——— Change in color: _____

Systemic

YES *NO*

——— ——— Fever/chills: _____

——— ——— Constitutional symptoms: _____

——— ——— Alleviated or aggravated by anything: _____

_____

ANY CURRENT TREATMENT:
YES *NO*

——— ——— Current treatment (e.g., prescription medications;

oral, injectable, topical; over-the-counter prepara-

tions; soaps, oils, shampoos, etc.): _____

_____

_____

_____ _____ Past evaluation or treatment (when, where, by whom,

diagnosis, biopsy, therapy, result): _____

_____

_____

PAST MEDICAL HISTORY:
YES   NO

_____ _____ Cutaneous: _____

_____

_____ _____ Noncutaneous: _____

_____

FAMILY HISTORY:
YES   NO

_____ _____ Psoriasis: _____

_____ _____ Seborrheic dermatitis: _____

_____ _____ Rosacea: _____

_____ _____ Atopic eczema: _____

_____ _____ Alopecia: _____

_____ _____ Cutaneous cancer: _____

OBJECTIVE DATA:

Age: _____

Sex: _____ Male _____ Female

General Appearance: _____

_____

SKIN EXAM: GENERAL
YES   NO

_____ _____ Skin color changes: _____

_____ _____ Vascular or purpuric changes: _____

_____ _____ Texture abnormality (moisture, temperature, rough,

etc.): _____

_____

_____ _____ Lesions (general configuration, distribution on body,

whether primary or secondary): _____

_____

_____

SKIN EXAM: REGIONAL

(Describe if abnormal, noting type, configuration and arrangement of lesions)

NAILS:
YES   NO

_____ _____ Hyperkeratotic: _____

_____ _____ Friable: _____

_____ _____ Pitting: _____

_____ _____ Onycholysis: _____

FINGER/HANDS/ARMS:
YES   NO

_____ _____ Hyperpigmentation: _____

_____ _____ Papule: _____

Skin Changes—Skin Conditions Worksheet

_____ _____ Scale: _____

_____ _____ Plaque: _____

_____ _____ Lichenification: _____

HAIR/SCALP:
YES *NO*

_____ _____ Alopecia: _____

_____ _____ Erythema: _____

_____ _____ Scale: _____

_____ _____ Plaque: _____

_____ _____ Pigmented papules: _____

FACE/EXTERNAL EAR/NECK:
YES *NO*

_____ _____ Central erythema on face: _____

_____ _____ Papule: _____

_____ _____ Pustule: _____

_____ _____ Vascular changes: _____

_____ _____ Scale: _____

_____ _____ Hyperkeratosis: _____

_____ _____ Nodule: _____

_____ _____ Tumor: _____

_____ _____ Lichenified plaque: _____

TRUNK:
YES   NO

_____ _____ Scale: _____

_____ _____ Papule: _____

_____ _____ Maculopapular:_____

_____ _____ Papulosquamous: _____

_____ _____ Zosteriform vesicles: _____

LOWER EXTREMITIES:
YES   NO

_____ _____ Scale: _____

_____ _____ Plaque: _____

_____ _____ Hyperpigmentation: _____

_____ _____ Vascular changes: _____

_____ _____ Ulcers:_____

FEET:
YES   NO

_____ _____ Vesiculobullous eruptions:_____

_____ _____ Scale: _____

_____ _____ Fissures: _____

_____ _____ Hyperkeratotic changes: _____

MOUTH:
YES   NO

_____ _____ Improperly fitting dentures: _____

_____ _____ Plaque: _____

Skin Changes—Skin Conditions Worksheet

——— ——— Dull white patches:————————————————

——— ——— Fissures: ——————————————————————

——— ——— Crusts:————————————————————————

GENITALS:
YES　　*NO*

——— ——— Papules:————————————————————————

——— ——— Plaque: ——————————————————————————

——— ——— Discharge: ——————————————————————

——— ——— Chancre: ————————————————————————

LYMPH NODE EXAM:
YES　　*NO*

——— ——— Enlarged/tender nodes: ————————————

———

LAB DATA: (DESCRIBE ALL FINDINGS)
　　　NOT
DONE　*DONE*

——— ——— Magnification of lesions: ————————————

——— ——— Illumination of lesions: ——————————————

——— ——— Diascopy of lesions: ————————————————

——— ——— Tzanck smear test (for differentiation of vesicular

herpetic lesions): ————————————————————————

——— ——— Darkfield examination (if the lesion is a painless ul-

cerated chancre): ————————————————————————

——— ——— KOH prep (if suspect monilia or tinea lesions): ———

——— ——— Culture (if lesions appear secondarily infected): ___

——— ——— Biopsy (in any lesion that has recently changed in size, color, appearance or with no known diagnosis):

———————————————————————————————————

——— ——— CBC with differential (if you suspect a skin manifestation of an underlying disease, or allergic reaction):

——— ——— VDRL (if you suspect syphilis): _____

——— ——— Platelets (if patient has purpuric lesions): _____

SKIN CHANGES—SKIN CONDITIONS WORKSHEET RATIONALE

SUBJECTIVE DATA:

Onset—Duration

Acute conditions usually last less than three weeks. They are more definite in onset and have a shorter duration. In the elderly, chronic conditions are more common, lasting longer than three months. They develop insidiously, making it difficult to pinpoint the time of onset. Subacute is considered between three weeks and three months.

Location—Distribution

Lesions occur locally, regionally, generally in a symmetrical or asymmetrical fashion. Identify the initial lesion and the subsequent pattern of eruption. Aids to diagnosis are the definitive patterns arising in specific anatomical regions.

Type and Character

Primary and secondary changes reflect the type of the lesions (see Appendix A). Ask about the wet, weepy or dry character of the lesions, including their roughness and their relation to the plane of the skin, such as elevated, level, depressed.

Course

The sequence of the condition can be continuous, flare up intermittently, or appear cyclically as with seasons. The lesions can subside quickly or slowly. Progression is manifested by the development of additional lesions, changing sequence in sites, and/or the coalescence of lesions.

Associated With
Occupation, leisure habits

Long-term exposure to carcinogenic precursors or agents are. hazardous to the skin. Inquire about variables such as working in the sun or near pitch or tar and exposure to chemicals, irritants, tobacco and/or their exhalants.

Season

Some conditions are more prevalent, exacerbate or remit at different times of the year. A contributing factor to dry skin is the dehydration that occurs in low-humidity heated residences in the winter. During the summer months, there is a greater exposure to allergens and chemical plant irritants. Summer is also a time when some improvement may be seen in psoriasis.

Immediate environment

Consider agents that cause allergic or contact problems such as animals, plants, metals or items used in hobbies.

Food

Alcohol, hot liquids, coffee and tea

may aggravate rosacea. Certain foods may cause allergic response, such as fruits, chocolate, or seafood.

Drugs

The elderly frequently take many drugs, swallowing many pills each day. As a result, a number of drug reactions or interactions can occur. A detailed history of all possible agents needs to be taken, including both prescribed and nonprescribed drugs. Inquire about sleeping agents, hypertensive drugs, nerve medications, vitamins, laxatives, headache remedies and recent vaccination or flu shots.

Relocation and travel

With retirement or death of a spouse, the elderly often relocate. This stressful event can precipitate neurodermatitis. Taking up winter resdence in southern climates can cause repeated exposure to intense sun.

Mechanical factors

Chronic irritation can occur from footwear, bed linen or clothing. Exposure to solvents or detergents can break down the protective sebaceous coating leading to drying of the skin.

Previous trauma

Due to isomorphic response, psoriatic lesions can arise at sites of previous or acute trauma (Koebner's phenomenon).

Associated Manifestations—Local
Pruritus

Pruritus is a disagreeable condition which can be felt as itching, burning, crawling or stinging in localized or generalized areas. It can range from mild to severe even to the point of disturbing sleep. Pruritus is caused by irritation or allergic sensitization which stimulates nonspecific itch receptors in the superficial dermis, releasing proteolytic enzymes. This is translated into a modified form of pain which is usually relieved by scratching. Causes for pruritus can be physiologic, idiopathic, specific cutaneous diseases, or underlying systemic diseases.

Pain, burning

Superficial pain can be due to secondary skin changes, i.e., fissures, which are aggravated by motion or moisture. Neuritic pain is found in approximately two-thirds of the patients afflicted by herpes zoster; over age 60 chronic postherpetic pain can result. Burning can occur in primary erythematous lesions or from secondary irritation caused by rubbing.

Color change

The skin is subject to hypo- or hyperpigmentation. Additional color changes may include local vascular changes such as erythema, telangiectasia or purpura.

Associated Manifestations—Systemic
Fever/chills, constitutional symptoms

Acute problems can manifest systemic symptoms like fever and chills. Constitutional symptoms such as weight loss may reflect underlying systemic disease, hormonal imbalances, or improper nutrition.

Alleviated By

Inquire about what has helped improve the condition. Dry lesions are often improved by hydrating agents and wet lesions by drying agents. Removal of the irritant or allergen such as change of detergent or season can help identify the precipitant.

Current Treatment
Prescription meds
Oral
Injectable
Topical
Over-the-counter agents
Soaps, oils, shampoos

Due to the chronicity of some conditions and living on fixed incomes, the elderly can resort to economical home remedies such as plasters, packs or a friend's supply of oral or topical agents. Soaps and oils such as mineral oil can act like drying agents. Commonly used OTC topical agents such as the caines medicaments can sensitize the lesion and even change its original appearance. Inquire about recent procedures or therapeutics prescribed by dentists or doctors.

Past Evaluation or Treatment

Long-term or intermittent therapy may have been employed for the more chronic lesions. Previous treatment modalities such as arsenic or radiation therapy may put the patient at risk for skin disease. Include duration, course, response to treatment and biopsy results.

Past Medical History
Cutaneous

Inquire about similar or apparently unrelated eruptions. Dates, duration, course, response to treatment.

Noncutaneous

A noncutaneous history of any systemic illness preceding, concurrent or subsequent to the initial onset should be ascertained. Inquire about allergy, venereal disease and diseases specific for dermatoses such as hyperlipidemia or diabetes.

Family History

Conditions that have a familial tendency are alopecia, atopic eczema, psoriasis, rosacea, and seborrheic dermatitis.

OBJECTIVE DATA:

Inspection and palpation are the principal modalities for the physical exam. Visual aids can include a pocket magnifier (2 to 7×) and transillumination. The patient should be completely disrobed. Adequate illumination is necessary, preferably natural daylight. Measuring lesions can be aided by a small, transparent ruler.

General Appearance

Observe the patient's nutritional state, degree of discomfort, hygiene and mental status.

Skin Exam

Initially conduct an overall low-power assessment. Generally survey: 1) changes in skin color; 2) vascular or purpuric changes; 3) the coolness or warmth of the tissue; 4) the type and degree of moisture (dryness, wetness or oiliness); 5) smoothness or roughness of the texture. Define lesions as primary or secondary, noting their color, size, shape, surface and relationship to the plane of the skin (see Appendix A). To assess the distribution, stand back from the disrobed patient to observe anatomical patterns. Configuration or arrangement of the lesions should be identified, such as annular, umbilicated zosteriform, polycyclic. Observe the lesions for a solitary, linear or grouped arrangement.

Nail Exam

In the elderly, the nails become more keratinized, resulting in thick, brittle nails with a tendency to peel and become distorted. Observe the nails for hyperkeratosis (fungal infections) and pitting, friableness, onycholysis (indicate psoriasis).

Fingers/Hands/Arms

Examine the dorsal aspects of the hands and wrists, the flexor and ex-. tensor surfaces of the elbows and the axilla for hyperpigmentation (lentigines), the lichenification (of atopic dermatitis or lichen simplex chronicus) and scaling (representative of psoriasis or lichen simplex chronicus). Observe fingers for verrucous papules.

Hair/Scalp

Anticipated changes are graying or lightening in color of the hair. It becomes thin, less kinky and wavy. Although there is a tendency for central alopecia, loss of 20 to 100 hairs daily is normal. Dryness of the scalp increases with age. Examine for hair texture, distribution and any patterns of alopecia. Observe for erythema or scales on the scalp and keratosis at the hairline (indicates seborrheic dermatitis). Psoriatic plaques can also be seen on the scalp.

Face/External Ear/Neck

Observe the more prominent epidermal sites for the superkeratinization of precancerous and cancerous lesions that arise from long-term sunlight exposure. Identify the active sebaceous gland areas, observing for the gritty, greasy scale of seborrheic dermatitis or the erythema of rosacea. Look for discrete vascular changes such as telangiectasia or venous lakes. Elevations above the skin can occur with skin tags and actinic keratosis. Lichenified plaques of lichen simplex chronicus can appear in the nuchal area.

Trunk

Seborrheic conditions are common on the presternal and interscapular areas. Typical distribution patterns of neurodermatitis (lesions in areas where patient can scratch) and herpes zoster (vesicular lesions unilaterally coursing along a nerve root) can be readily observed on the trunk. Isolated cherry angiomas can arise on the lower thorax. Monilial and bacterial infections can be observed under the pendulous breasts of women.

Lower Extremities

The anterior tibial region is a common site for dry, scaly conditions of xerosis and lichen simplex chronicus. Psoriasis can often be seen on the knees. Vascular changes (discoloration) in the lower extremities contribute to the presence of stasis dermatitis, purpura and venous stars.

Feet

Trauma by footwear promotes hyperkeratotic changes on the prominences of the feet, giving rise to corns and calluses. Examine instep and plantar surface for various stages of athlete's foot or plantar warts. Dry, brittle toenails can harbor fungal infections.

Mouth

Edentulous patients may struggle with dentures that become loose with weight loss or loss of muscle tone. Examine carefully the buccal mucosa, gums, tongue and inner aspect of the lips for the dull white patches of leukoplakia. Macerated fissures angulating at the corners of the mouth may indicate perlèche which can become crusted by secondary invasion of fungus or bacteria.

Genital Exam

Look for the discrete gray-white plaques of leukoplakia on the inner surfaces on the labia and perineum. Fungal infections (monilia) and venereal lesions (chancre, verrucous lesions) should be identified.

Lymph Node Exam

Regional adenopathy can occur with secondary infection of cutaneous lesions, metastases of cutaneous cancers, and with venereal disease.

LAB DATA:

Visual Aids

Magnification

Pocket magnifiers (2 to 7×) can be used to assess the more discrete differentiating characteristics of lesions like the raised border of basal cell carcinoma.

Illumination

Sidelighting of lesions in a darkened room is helpful to detect surface configurations, elevations, depressions or the subtle extensions of eruptions.

Diascopy

Diascopy permits the differentiation of erythematous macules from purpura. Firmly press a glass slide over the lesion. The capillary dilatation of erythema will blanch.

Tzanck Smear Test

This test is used to determine the presence of giant epithelial cells or multinucleated giant cells in vesiculobullous lesions like herpes zoster. Using a #15 scalpel blade, gently open the vesicle and scrape the base. Smear specimen on a slide and prepare with Giemsa's or Wright's stain.

Darkfield Examination

This test is used to detect the presence of Treponema pallidum in syphilitic lesions. While wearing gloves, extract the serum from a freshly abraded genital lesion and place on slide with slipcover.

KOH Preparation

To detect the presence of fungi or yeast in vesiculobullous or papulosquamous lesions, scrapings should be taken from the active border of the lesion, prepared with KOH, coverslipped and heated. Observe for branching hyphae or collections of spores.

Culture

For detection of bacteria or fungus, extract a specimen from the active part of the lesion. Swab on medium.

Biopsy

Histological diagnosis is indicated for suspicious eruptions. After preparing with alcohol, inoculate the area with 1 percent Xylocaine. Rotate a sharp 3 to 4 mm Keyes dermal punch or an Orentreich punch through the entire thickness of the epidermis and dermis. As a general rule, biopsy should be deep enough to include fat, and as the punch reaches this point there will be a definite give. Stop the bleeding with pressure, absorbable gel foam plug or suture. Expertise in procedure is required for facial lesions. Biopsy specimen and history of lesion need to be sent to a pathologist.

Blood Tests

CBC with differential can be done on patients with constitutional symptoms or where there is suspicion of systemic disease. VDRL for syphilis is drawn at a minimum of one week after the appearance of the lesion. Platelet tests and coagulation studies should be done in purpuric conditions.

ASSESSMENT:

I. *Common Skin Changes in the Geriatric Patient*

With advancing age, the skin can reflect changes that are anticipated and require minimal or no treatment. These changes are usually asymptomatic, but the patient is often concerned about the appearance, mechanical annoyance, or the pathological implications of these slowly developing lesions. It is important to differentiate some of these changes from cutaneous cancers such as basal cell carcinoma or malignant melanoma. For any skin change, it is helpful to have a pictorial atlas of dermatological diseases to confirm the appearance of the clinical lesion.

Lentigines (Liver Spots)

Lentigines are a solitary or group of sharply circumscribed, lightly pigmented to brown macules, somewhat variegated, and are found on the dorsal surface of the hands, wrists, forehead, and cheeks. They are benign hyperpigmented lesions nevoid in character, which result from an inability of the melanocytes to produce an even distribution of pigment in skin; usually they are caused by chronic sunlight exposure. These nonfading lesions slowly increase after the fourth or fifth decade and may be of cosmetic or pathological concern. Lentigines need to be differentiated from malignant melanomas. Lentigines are usually round, macular and tan to brown in color while malignant melanomas vary in size and color and are not restricted to sun exposure areas. Lentigines are different from freckles, which tend to fade when protected from sunlight.

Senile Purpura

Senile purpura are caused by the fragility of blood vessels resulting from apparent loss of their connective tissue support. They can result in spontaneous petechiae occurring on exposed portions of the hands. These lesions are macular, less than three cm in diameter, and are often located on the exposed portions of the hands.

Senile (Cherry) Angioma

A senile angioma is a localized overgrowth of dilated capillaries which can appear in the third decade, but is seen more commonly in the middle years. By the age of 80, close to 100 percent of the population develop them (Tindall, 1971). Senile angiomas classically begin with a gradual appearance of one or more bright red papules 1 to 3 mm in diameter, located primarily on the upper chest and trunk; singular round nodules of a bluish-red color may arise on the lip. Senile angiomas are asymptomatic but may bleed when traumatized.

Venous Lakes

Venous lakes are deep blue cutaneous nodules, venous in character, which tend to arise in exposed regions or areas of trauma. The patient may be concerned about their appearance. Venous lakes begin with the gradual onset of singular or multiple small, irregular, blue-black to gray papules which can resemble a soft blood blister, located on the face, ears, and neck. Occasionally, the lesion may thrombose and involute. Solitary lesions may resemble basal cell carcinoma or malignant melanoma that can be differentiated by biopsy.

Acrochordon (Skin Tag)

The acrochordon is a pin to a pea-sized soft, flesh-colored, pedunculated papule located on the front or side of the neck, axilla, and upper part of the trunk. It is a common, benign, dermatologic finding which rarely causes difficulty unless located in an area of chronic irritation such as from a necklace or a stiff collar of a shirt.

Venous Star

The venous star is a few to several centimeters, linear, irregular, cascading or spider-shaped, blue lesion often found on the legs; there is a negative blanching sign. The venous star is a vascular lesion that results from increased pressure in the superficial veins and is commonly associated with varicosities. Venous stars have a gradual appearance, increasing in number with age. Cosmetically, the appearance of large or multiple lesions is distressing particularly in women.

Angiokeratoma

Angiokeratomas are scattered, multiple 2 to 3 mm, purple-red vascular papules with a somewhat warty appearance. These dilated vascular lesions of the scrotum are found in middle-aged and elderly men; they tend to appear gradually and are asymptomatic.

II. Skin Conditions Common to the Geriatric Population

Xerosis (Dry Skin)

Xerosis is primarily a noninflammatory dermatosis related to a decrease in sebum production and a loss of water from the stratum corneum. It is more prevalent in environmental or climatic conditions that have high temperatures and low humidity (e.g., in heated residences during winter or arid parts of the country). Exposure to agents like strong soaps, alcohol rubs, excessive soaks or solvents can remove the protective sebum and inflame the skin. Mechanical irritation may accentuate the condition.

Xerosis usually involves the lower legs but also can be diffuse. The skin initially has a dry, fine, scaling appearance with a tendency to flake. With progression, checkered fissures and erythema can develop. Mild to severe pruritus is a predominant feature leading to scratching and subsequent excoriations. Without treatment, eczematoid changes may occur; secondary infections which can be confirmed by KOH prep or culture may develop.

Senile Sebaceous Adenoma

Senile sebaceous adenomas are benign lesions formed by hypertrophic sebaceous glands located on the forehead and cheeks. The color and shape of the adenomas can be confused with basal cell carcinoma, particularly if the lesion is singular; the patient may be concerned about the cosmetic effect or the presence of malignancy.

They begin with a gradual appearance of a few to many soft, small, flat-topped, yellow or pearly-colored papules varying in size from 1 to 8 mm and are characterized by a minute central depression from which sebum can be expressed.

Senile Seborrheic Dermatitis

Senile seborrheic dermatitis is a common papulosquamous disorder characterized by diffuse, fine, whitish, gritty, oily uninflamed adherent scales overlying a dull yellow-red skin. This condition has a tendency to become chronic and to recur. Lichenification, fissuring and excoriations may be apparent.

There appears to be a genetic disposition with an interplay of hormones, nutrition, infection, and emotional stress contributing to its development. Patients who are inactive or have central nervous system disease appear especially susceptible.

Senile sebaceous dermatitis develops in active sebaceous gland areas, where the natural oils, particularly fatty acids, are trapped under the outer layer of scaly skin. This reaction can be aggravated by bacteria evidenced in mild symptoms. The incidence is greater in men because they retain their sebaceous gland activity longer than women.

This condition needs to be differentiated from psoriasis, contact dermatitis, intertrigo, and fungal infections. Aids to diagnosis are the presence of a less discrete outline than seen in psoriasis and the distribution which is predominantly on the scalp, but also the facial folds, eyebrows, retroauricular, sternal and pubic regions. Secondary infection with regional node involvement can occur.

Moderate to marked pruritus and burning may be present. Emotions, cosmetics, hair sprays, and perspiration aggravate the condition.

Lichen Simplex Chronicus

Lichen simplex chronicus is a chronic, localized pruritic neurodermatitis perpetuated by repeated trauma, particularly rubbing and scratching (scratch-itch cycle). This condition initially appears as well-localized, singular, distinct, pink, rectangular papules several cm in diameter. It progresses to dry, lichenified lesions that are centrally brown with a whitish scale, which exaggerates the lines of the skin, giving a cross-hatched appearance.

Lichen simplex chronicus is marked by remissions and exacerbations. It is located primarily on the nape of the neck, extensor forearms, wrists, anterior tibial regions, ankles or genitals, and it may originate at the sites of normal skin or a previous dermatitis. It is common in women over 40 and persons of Oriental extraction. It needs to be differentiated from other conditions that arise in the same anatomic areas or that have a plaque appearance (e.g., contact dermatitis, stasis dermatitis, psoriasis and seborrheic dermatitis).

Rosacea

Rosacea is a chronic inflammatory disorder of the facial sebaceous glands in middle-aged and older persons, characterized by a vascular component (erythema and telangiectasias) with or without an acneform component. Localized in the middle half of the face, it initially appears as a transient flush over the cheeks, nose, and sometimes central forehead and chin. Rosacea progresses to persistent erythematous papules and pustules as well as telangiectasias. A disfiguring enlargement of the nose (rhinophyma) can occur as a late sequela in males. The erythema will blanch on diascopy.

Rosacea can present with ocular lesions such as blepharoconjunctivitis. It is more common in women and Caucasians. Patients are concerned about the insidious onset of an irritated, red face and appearance.

Perlèche

Perlèche is a commissural dermatitis of the mouth that can be mistaken for vitamin B_2 deficiency (riboflavin).

Poorly fitting dentures, loss of teeth or loss of facial muscle tone make the corners of the mouth droop and saliva drains out onto the skin. The resultant macerated skin is prone to secondary bacterial or mycotic infections which can be diagnosed by KOH and/or culture. Painful fissuring occurs and the patient frequently licks the lesion to temporarily allay the burning discomfort.

It is characterized by soggy, white, angular lesions located at the commissures of the mouth that can progress to fissures, yellow crusts and possible submental node involvement.

Tinea Onychomycosis (Nails)

Tinea onychomycosis is a chronic, noninvasive, fungal infection of the nails which results in a dystrophic, thickened nailplate and an increase in keratin under the nail. This infection exists as a painless disfiguration of the nails except when irritated by footwear or pressure. Initially the infection appears on the terminal and lateral margins of one or two nail beds; they appear as opaque, white or silver patches which later change to yellow, then brown in color. The nails become thick, friable, even pithy and as the hyperkeratosis progresses the nail can separate from its bed. These subungual changes can appear identical to psoriasis. Nail changes resulting from contact with alkalies and other chemicals can be confused with tinea onychomycosis. Development of secondary monilial infections is possible, particularly in diabetics.

Scrape the debris from under the nail plate and prepare with KOH. Fungi may also be cultured using Sabouraud's medium.

Tinea Pedis (Athlete's Foot)

Tinea pedis is an extremely common, acute or chronic fungal infection affecting over one-half of the population at some time in their lives. There is a higher incidence in men. The presenting symptoms can be pruritus, stinging or burning. In the acute phase, vesiculobullous lesions can appear in the instep or plantar surface. The lesions can scale and become subject to secondary infection. Chronic forms present as intertriginous scales and fissures associated with maceration. Chronic hyperkeratotic scaling can develop unilaterally on the heel and plantar surface. Scrape the active margins of the lesions and prepare with KOH. Culture on Sabouraud's medium may prove informative.

Heredity plays a part as well as sweating, type of footwear and immunologic factors. The anatomical location and nature of tinea pedis requires a differentiation from other conditions such as psoriasis, contact dermatitis or atophic dermatitis.

Verruca (Warts)

Verrucae are rough, hyperkeratotic,

verrucous yellow to brown papules that can be solitary or multiple and are usually asymptomatic. They may arise at sites of recurrent irritation or trauma as on a finger from sewing or plantar surface from improper weight bearing. Verrucae on the fingers tend to plane while planter warts may have a mosaic pattern and are tender on pressure. Oblique transillumination is helpful in visualizing flat warts.

Warts are presumably due to a virus that incubates from 2 to 18 months before developing into a lesion. Reinfection is possible and individual resistance to the virus is highly variable. The lesions can occur anytime in the lifespan and in immunosuppressed patients. Rough, raised appearing warts need to be differentiated from corns; warts can be positively identified by paring away the keratotic surface with a sharp scalpel and observing the pinpoint bleeding from capillaries. Corns and calluses are avascular.

Pruritus Vulvae and Ani

Existing in the anogenital region, this condition is caused by a number of primary and secondary cutaneous conditions and secondary gynecological problems such as senile atrophy and vaginitis. Pruritus of the anogenital area can be moderate to severe, is chiefly nocturnal and can lead to excoriations. Perform a complete cutaneous inspection for primary and secondary lesions. Moist lesions appear soggy and gray-white. Chronic conditions appear lichenified with accentuated natural markings. Gynecological exam should include Pap smear, wet prep for yeast and trichomonas. Culture cutaneous and mucous membrane lesions for fungus.

Examination of the feces may reveal parasites. Urinalysis and blood sugar may detect diabetes. Improper hygiene, moisture, incontinence, irritation, and obesity folds aggravate the condition. Self-treatment can alter the clinical appearance of the original lesion. Diabetes mellitus should be ruled out.

Cellulitis

Cellulitis is a diffuse, edematous, spreading, erythematous infection involving the deeper tissues, caused by a number of organisms (usually Streptococci). It needs to be differentiated from the more superficial circumscribed erysipelas. Pain, limited function, constitutional symptoms, and regional adenopathy can result along with leukocytosis. Lymphangitis requires prompt treatment.

III. Cutaneous Cancers
A. Precancerous conditions
Precancerous lesions are confined to the epidermis and may or may not evolve into cancerous conditions. Examination of lesions is aided by a hand lens. In some instances, a biopsy is needed.

Seborrheic Keratoses

Seborrheic keratoses are discrete, elevated, segmented lesions scattered mostly on the trunk, with some on the neck and hairline. Initially, the lesions appear as slightly raised, yellow plaques covered with a greasy scale, much resembling a drop of candle wax. They can slowly mature into brown-black verrucous lesions, finally achieving a granular appearance. At this stage, they can be pulled off by a fingernail only to appear again. Close to 90 percent of the older population develop seborrheic keratoses. Concern may be expressed about their appearance or possibility of malignancy. Having only a slight potential for malignancy, these noninvasive tumors arise from the epithelium which gives them a pasted-on appearance. With age, keratoses gradually increase in size and number. A rapid onset, within two months, of many keratoses can be associated with an internal malignancy. They usually can easily be differentiated from a malignant melanoma by inspection.

Actinic (Solar) Keratoses

The most common precancerous lesions found on chronically sun-exposed areas, actinic keratoses appear as multiple, well-circumscribed, flesh-colored, slightly reddened or light brown macules or papules with an adherent scale. The incidence is greater in fair-complexioned people. It is considered a low-grade cancer, but estimates are as high as 20 percent that these lesions will evolve into squamous cell cancer.

They vary in size up to one cm, have a sandpaper consistency, and are located on face, neck, dorsa of forearms and hands, and outer border of the ears and lips. Associated actinic changes of wrinkling, telangiectasia, and diffuse, yellow papules can occur. These nontender lesions are often felt better than they are seen. Tenderness at the base may indicate malignancy. If actinic keratosis progresses to squamous cell, the tissue is friable and tears readily. Diagnosis can be confirmed by biopsy.

Keratoacanthoma

Keratoacanthomata are rapid growing, self-healing lesions that arise on exposed skin. They are found only in Caucasians and are more common in men by a 2:1 ratio.

Located most often on the cheeks and nose, the mature lesion is a flesh-colored or slightly reddened, dome-shaped tumor with a central crater filled with fibrous keratinous debris. Keratoacanthomata grow rapidly to 1 to 4 cm in six weeks and then spontaneously subside in six months to one year.

Solitary forms are usually seen between ages 60 and 65; multiple forms occur earlier. There is a familial tendency with a greater incidence in pitch and tar workers, smokers, and those living in heavily polluted areas. Keratoacanthomata often arise at sites of previous trauma or secondary to other skin lesions such as eczema, seborrheic dermatitis, or psoriasis. Frequently, they can be mistaken for squamous cell carcinoma, or squamous cell carcinoma may be present at the base of the lesion.

Leukoplakia

An equivalent of actinic keratosis, leukoplakia arises on the mucous membranes secondary to chronic irritation from tobacco smoking, poor dentition, or a focal infection.

Located on the buccal surface, gums, dorsum of the tongue, inner aspects of the lips and vulva, the lesion initially appears dull white to silver and smooth as if white enamel has been spilled on the mucosa. If the lesion progresses, it thickens to raised verrucous patches, having a stuck-on appearance. On the vulvar mucosa, fissures and ulceration can occur. When found on the vulva, 50 percent of the cases are precancerous. Oral lesions are usually nontender elevations, sometimes rough in character, which may be felt by the tongue.

B. Cancerous conditions
Asymptomatic, often located in obscure areas, skin cancer can be overlooked. Predisposing factors include long-term sunlight exposure, heredity, and past treatment with radiation and arsenic.

The most frequently encountered cutaneous cancers are basal cell carcinoma, squamous cell carcinoma, and malignant melanoma. A guide for examining the lesions is as follows: draw an imaginary line from the commissures of the mouth to the ear lobe, two-thirds of the skin cancer lesions located superior to this line are usually basal cell and two-thirds located below are usually squamous cell.

Basal Cell Carcinoma (Epithelioma)

Basal cell carcinoma is a very low-grade, locally invasive tumor that rarely metastasizes. It is a slow-growing, nontender, discrete, flesh-colored papule with a raised, pearly opalescent border. The consistency is waxy, friable and fine telangiectasias cover the umbilicated surface. Central ulceration and crusting can form. Ninety percent of basal cell lesions are found on the head and neck, primarily on the T-zone of the face including the forehead, eyelids, cheek, nose, and lips. Diagnosis is often made by inspection. The tumor reflects the proliferation of the basal cell layer of the epidermis. It arises on sun-damaged skin after the fourth decade, predominantly in fair-skinned people. The average age of onset is 57.3 years (Tindall, 1971).

Squamous Cell Carcinoma

Squamous cell carcinoma is an epidermal carcinoma, which is locally infiltrative and can metastasize to regional lymph nodes. This lesion is a solitary, flesh-colored nodule with a warty, dirty, or scaly appearance which can slowly progress to ulceration. It lacks the pearly border seen in basal cell carcinoma. Often located on the lower lip and neck, regional adenopathy may be present.

The onset is between 50 and 70 years, with the average age being 66.2 years (Tindall, 1971). Predisposing factors include previous actinic keratoses, exposure to radiation, immunosuppressive therapy, and carcinogens such as tars, benzines, and arsenicals.

Malignant Melanoma

Malignant melanoma is a highly malignant cutaneous cancer that can arise from a preexisting nevi—circumscribed polychromic (red, white, blue mixed with brown) macules and papules. They can be friable with a tendency to bleed. They can be located anywhere, but those on the head and neck have a higher incidence of malignancy. Regional adenopathy can occur. Peak incidence is in the seventh decade. If the person is fair-skinned and had chronic sunlight exposure, it can appear in the fifth decade. The patient may identify a change in size, shape, or color of a mole, with bleeding or itching.

IV. Incidental—Inveterate Conditions

The elderly are subject to conditions also found in younger age groups. Some of these appear incidentally while many others have been firmly established at an earlier age. (Cited is a general discussion of some of the entities. A more complete discussion can be found in Hudak et al., 1976.)

Drug Eruptions

Ingesting a multiplicity of drugs makes the elderly patient subject to a variety of drug reactions. Widespread symmetrical erythematous, urticarial, or purpuric rashes can manifest a reaction to drugs.

Herpes Zoster

The varicella zoster presumably causes this painful, multiphased disease marked by grouped vesicles coursing unilaterally along a nerve, usually on the face or trunk. Regional lymph nodes can swell. Chronic postherpetic pain can occur after 60 years. In any one year, persons over 70 are five times more likely to develop zoster than a middle-aged person (Tindall, 1971). Involvement of the ophthalmic branch of the fifth nerve can cause damage of the cornea.

Contact Dermatitis

Elderly persons' dry skin predisposes them to react to allergenic or highly irritating substances. These provoke well-patterned vesiculobullous eruptions. Common offenders are nickel, jewelry, clothing, cosmetics, soaps, dermatologic agents, or items used in new or old hobbies.

Neurodermatoses

Neurodermatoses represent a range of eczematous dermatoses that have a common histologic picture of eczematous eruptions. Pruritus is a common feature with a personal or family history of allergy, or a cutaneous reaction to emotional problems. Distribution of lesions is classically within scratching reach of the patient. The scratch-itch cycle aggravates the condition.

Psoriasis

Psoriasis is a chronic condition with a 30 to 40 percent familial incidence affecting 1 to 2 percent of the population (Fitzpatrick et al., 1971). This papulosquamous condition is marked by a rapid turnover of epidermal cells evidenced by sharply marginated, silvery plaques commonly found on the extensor surfaces of extremities, scalp, sacrum, and nails.

Stasis Dermatitis

Secondary to a variety of causes, peripheral edema is a common finding in the elderly. Prolonged, passive congestion interferes with the nutrition of the skin, resulting in stasis dermatitis (atrophic, pigmented skin with pruritus, eczematous changes and ulcers).

Syphilis

Although an uncommon finding in the aged, development of secondary syphilis is evidenced by a bilateral nonpruritic, nonscaling macular rash located on the trunk and proximal extremities. There may be a history of symptoms and/or a previous history of a chancre.

PLAN:

I. Common Skin Changes

Therapy is generally directed toward reassuring the patient that these changes are anticipated with age and do not require specific treatment. Those causing cosmetic distress can be referred for eradication. Any suspicious skin change (nonclassic lesion, lesion growth or change, unusual presentation) should be referred to a physician/dermatologist for examination/biopsy.

Lentigines (Liver Spots)

Any suspicious lesion should be referred for evaluation. Treatment is not indicated for the characteristic lentigines. Ablative procedures are discouraged, since the exact nature of these lesions is not well understood.

Senile Purpura

No treatment indicated.

Senile (Cherry) Angioma

No treatment required. Electrodesiccation leaves only a tiny scar.

Venous Lakes

Solitary lesions should be referred for biopsy to rule out pigmented basal cell carcinoma or malignant melanoma. No treatment is required for venous lakes. Electrodesiccation can be used for cosmetic improvement.

Acrochordons (Skin Tags)

Irritation may be sufficient to occlude vascular supply to the tag, resulting in spontaneous loss of the lesion. Cosmetic removal can be achieved by light desiccation.

Venous Star

Support stockings and periodic elevation will decrease the pressure in incompetent varicose veins.

Angiokeratoma

Treatment is not indicated. Eradication is possible by desiccation, but new lesions are likely to appear.

II. Skin Conditions Common to the Geriatric Population
Xerosis (Dry Skin)

The skin is capable of absorbing four times its own moisture. The aim of therapy is to hydrate the skin and then apply agents that have a sebumlike action which will retard the loss of moisture.

Soak or submerge the affected area in plain, lukewarm water for 10 to 15 minutes. Blot the skin dry without rubbing and apply an agent that can form a continuous protective layer, such as solidified petroleum, zinc oxide paste, petroleum-containing silicone or vegetable oils. Eucerin is a popular inexpensive water-and-oil agent that is not quite as greasy or occlusive as Vaseline. Some OTC preparations like CZO, and Quotane also include antipruritics to soothe the irritation. Thickened keratin can effectively be dissolved by 5 to 10 percent urea agents or lactic acid preparations which produce a smooth, moist skin. For cleansing, only superfatted or mild deodorant soaps are recommended.

Alert the patients that many over-the-counter preparations are ineffective or may aggravate the condition. Instruct them to carefully read labels. Popular skin aids such as vanishing creams, hand and baby lotions provide a noncontinous layer which permits the loss of moisture. The efficacy of bath oils is questionable. When added to bath water, oil droplets suspend in the water and are not absorbed by the skin. If used, the patient should soak for 5 to 10 minutes in the water before adding a nonperfumed oil and then pat the skin dry. In using bath oils, slipping accidents can be averted by placing a towel in the bottom of the tub.

Debate currently exists over some other popular dry skin agents. Some authorities state that lanolin can sensitize the skin and mineral oil can act as a drying agent. Glycerin, vitamin A and estrogen hormone preparations are also of questionable value.

Senile Sebaceous Adenoma   Suspicious lesions (especially angular) should be referred to a dermatologist for eradication.

Senile Seborrheic Dermatitis

With a tendency for lifelong recurrences, therapy is symptomatic.

Antiseborrheic preparations have antiseptic properties which reduce the microbial flora on the scalp. Agents containing sulfur, salicylic acid or resorcinol have an added keratolytic action that debrides the scale. Some preparations also have additional surfactants which will affect the surface tension permitting better penetration and removal of the sebum. Prescribe weekly or greater use of alternating antiseborrheic shampoos. Allergy and refractory response can occur which will require a switch to another agent or to a mild, more neutral shampoo. Mild deodorant or superfatted soaps should be used for general cleansing.

Topical corticosteroid therapy consisting of less than 1 percent hydrocortisone in the form of lotions, creams or solutions can be applied to eczematous areas. Fluorinated steroids applied to the face can stimulate acne and should be avoided. Antibiotics can be prescribed for secondary infections. Advise avoidance of irritants and modification of stressors. Counsel concerning the regulation of lifestyle by balancing work, sleep, recreation and nutritional habits. Modification of dietary fats is of little proven value.

Lichen Simplex Chronicus

Topical steroids can be applied three to six times daily. Protect the treated area at night with Saran Wrap. An unrelenting case can be referred to a dermatologist for intralesion steroid injections that are done weekly for three to four weeks.

The area needs to be protected from trauma. Counsel regarding the management of stressful situations and avoidance of the trigger for the scratch-itch cycle. Sedation may be of help.

Rosacea

Since there is an apparent relationship between rosacea and the other sebaceous conditions like seborrheic dermatitis and acne vulgaris, the treatment plans are similar. Since resorcinol and salicylic acid have been shown to aggravate the erythema, use of antiseborrheic and topical drying agents are limited to the sulfur-based preparations. Concentrations up to 15 percent of precipitated sulfur can be applied to the face. Acneform lesions are treated with broad spectrum antibiotics which reduce the normal flora and diminish the erythema. Initially, doses of tetracycline or erythromycin (0.5 to 1.0 gm per day) are taken on an empty stomach. With clinical improvement of the lesions, maintenance doses of 250 mg daily can be ordered. Ultraviolet light is of little value in treating rosacea. Topical steroid creams should be avoided because of an increase in the rosacea flush and skin thinning. The patient should be advised that the erythema can be stimulated by vasodilators (i.e., heat, excessive sunlight, hot liquids, highly seasoned foods and alcohol).

Perlèche

Refer to an orthodontist to correct the underlying problem of poorly fitting dentures. If the patient is on limited income, consult social service agencies for financial aid in paying for the dentures.

To crusted lesions, apply an antimicrobial/antifungal cream sparingly four times per day. In the absence of infection, apply a heavy coat of Vaseline at bedtime to protect the area from being moistened or licked during sleep.

Advise the patient to avoid moistening lesions with his or her tongue. The patient should wear dentures at all times to maintain anatomic correction of the lips. Avoid transmission of secondary infection by separate use of cups and towels.

Tinea Onychomycosic (Nails)

Cure of this chronic condition is difficult, and fungal infections of the nail are least responsive to griseofulvin therapy. In the face of prolonged therapy, the toxic effects of this drug require periodic monitoring of organ system functioning including renal, hepatic and hematopoietic. Griseofulvin decreases the activity of warfarinlike anticoagulants and the patient should be advised of photosensitivity reactions. Taking griseofulvin with a fatty meal contributes little to the therapy. Candida or bacterial infections will not be eradicated with this drug.

Treatment for the fingernail requires .05 to 1 gram of griseofulvin daily for four to six months or until the infection subsides. A divided daily dose of 500 mg is recommended. For topical measures, see toenail.

Local measures for the treatment of toenail tinea is the treatment of choice. The goal of therapy is to reduce the nail so that shoes can be comfortably worn. Locally, debride or pare the thickened nail. Then apply local antifungal/drying agents to the nail (i.e., 2 percent miconazole nitrate cream, a tannic acid/boric acid/salicylic acid solution, or 1 percent clotrimazole cream) twice daily. More refractory cases may require a referral to a podiatrist for surgical removal of the nail. Griseofulvin in full, daily doses can be given, but a cure is rarely achieved.

Secondary Infection: For candida infections, apply astringent compress such as aluminum acetate; follow this with application of a nystatin cream. Rule out the possibility of diabetes mellitus.

Tinea Pedis (Athlete's Foot)

Appearance of the lesions guides the treatment plan. Avoid overtreatment.

For acute inflamed vesicular lesions, soak the area in Burrow's solution for 20 minutes two to three times daily. In the presence of secondary infection, use 1:10,000 potassium permanganate one to two times daily. Avoid topical preparations during this phase.

For subacute lesions, apply 2 percent miconazole cream or 1 percent clotrimazole cream twice daily.

For chronic lesions, use sulfur-salicylic acid ointment, tolnaftate solutions, or 1 percent haloprogin cream as needed. Sedation may be used with severe pruritus.

Griseofulvin therapy has been relatively ineffective and should be used only in the most severe cases.

Tinea requires considerable time to subside and can recur in those with a predilection for the condition. Follow-up should be made on a regular basis, until the inflammatory phase is under control.

Strict food hygiene is required if antifungal agents are to be effective. Carefully debride thickened or dead tissue after soaks or bath. Advise the patient to dry his or her feet carefully and to wear clean cotton socks daily. Open-toed shoes or sandals are preferred footwear. Avoid footwear that promotes sweating (e.g., vinyl shoes). Rotate shoes and avoid prolonged wearing of boots. Cotton can be placed between toes at night.

Verruca (Warts)

In time, warts may resolve spontaneously. Treatment is indicated for warts that cause functional or cosmetic impairment.

Finger: Freeze with liquid nitrogen. A blister will erupt that will eventually resolve.

Plantar: Treatment consists of applying a keratolytic agent followed by mechanical paring. Forty percent salicylic acid plaster pad is cut to cover only the lesion. The pad is worn for five to seven days before the lesion is trimmed. Continue the procedure until wart has completely regressed. Counsel the patient about its contagious property and to avoid scratching the lesions.

Pruritus Vulvae and Ani

The underlying etiology must be identified and treated accordingly (e.g., vulvar pruritus is frequently cleared by treating the vaginal infection, and pruritus ani is cleared by treating the hemorrhoids, incontinence, etc.). Remove any precipitating or irritating causes such as incontinence. Soothing compresses or colloidal sitz baths with the avoidance of soap can be helpful. Topical agents should have a cream base rather than an ointment. Vioform-hydrocortisone cream can be effective.

Ascertain the hygiene habits and counsel the patient accordingly. Cotton underwear will permit a better exchange of air and should be changed daily. The condition may persist or recur. Scratching should be avoided.

Cellulitis

Consult with or refer to the patient's physician. Rest and elevate involved area, apply hot packs and treat pain and fever symptomatically with aspirin. Oral antibiotic therapy may include a course of penicillin or erythromycin.

III. Cutaneous Cancers

Prevention is the best cure. Sunscreens containing 5 percent para-aminobenzoic acid (PABA) should be applied an hour before sun exposure. Avoidance of the intense short wave-length ultraviolet sun rays during the midday hours is recommended. For travelers to climates with intense sun added protection can be achieved by daily applications a week prior to departure.

A. Precancerous conditions

Seborrheic Keratoses

Suspicious lesions or the rapid onset of multiple lesions should be referred to a dermatologist. Early, flat lesions can be rubbed off with castor or olive oil by lightly abrading with a gauze pad.

Mature lesions located at sites of constant friction may be prone to infection. These may be removed by curettage (after consultation with or referral to the patient's physician).

Actinic (Solar) Keratoses

Solitary lesions can be referred to a dermatologist for eradication. The presence of a few lesions can be treated with liquid nitrogen. Referral to a dermatologist is indicated. Multiple lesions are sometimes treated with topical fluorouracil lotion. Duration of therapy is 10 days to four weeks until an inflammatory response is achieved, appearing as an irritated or raw, denuded area.

Complete healing may not be evident for one to two months. The patient's adherence to therapy should be closely monitored as the inflammatory reaction from the fluorouracil therapy affects compliance. Occlusive dressings increase the reaction; dressings used for cosmetic reasons should be limited to porous gauze.

Follow-up should be done during therapy and for six to 12 month intervals because of the potential of developing squamous cell cancer. Advise the patient to observe the present lesions and the development of any new lesions. Prevention should include the use of PABA sunscreen, protective clothing and avoidance of midday hours of intense sunlight.

Keratoacanthoma

Observe bimonthly for spontaneous regression. Refer for pathologic confirmation if nonhealing.

Leukoplakia

Conservative treatment for the early nonthickened lesions is removal of the irritant. Recommend that the patient stop smoking, utilize proper dental hygiene, and avoid highly seasoned food. Prescribe a soothing mouthwash and bland dentifrices. Thick or ulcerated lesions should be referred for further evaluation.

B. Cancerous conditions

Basal Cell Carcinoma (Epithelioma)

Although a low-grade tumor, slow in growth, it can be invasive and cause marked local destruction. Refer promptly to a dermatologist for electrodesiccation, curettage, excision, x-ray therapy, or chemosurgery; 5-FU treatment is ineffective as it does not erradicate the borders of the lesion.

Squamous Cell Carcinoma

Prompt referral to a dermatologist for evaluation and treatment is indicated. For lesions less than 2 cm without regional node involvement, the cure rate is as high as in basal cell carcinoma. Recommend 5 percent para-aminobenzoic acid sunscreen preparations for skin and lips.

Malignant Melanoma

Prompt referral should be made to a dermatologist/surgeon for diagnosis and treatment. Wide excision of the lesion with or without regional lymphadenectomy should be done.

IV. Incidental—Inveterate Conditions

Drug eruptions
Herpes zoster
Contact dermatitis
Neurodermatoses
Psoriasis
Stasis dermatitis
Syphilis
Erythema multiforme
Herpes simplex

These conditions are either incidental (common to any age) or inveterate (conditions that originated earlier in life but may continue to remain a skin problem). For further assessment and plan of these conditions, see Hudak, and associates' chapter on Rash-Skin Problems (1976).

APPENDIX A

Table 7-1. Primary Lesions of the Skin

Type	Description	Examples
Macule	*Flat, circumscribed, nonpalpable area of color change ranging in size from less than 1 mm to several cm*	*Lentigines, petechia*
Papule	*Circumscribed, solid, palpable, lesion less than 1 cm that may be elevated, depressed or level with the skin.*	*Senile angioma, venous lakes, verruca*
Nodule	*A larger papule, 1 to 2 cm in size, extending deeper in the skin and may involve the subcutaneous tissue*	*Pigmented nevi*
Tumor	*A larger nodule which is over 2 cm, often used in designating neoplastic lesions whether benign or malignant*	*Keratoacanthoma, basal cell carcinoma*
Vesicle	*Circumscribed, fluid-containing lesion less than 1 cm in size*	*Herpes zoster, contact dermatitis, blister*
Bulla	*Large, circumscribed, fluid-containing lesion greater than 1 cm*	*Herpes zoster, athlete's foot, second-degree burn*
Pustule	*A vesicle that contains a purulent exudate*	*Acneform component of rosacea*

Table 7-2. Secondary Lesions of the Skin

Type	Description	Examples
Scale	Accumulated, dry or greasy, laminated debris from the stratum corneum	Seborrheic dermatitis, actinic keratosis
Plaque	Large, elevated scale	Psoriasis, lichen simplex chronicus
Crust	Residual of serous, sanguinous, or purulent exudate from diseased or ulcerated skin that is mixed with debris	Vesicular lesions, perlèche
Fissure	A linear cleft into the epidermis or epidermis and corium	Perlèche, athlete's foot
Excoriation	Superficial abrasion of the epidermis induced by mechanical irritation	Xerosis, pruritus vulvae
Ulcer	Circumscribed destructive lesion involving the corium or deeper tissue	Basal cell carcinoma, stasis ulcer
Lichenification	Plaquelike thickening of the skin which accentuates the normal markings	Lichen simplex chronicus, neurodermatosis
Scar	Permanent formation of new connective tissue lacking the normal markings	Acneform component of rosacea, herpes zoster
Atrophy	Almost transparent thinning of the skin with or without loss of normal skin markings	Senile atrophy, basal cell carcinoma

Appendix B

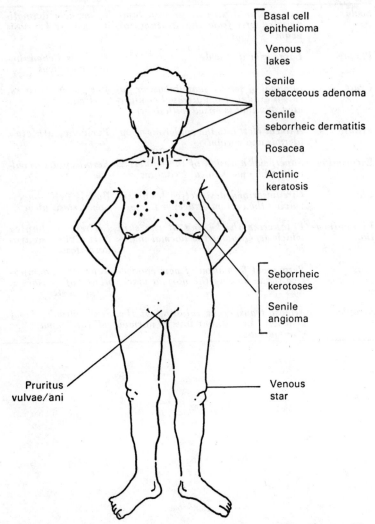

Figure 7-1. *The Distribution of Common Geriatric Skin Changes/Conditions*

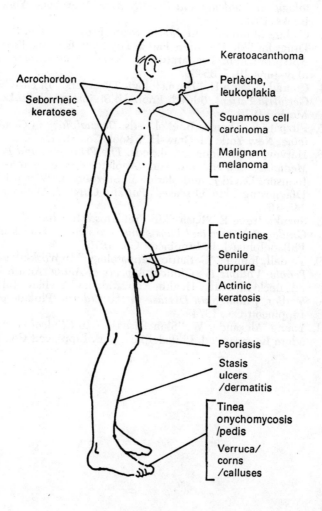

Keratoacanthoma

Perlèche, leukoplakia

Acrochordon

Seborrheic keratoses

Squamous cell carcinoma

Malignant melanoma

Lentigines

Senile purpura

Actinic keratosis

Psoriasis

Stasis ulcers /dermatitis

Tinea onychomycosis /pedis

Verruca/ corns /calluses

REFERENCES

1. Brotman, H. B. "The Fastest Growing Minority: The Aging." *American Journal of Public Health*, 64, March 1974, 249–252.
2. Burnett, Joseph W. and Harry M. Robinson, Sr. *Clinical Dermatology for Students and Practitioners*. New York: York Medical Books, 1978.
3. Collar, Maureen and Marie Scott Brown. "Over-the-Counter Drugs for Skin Disorders Part 2: Dry Skin, Eczema, Psoriasis, and Antiseborrheic Preparations." *Nurse Practitioner*, 2:14–16, May–June 1977, 35–36.
4. Conrad, Adolph H. "Dermatologic Disorders." In *The Cure of the Geriatric Patient*, 5th ed. Franz U. Steinberg ed. St. Louis: C.V. Mosby, 1976.
5. Fitzpatrick, Thomas B. et al., eds. *Dermatology in General Medicine*. New York: McGraw-Hill Book Co., 1971.
6. Harvey, A. McGehee et al., eds. *The Principles and Practice of Medicine*, 19th ed. New York: Appleton-Century-Crofts, 1972.
7. Johnson, David P. and Marion B. Sulzberger. "Visual Pointers to Diagnosing Skin Disease." *Patient Care*, 7, October 1, 1974, 142–167.
8. Suzuki, Irene E. "Rash-Skin Problems." In *Clinical Protocols: A Guide for Nurses and Physicians*. Carolyn M. Hudak et al., eds. Philadelphia: J. B. Lippincott Co., 1976.
9. Tindall, John P. "Geriatric Dermatology." In *Working with Older People: Volume IV, Clinical Aspects of Aging*. Austin B. Chinn, ed. Rockville, Md.: Health, Education and Welfare, July 1971.
10. Verbor, Julian. *Skin Disease in the Elderly*. Philadelphia: J. B. Lippincott Co., 1974.
11. Young, Alexander W. "Skin Disease." In *Clinical Geriatrics*. Isadore Rossman, ed. Philadelphia: J. B. Lippincott Co., 1971.

Protocols for Chronic Conditions Common to the Elderly

Chapter 8

Constipation

OVERVIEW

Constipation is probably the most common problem encountered by the geriatric nurse practitioner in any setting. The term constipation has different meanings to different people. For some, the term may mean a decrease in the frequency of their normal pattern; for others, it may mean an increased difficulty in passing stool. If the *patient's* definition of constipation represents an acute onset of a decrease in the frequency of stools, then this change in bowel habits represents true constipation (Benson, 1975). An acute onset of true constipation is more ominous than chronic constipation and warrants a more complete work-up. Therefore, it is imperative that the primary health care provider understand the normal process of defecation and the factors that contribute to constipation in the aged; it is also important to ascertain the etiology of an acute onset of true constipation and institute appropriate intervention.

Defecation in the aged should not be a difficult process; it is a normal process that results from several activities. Movements of the colon related to the process of defecation begin when food passes through the ileocecal valve. The mixture of digested food, enzymes, etc. called chyme, fills the cecum and ascending colon, and through peristaltic contractions fills the remaining parts of the colon. The urge to defecate then results from filling of the sigmoid colon and rectum with feces, producing distention of their walls and stimulating pressure receptors. This pressure sensation results in the opening of the sphincters and expulsion of feces through the anus. In addition to the physiological activities related to defecation, the process of elimination is aided mechanically by the contraction of the diaphragm and abdominal muscles which increase intraabdominal pressure and aid in the passage of feces.

Constipation should be considered a symptom rather than a disease (Benson, 1975), and can result from several factors, including: 1) *poor bowel habits*, 2) the formation of *dry, hard stool* that is difficult to pass or 3) it may be *a complaint in patients who are having normal physiological response* but have a misunderstanding of the definition of true constipation. Constipation secondary to *poor bowel habits* occurs when patients ignore the urge as a result of social conditions, immobility, or painful perianal disease. When the urge to defecate is ignored the stool is returned to the sigmoid and descending colon until pressure receptors are stimulated at a later time by distention. Constipation caused by the delayed passage of stool through the colon leading to the formation of *dry, hard stools* that are difficult to pass can result from several causes: 1) organic illnesses (i.e., hypothyroidism, hypercalcemia, hypokalemia, strictures or tumors), 2) lack of proper fiber in diet, 3) lack of proper fluid intake, 4) anorexia secondary to depression and 5) drugs, particularly iron preparations, anticholinergics, antihypertensives, analgesics and/or certain antacids containing calcium or aluminum. Finally, the patients may complain of constipation when in fact they are having normal bowel movements (i.e., the change in pattern is less frequent than the patients feel is normal). Thus, constipation may be a *complaint in patients who are having a normal physiological response*. In this case the complaint most commonly arises from the belief that a normal bowel pattern involves a daily evacuation. Patients who feel they do not meet this criteria may erroneously complain of constipation.

Whatever the origin, any elderly patient who continues to complain of true constipation after all preliminary measures to correct it have been utilized (e.g., increase fiber content of diet, increase fluid intake) should have a thorough work-up to identify the cause with appropriate treatment instituted. Through accurate identification, treatment and correction (as far as possible) of the underlying causes of constipation, the quality and perhaps quantity of the aged individual's life can be improved.

CONSTIPATION WORKSHEET

To be used for patients with a report of a change in bowel patterns: 1) the passage of hard, dry stools that requires undue straining, 2) an acute onset of absolute absence of stool passage (obstipation) or 3) a decreased frequency in passage of stool.

What you cannot afford to miss: organic illness of any origin that is contributing to constipation, or a bowel obstruction.

Chief Complaint: _____

SUBJECTIVE DATA:

Onset: _____

Frequency of stools: _____

Duration of problem (mos., yrs., etc.): _____

Course (better, worse or same): _____

Description of stools (note any change in color, size, etc.):

past _____

present _____

Patient's definition of constipation: _____

Difficulty in passing stool, gas: _____

Characteristics of patient's toilet habits (length of time on toilet, how

often does he try, etc.: _____

HEALTH HABIT HISTORY:

Daily exercise: _____

Daily fluid intake: _____

Daily food intake (list average 24-hour dietary history): _____

Constipation Worksheet

(Describe All Positives)

PAST MEDICAL HISTORY:

YES   *NO*

_____   _____   Past medical diagnosis: _____

_____

FAMILY HISTORY:

YES   *NO*

_____   _____   Family history of diabetes, ulcerative colitis, polyps

or cancer of the colon: _____

_____

Has the patient experienced any of the following? (Describe All Positive Reponses):

YES   *NO*

_____   _____   Absence of urge to defecate: _____

_____   _____   Laxatives used (what kind, effectiveness, past or cur-

rent use, etc.): _____

_____   _____   Enemas or suppositories used: _____

_____   _____   Digital stimulation: _____

_____   _____   Any recent major life changes (i.e., retirement, insti-

tutionalization, death of loved one, spouse, etc.): ___

_____

_____

_____ _____ Other medications (prescription and over-the-

counter): _____

Has the patient noticed any of the following associated with the
onset of constipation? (Describe All Positive Responses):

YES   *NO*

_____ _____ Intolerance to cold: _____

_____ _____ Mucus or bloody stools: _____

_____ _____ Alternating periods of diarrhea and constipation: ___

_____ _____ Abdominal pain or distention: _____

_____ _____ Nausea or vomiting: _____

_____ _____ Unexplained weight changes: _____

_____ _____ Large diameter or pencil-thin stools: _____

_____ _____ Depression or anxiety: _____

_____ _____ Bloating sensation: _____

_____ _____ Decreased mobility, ability to walk or exercise: ___

_____ _____ Malaise: _____

_____ _____ Anorexia: _____

_____ _____ Weakness: _____

_____ _____ Low back pain: _____

_____ _____ Tenesmus: _____

_____ _____ Fecal incontinence: _____

Constipation Worksheet

_____ _____ Anal pain: _____

_____ _____ History of hemorrhoids, fissures, fistulae:_____

OBJECTIVE DATA:

A screening physical exam and lab should be done if the patient has not been thoroughly examined in the last six months. Particular attention must be paid to the following areas. (Describe All Abnormal Results):

AB- NOR- MAL	NOR- MAL	

_____ _____ Screening exam: _____

_____

_____

_____

_____ _____ Abdominal exam: _____

_____

_____ _____ Rectal exam:_____

_____

LAB DATA:

	NOT	
DONE	DONE	

_____ _____ Hemoccult X3: _____

_____ _____ Hematocrit: _____

The following lab data should be obtained if the patient has not responded to nutritional or bowel habit teaching, or their constipation represents a significant change in the patient's normal bowel pattern:

——— ——— Urinalysis: _____

——— ——— Electrolytes: _____

——— ——— SMA 12: _____

——— ——— Abdominal x-ray: _____

The following lab tests should be ordered for the patient with unresolved constipation or a documented presence of blood in the stools:

——— ——— Barium enema: _____

——— ——— Proctoscope exam: _____

——— ——— Sigmoidoscope exam: _____

CONSTIPATION WORKSHEET RATIONALE

It is imperative that you determine whether the complaint of constipation represents a change in bowel habits and if this change has an acute or chronic onset. The assessment and plan will depend on this. The goal for therapy will be the passage of soft-formed stools without the need to strain ranging from three times a week to three times a day.

SUBJECTIVE DATA:

Description of Stool (pattern, character, etc.)

The past and present history of the frequency of defecation, and the character of the stool will aid in making an accurate assessment and in determining if a recent onset of true constipation does exist. A history of a recent onset of constipation associated with a change in character of the stool (e.g., bloody, pencil thin) is a more ominous sign. Recent difficulty in passing stool or gas may indicate a bowel obstruction.

The time span of the problem (i.e., acute or chronic) and the course (i.e., is the constipation getting better or worse) will give important diagnostic clues as to whether the problem is acute and serious or of a chronic nature.

Health Habit History

A complete dietary and exercise history will give important diagnostic clues as to the etiology of the patient's constipation.

Past Medical Diagnosis

It is particularly essential to obtain a past medical history of: diverticular disease, bowel surgery, irritable colon syndrome, anal fissure, anal abscess, hemorrhoids, hernia, ulcerative colitis, rectal prolapse, hypothyroidism, depression or psychosis, Parkinson's disease, diabetes, or cancer; any of these diagnoses may be related to the current problem of constipation.

Family History

It is important to note a history of ulcerative colitis, polyps of the colon or cancer of the colon because they have a familial incidence and are considered to be somewhat premalignant conditions.

Urge to Defecate

An absence of the urge to defecate may indicate: 1) an organic etiology, 2) constipation secondary to a longstanding laxative abuse which may result in colon atony, or 3) a failure to answer the urge over a long period of time. A history of a patient not responding to the urge indicates a future need for education in bowel retraining.

Laxatives Used

Chronic laxative abuse leads to atony of the musculature with a resultant decreased awareness of the presence of stool in the ampulla. A decreased awareness of rectal sensations results in a decreased urge to defecate with consequent constipation.

Recent Life Changes

Any significant life stress or loss can result in depression, and càn cause the patient to present with the chief complaint of constipation.

Medication Use

Certain antacids (Amphojel and Basaljel), some diuretics (those that cause K+ depletion), opiated analgesics and tranquilizers may cause constipation. Antihypertensive agents, antispasmodics, anticholinergics and anticonvulsants are infrequently the cause of constipation.

Associated Symptoms
Intolerance to cold

Intolerance to cold associated with weight gain, hoarseness, slowed mentation, edema, etc. may indicate hypothyroidism as cause of constipation.

Mucus or bloody stools

Pure mucus in the stools is most often a sign of a functional disorder of colon motility, although it may be seen in inflammatory bowel disease (i.e., ulcerative colitis). Blood in stools may be due to hemorrhoids, fissures, ulcerative colitis, diverticulitis, cancer of colon, an impaction or a foreign body.

Alternating periods of diarrhea and constipation

A history like this may indicate the presence of stenotic lesions, tumors, irritable colon syndrome, or fecal impaction.

Abdominal pain

Usually, abdominal pain arising from the colon will present as pain in the affected region. Pain in the left lower quadrant that is increased by defecation may be secondary to diverticulitis. Abdominal pain in the left lower quadrant that is increased with periods of emotional stress and decreased by defecation, and associated with a long history of such episodes indicates irritable or spastic colon.

Nausea and vomiting

These symptoms associated with constipation may be indicative of diverticulitis or bowel obstruction. In a distal bowel obstruction, the vomitus may contain fecal matter.

Unexplained weight changes

Weight loss may be secondary to: 1) depression, 2) malignancies or any chronic illness, or 3) poor nutrition secondary to edentulous state, lack of money, poor vision or immobility preventing food preparation. Weight gain may indicate hypothyroidism or depression. (Although weight loss is much more common in depression, weight gain is occasionally seen.)

Change in diameter of stools

The most common causes of thin stools are irritable colon, diverticular disease, hemorrhoids and rectal cancer.

Depression and anxiety

Constipation is often a symptom of depression. Therefore, ascertain a mental health history with past and present coping strategies, and look for other vegetative signs of depression (i.e., anorexia, sleep disturbances).

Bloating sensation

May occur in association with symptoms of irritable colon or bowel obstruction.

Decreased mobility

Decreased activity in the elderly may contribute to constipation.

Malaise, anorexia, weakness

Vague nonspecific complaints can be indicative of either functional or organic problems. Colon cancer, associated with blood loss and anemia, may present with weakness and malaise.

Low back pain

Irritable colon syndrome may be associated with complaints of low back pain. The pain may also be secondary to rectal problems that irritate the sacral plexis.

Tenesmus

Tenesmus (an uncomfortable feeling of the need to defecate associated with straining but an unsuccessful effort to defecate) may contribute to the development of hard fecal matter. Prolonged tenesmus in itself may lead to prolapse (due to the straining). The stimulation causing tenesmus is usually secondary to an inflammation.

Fecal incontinence

Fecal incontinence may be secondary to neurogenic causes or a longstanding failure to respond to the defecation urge (due to immobility, etc.). When due to neurogenic diseases, the patient will usually state that he or she involuntarily passes one to two formed stools per day.

Fecal incontinence consisting of the passage of semisolid feces and associated with passing mucoid matter several times per day may be due to the Terminal Reservoir Syndrome. In this condition, large masses of stool collect in the rectum and back up into the colon. This frequently occurs as a result of the rectal muscles becoming insensitive to distention from the patient's failure to respond to the urge (perhaps due to social, economic or mobility reasons). As the stool collects higher up in the colon, the fecal mass irritates the colon mucosa and causes an outpouring of mucus; the mucus passes the mass, softens it to some degree, and results in the passage of liquid stool and a soiling of clothes.

Anal pain, hemorrhoids, fissures

Any of these may cause pain associated with the passage of stool, thus the patient may not heed the urge to defecate and as a result experience constipation.

OBJECTIVE DATA:
Abdominal Exam

A thorough abdominal exam (with special attention to inspection, auscultation, percussion and palpation) is essential to rule out organomegaly, masses and/or tenderness. Stool should be felt for in the transverse and descending colon. The character of the bowel sounds should be noted. Any ascites, herniations or pronounced peristaltic waves should be carefully noted. Hepatomegaly may be secondary to an invasive neoplasm of the colon.

Rectal Exam

Special attention should be given to looking for fissures, rectal spasms, masses, tenderness, sphincter tone, the presence or absence of stool in the rectum and hemorrhoids, and the prostate should be carefully palpated in males. A careful palpation of the rectal wall for masses should be done because approximately one-half of all rectal carcinomas are within the reach of the examining finger.

Laboratory Data
Hemoccult x 3

In any patient with a complaint of constipation, a stool hemoccult should be done on three consecutive days to rule out the presence of blood. Blood present in the stool may be due to ulcerative colitis, diverticulitis, cancer of the colon, hemorrhoids, fissures or upper GI sources of bleeding. All patients with blood in their stools who do not have hemorrhoids or healing perianal disease should have a proctosigmoidoscope as part of their initial evaluation.

Hematocrit

A hematocrit should be done as routine screening to look for *anemia* (seen in cancer of the colon, ulcerative colitis or upper GI bleeds).

Urinalysis

The urinalysis, a routine screening procedure, may pick up a urinary tract infection due to fecal incontinence and contamination in females.

Electrolytes

Electrolyte disturbances may be seen in ulcerative colitis and iatrogenic causes of constipation (e.g., secondary to diuretics, etc.).

SMA 12

Biochemical assays may show an increased alkaline phosphatase (i.e., a colon cancer that has metastasized to the liver) or hypercalcemia (any cause may be associated with constipation).

Abdominal x-ray

An x-ray should be done on elderly patients complaining of an acute onset of constipation and/or when the physical exam shows abdominal tenderness, distention or increased/absent bowel sounds; an x-ray will help to rule out a bowel obstruction. On the x-ray you are looking for large dilated segments of the colon.

Barium enema, proctosigmoidoscope

These procedures should be done in cases of an acute onset of a change in bowel habits, blood in the stool, or when there is no evidence of perianal disease; their purpose is to help rule out the organic causes of constipation.

ASSESSMENT:

The following are common causes of constipation:

Anal disease

Anal disease may contribute to constipation because the pain associated with these conditions may cause the patient to ignore the urge to defecate. In addition bloody stools may frequently be associated with fissures, fistulas, hemorrhoids, etc. The patient should be followed closely for the presence or absence of blood in the stools after healing his or her anal disease. If blood persists, a complete work-up should be done to rule out other causative diseases such as cancer. When fistulas are found, one must consider diseases which may have prompted their formation (e.g., cancer, ulcerative colitis, etc.).

Atony of colonic musculature

Atony of the colonic musculature as a cause of constipation should be suspected when there is a history of laxative abuse and the physical findings are essentially negative.

Inadequate fluid intake

Inadequate fluid intake should be suspected as a contributing cause of constipation with negative subjective and objective findings except for a history of poor fluid intake. With inadequate fluids the necessary amount of water and electrolytes are reabsorbed into the systemic circulation, resulting in the formation of hard, dry stools.

Lack of proper dietary regimen

Again, a history of a poor diet in combination with a negative history and physical should suggest constipation secondary to lack of fiber, improper diet, etc. as a cause for the constipation. There may be many causes for constipation of this type: inadequate number of teeth or teeth in poor repair, ill fitting dentures, lack of income, presence of disability that precludes preparation of food or poor life-long eating habits, etc.

Immobility

The absence of positive history or physical findings except a condition of immobility should implicate lack of exercise as a contributing cause for the constipation. The increased incidence of disabling conditions in the elderly makes immobility a major cause of constipation. Immobility or decreased exercise decreases peristalsis and as a result may contribute to the development of constipation.

Iatrogenic

Certain antacids, diuretics, opiated analgesics and tranquilizers may contribute to the formation of constipation (see Subjective Data 'Medication Use' rationale section).

Depression

Depression should be suspected as the cause of the constipation if the patient has functional complaints with a negative physical exam and a positive history of unresolved grief, loneliness, etc. The patient may be complaining of mood disturbance, feelings of helplessness or hopelessness, anorexia, difficulty sleeping, weight loss (or other biologic signs of depression).

The following possible assessments are organic illnesses that may contribute to the complaint of constipation:

Hypothyroidism

Suspect constipation as a result of abnormal thyroid functioning if it is associated with weight gain, dry skin, coarse hair, slowed reflex response or confusion. Thyroid tests will be diagnostic (i.e., T4, TSH).

Automatic neuropathies

Neurologic abnormalities such as CVA or Parkinson's disease may be a contributing cause of the constipation. These conditions would present with an abnormal neurologic exam.

Hypercalcemia

Hypercalcemia may be detected by abnormal serum calcium levels. Constipation may be caused by hypercalcemia due to any etiology (e.g., multiple myeloma, milk alkali syndrome, sarcoid, hyperparathyroidism, etc.).

Diverticular disease

The associated constipation may be of an acute nature. Suspect if the physical exam shows left lower quadrant pain and tenderness with some guarding. The pain may be increased with defecation. Associated symptoms include fever, leukocytosis and blood in the stools.

The following causes of constipation are the most worrisome:

Cancer of the colon

The patient may have generalized nonspecific complaints such as weakness, weight loss, etc. Suspect cancer of the colon as a cause of the patient's constipation if associated with hemoccult positive stools and the above symptoms.

Bowel obstructions

The patient usually complains of an acute onset of abdominal pain, distention, nausea, vomiting, the absence of flatus and sometimes vomitus of fecal matter.

PLAN:

Anal disease

The treatment for hemorrhoids includes: (1) warm sitz baths and (2) suppositories that have a soothing, lubricating or antiinflammatory effect on the mucous membranes and may provide local relief of symptoms. Fistula and/or fissure treatment may include sitz baths and/or referral.

Atony of colonic musculature

Management plan should follow the outline *Plan for General Causes of Constipation.*

Inadequate fluid intake

Management plan should follow the outline *Plan for General Causes of Constipation.*

Lack of proper dietary regimen

Management plan should follow the outline *Plan for General Causes of Constipation.* Referral to appropriate community resources may be indicated.

Immobility

Management plan should follow the outline *Plan for General Causes of Constipation.*

Iatrogenic causes

Once the responsible drug has been identified, appropriate medication change may need to be instituted.

Depression

Refer to the depression protocol for differential diagnosis and management of the patient with depression.

Hypothyroidism	Obtain a T4 and TSH level. Consult and/or refer for medical management.
Automatic neuropathies	The underlying disorder must be treated with the proper therapeutic regimen through consultation and/ or referral. The patient should be referred with any unexplained abnormal neurologic exam findings.
Hypercalcemia	If hypercalcemia is found refer to a physician for a thorough work-up.
Diverticular disease	Treatment, if an acute onset, frequently requires hospitalization and usually consists of a liquid diet to quiet the GI tract. Chronic diverticular disease should be treated with a high bulk diet, stool softeners and sometimes a broad spectrum antibiotic.
Colon or rectal cancer	Diagnostic tests include a barium enema and proctosigmoidoscope. Refer to a physician.
Bowel obstruction	Refer immediately.

PLAN FOR GENERAL CAUSES OF CONSTIPATION—PART I

Once all organic causes of constipation have been ruled out and the patient's constipation has been determined to be of a chronic nature:

1. *Teach patient (or staff of health care facility) to keep a complete food diary for three days.*	The food diary will be an evaluative tool in counseling the patient. Use Food Diary Check List, Addendum 1. Evaluate the patient's food intake from the diary at the next visit. The Food Diary may be used as an evaluative and/or educational tool at each return visit.

2. *Teach patient (or staff) to keep a bowel flow sheet.*

   This will serve as an evaluative tool and as a method of monitoring progress toward a bowel routine. Use Bowel Flow Sheet, Addendum 2.

3. *Encourage* A.M. *and* P.M. *walks for ambulatory patients and for bedbound and nonambulatory patients do passive ROM and pelvic tilting exercises.*

   Exercise encourages peristaltic waves to propel bowel contents.

4. *Encourage the following foods in the patient's diet:*
   Breads and cereals

   The general principle of decreasing white flour and sugar intake while increasing the following roughage foods should be adhered to in the mobile elderly. Encourage such roughage foods as whole wheat bread, bran muffins, All Bran, Shredded Wheat, Roman Meal cereal, and bran.

   Fruits

   Rhubarb is an anthraquinone laxative which is not used in the United States but is widely used in Europe. It is very potent, and in its natural state has an emetic quality if sufficient amounts are ingested. However, as a food it is a useful adjunct for its fiber and laxative properties.

   Prunes are a useful adjunct in increasing peristalsis. Use rhubarb and prunes three times a week and supplement with fresh apples, oranges, and bananas in order to have a daily diet that contains three servings of fruit.

   Vegetables

   Fresh vegetables add fiber content to the diet. Fresh ground carrots, cabbage, greens and potatoes with the skin are particularly good.

Meats and eggs

Use fish, fowl and beef ad lib.

Milk and dairy products

Use milk and cheese in moderate amounts because they have a constipating effect. The patient should have ⅓ cup of unpasteurized yogurt per day; yogurt promotes the increase of normal flora and deters the growth of flora that thrive on refined polysaccarides and form gas. It is known that the anthraquinone family of laxatives is not potentiated in the colon unless the bacterial flora are present in sufficient kind and numbers.

Beverages

In order to promote an adequate intake of fluids, the patient should drink one 8-ounce glass of water with each meal, two glasses of juice per day and two cups of senna tea (once in the A.M. and once in the evening).

Senna tea has been used for over 2700 years for its laxative properties. It is said to have no toxic effects except in grievously prolonged overdoses. In that rare case, the side effects are related to electrolyte loss and other predictable laxative abuse symptoms. Senna tea is only slightly absorbed systemically, and seems to be effective in small doses by acting locally on the colon to encourage peristalsis.

In the mobile elderly, the evening tea should be taken with a bran muffin, raisin whole wheat cookie or piece of whole wheat toast (this adds fiber to the diet).

5. *The patient should be counseled at length to ensure an understanding of the mechanism of simple constipation.*

The following Patient Education Handout can be used as a teaching outline and/or handed directly to the patient. See Addendum 4.

6. *The proper use of the toilet should be taught.*

The patient should be taught to use the toilet immediately after breakfast for 15 to 20 minutes. It is also helpful to elevate the feet on a small footstool to flex the thighs and increase intraabdominal pressure. This is particularly helpful for those patients with a decreased abdominal musculature. The forward thrust of the body with flexed thighs allows the diaphragm to help in expelling stool.

Avoid using the bedpan; use the commode when at all possible. The bedpan forces extension of the legs and hyperextension of the abdomen and causes the expulsion of feces to be borne without muscular help, thus requiring a greater straining effort.

PLAN FOR GENERAL CAUSES OF CONSTIPATION—PART II

If after three weeks the stools have not attained a soft formed consistency, and/or they are still passed with difficulty (and the patient has followed previous steps), then the following additional management is indicated:

1. *Continue to have the patient use the toilet for 15 to 20 minutes with the feet slightly elevated; add a gentle digital stimulation with a gloved finger and a water soluble jelly for 1 minute.*

2. *Add Senokot tablets 1 to 4 per day, or Senokot granules 1 to 3 teaspoons per day or Senokot syrup 1 to 3 teaspoons per day.*

   Be very careful to titrate the doses based on individual responses.

3. *Add Serutan 1 teaspoon in juice twice a day.*

   Serutan is the bulking agent of choice for two reasons: it is without dextrose, so, unlike Metamucil and many others that are 50 percent dextrose, it is usable for diabetics. Second, it is also a combination of psyillium and methylcellulose which gives it a lower swelling factor than other bulking agents. This characteristic makes it less likely to cause a bolus in the esophagus or gut of debilitated patients. The dispersal into juice is also an important precaution for the prevention of an obstruction.

4. *Fecal impactions should be gently removed digitally and followed by a Dulcolax or Senokot suppository. Enemas or other laxatives are not recommended.*

   See drug Addendum 3.

ADDENDUM 1
Food Diary Check List

Date:	B	L	D	B	L	D	B	L	D	B	L	D	B	L	D	B	L	D
Fruit																		
Vegetable																		
Meat, egg																		
Whole wheat bread																		
Milk, cheese																		
Yogurt																		
Senna tea																		
8 oz. Water																		

The patient should check if a food was eaten from each food group under the appropriate meal: Breakfast (B), Lunch (L) and Dinner (D).

ADDENDUM 2

Bowel Flow Sheet

Date:										
Bowel movement										
Time of stool										
Amount: small (1), medium (2) or large (3)										
Consistency: unformed (U), soft (S) or hard (H)										
Any urge to defecate										
Continent (C) or incontinent (I)										
Digital stimulation needed										
Bedpan (B), commode (C) or toilet (T) used										
A.M. and P.M. walk										

The patient should check the appropriate box under the correct date. Check indicates an affirmative answer.

ADDENDUM 3
TYPES OF LAXATIVES AND THEIR MODE OF ACTION

A. STIMULANTS

1. *Anthraquinone glycosides* (acts in 6 to 24 hours) includes senna and cascara.
   Characteristics:
   —active in small amounts and are virtually unabsorbed systemically
   —chemically active only at the colon and are activated by bacterial activity
   —side effects (seen only in high dosages for prolonged use): gripping, loose stools and melanosis
   —most physiologic of known laxatives
   —they have a high regulative and restorative value with the spasmolytic action of the bowel maintained.

2. *Anthraquinone aglycone* (acts in 4 to 12 hours) includes: Doxidan, Doxan, Dorbantyl, Dorbane, Modane (some of these are combination laxatives)
   Characteristics:
   —is systemically absorbed in the duodenum
   —has poor peristaltic and laxative action except at high dosage

3. *Phenolphthalein* includes: Agoral, Evac-U-Gen, Ex-lax, Phenolax, and (in combination with other ingredients) Alophen, Caroid and Bile Salts.
   —high allergic potential with symptoms such as pruritus, rhinitis, asthma and urticaria
   —absorbed and circulated systemically

4. *Bisacodyl Dulcolax* (artificial stimulant)
   Characteristics:
   —not electrolyte disruptive in therapeutic doses
   —affects peristalsis
   —available as tablet or suppository
   —detergent lubricant

5. *Diocytyl sulfosuccinate* (wetting agent and softener) includes: Colace, and Surfak; in combination with other ingredients includes: Milkinol, Peri-Colace, Dialose, Doxan, Doxidan and Dorbantyl

—inhibits or destroys completely the glucose active transport system

—competes with bile for fat soluble vitamins

—disrupts the energy balance causing fatigue and weakness by preventing absorption of nutrients

6. *Mineral Oil* in combination with other ingredients includes: Haley's M-O, Kondremul, Milkinol, and Petrogalar
Characteristics:

—same mechanism as above drug

—has the added danger of oral aspiration and lipid pneumonia

B. BULK AGENTS (Work from 12 to 24 hours up to three days) members contain psyllium, carbomethylcellulose, methylcellulose, pectin, karaya, agar or guar
Characteristics:

—works for 12 to 24 hours up to three days

—may cause GI obstruction if taken without sufficient liquid; because of this it *should not be used in the immobile aged*

—may contain 50 percent dextrose or substantial amounts of sodium (Metamucil and Hydrocil contain dextrose)

—other products that include another ingredient are: Casyllium, and Dialose Plus.

—are largely unabsorbed and do not cause loss of fluid from the colon

—Effersyllium is a useful bulk agent because it has a lower NA$^+$ content than others

C. SALINE CATHARTICS includes Milk of Magnesia, Haley's M-O and Magnesium Citrate Solution
Characteristics:

—magnesium salts are dangerous to those in renal failure

—some contain sodium and should not be used by persons with cardiovascular disease

—can cause dehydration by drawing excessive body fluid through the bowel, produce watery stools and temporarily disrupt normal bowel peristalsis; long-term usage may cause an electrolyte imbalance

D. ENEMAS
Characteristics:

—soap may cause bowel necrosis if it is not immediately evacuated

—destroys the mucoid secretion function of bowel

—evacuates so completely that it may take two to three days to accumulate enough stool to have an urge to defecate

—tap water enema can cause water intoxication and severe electrolyte loss

ADDENDUM 4
PATIENT EDUCATION HANDOUT

A. What Is Constipation?
Constipation is a disruption of the consistency of a bowel movement. This disruption causes the stool to become hard, dry and difficult to pass.

B. How Often Should I Have a Bowel Movement?
This varies from person to person—as long as the movement is not hard, dry or difficult to pass, it is normal no matter how long the time between movements. A normal range is from three days to three times a day:

1. 90 percent of people have one bowel movement a day.
2. 5 percent of people go longer than three days.
3. 5 percent of people go as often as three times a day.

C. What Causes Constipation?
One or several factors may be involved:
1. Not eating enough
2. Not eating enough fibers
3. Not getting enough exercise
4. Not going to the toilet when you feel the urge to pass a stool
5. Not staying on the toilet 20 to 30 minutes
6. Not bending your legs and thrusting forward with abdominal pushing in order to expel feces
7. Poor fluid intake
8. History of laxative abuse

D. What Changes Do I Have to Make in My Diet to Decrease Constipation?
You should eat plenty of: 1) whole wheat bread and bran muffins, cereal; 2) stewed rhubarb and prunes with other fresh fruits such as apples, oranges and bananas; and 3) vegetables, especially raw carrots, celery, cabbage, and leafy green vegetables.

E. Why Is Exercise Important?
Exercise, along with eating, begins the peristalsis or gentle gut motions. These occur two to three times a day and move the chyme (food mixed with water) into the colon. Unless there is bulk in the diet, the food moves along sluggishly and does not stay wet. The water is absorbed and hard stool fills the rectum.

Bulky foods encourage the peristaltic action to push the food through the bowel, while refined foods without bulk cause a decreased gut action. When the food stays for a long time in the bowel there is more time for the bacteria to form gas and for the slow movement to cause a hard stool.

F. Why Can't I Use Enemas and Laxatives?
Enemas cause large amounts of water to flow into the colon. This dilute water when it is expelled takes important electrolytes from your bowel and leaves the bowel lazy and noncontractile. It inflames the lining and can eventually destroy the nerves that make you want to defecate, thus leaving you chronically constipated. Enemas are dangerous and should be avoided. Many laxatives also deprive your body of its fluid and cause pain with cramping and watery stools.

In Summary:

It is really best to control constipation by improving your eating habits, exercising more and going to the bathroom immediately when you have the urge. Allow yourself enough time to relax; when you feel an urge, press forward, tense your abdomen and push.

REFERENCES

1. Benson, John A. "Simple Chronic Constipation." *Post Graduate Medicine*, Vol. 57, No. 1, January 1975, pp. 55–59.
2. Berman, Phillip. "The Aging Gut: Part II—Disease of the Colon, Pancreas, Liver, Gallbladder, Functional Bowel Disease and Iatrogenic Disease." *Geriatrics*, 1972, pp. 117–126.
3. Brocklehurst, J. C. *Textbook of Geriatric Medicine and Gerontology*. London: Churchill-Livingston, 1973, pp. 346–363.
4. Brown, Marie Scott. "Over the Counter Gastro-Intestinal Drugs: Part II—Laxatives." *The Nurse Practitioner*, July–Aug. 1976, pp. 15–20.

5. Fairburn, J. W. "The Anthraquinone Laxatives." *Pharmacology*, Vol. 14, Supplement 1976, pp. 1–105.
6. Jones, Sir Avery Francis and Edward W. Godding, eds. *Management of Constipation*. Oxford: Blackwell Scientific Publications, 1972.
7. Sklar, Manuel. "Functional Bowel Distress and Constipation in the Aged." *Geriatrics*, Sept. 1972, pp. 79–86.

Chapter 9

Depression

OVERVIEW

Depression is a clinical entity that causes a great deal of human suffering. The only mental illness that necessitates more hospitalizations is schizophrenia. In the United States in 1970, 251,000 individuals were hospitalized with an admitting diagnosis of depression, 200,000 people received outpatient therapy for depression, and it is speculated that 2 to 4 percent more of the population should be under therapy for their depression. Moreover, 1 in every 200 depressed patients will commit suicide (Schuyler, 1974).

This protocol will include a definition of depression, the symptomatology, causes, modes of therapy, and a brief discussion of suicide. The biological theories for causes of depression will not be discussed because of limited space. The following protocol will aid the primary health care provider in identifying the common condition of depression and assist him or her in separating it from organic illnesses which may present in a similar manner.

The National Association for Mental Health defines depression as "an emotional state of dejection and sadness ranging from mild discouragement and down-heartedness to feelings of utter hopelessness and despair" (Schuyler, 1974). The most common symptomatology of depression can be divided into three areas: physical, emotional and psychic. The physical symptoms that occur most frequently are fatigue, insomnia, anorexia, constipation, weight loss and abdominal discomfort. Emotional manifestations of depression are usually an alteration in mood (the patient feels sad, cries or expresses the desire to cry) and fear, which at first may be directed at an identifiable source, but eventually progresses to a fear of fear itself. The patient may exhibit slowed mentation, difficulty expressing thoughts and an incapacity to make decisions. While most patients who are depressed will be withdrawn, frequently the underlying depression can be masked by anxiety, irritability and an inability to sit still. Guilt, self-reproach and self-accusation are common in depression. In addition, the person will express feelings of hopelessness, helplessness, and, depending on the depth of depression, may not foresee any relief from suffering in the future. The psychic symptoms include psychomotor retardation, loss of interest in self and others, death wishes and ultimately delusions, hallucinations and paranoid ideation in psychotic depression.

The causes of depression in the aged population are similar to the causes in a younger age group. However, some depression in the aged is an exaggeration of grief or mourning secondary to a loss. Because elderly persons are subjected to more change and loss than in any other period of life, they are called upon to make more and more adaptations. Enelow (1970) feels that loss in the aged can be categorized into three main areas: biological, psychological and social. The biological losses are secondary to the normal aging process, which may occur more rapidly in the presence of debilitating chronic illnesses. Whatever the underlying etiology of biological aging, the changes incurred pose a real and pervasive threat to the person's mental integrity. The psychological losses are centered on a decline in mental abilities such as memory, concentration and slowed reflex responses. This is particularly distressing to an individual who has depended on intellectual capacities to bolster self-esteem. The sociological losses are closely linked to the psychological ones. Elderly persons may be forced to retire from their jobs, and thus may suffer a blow not only to their self-images but also to their pocketbooks. In addition, the aged may lose friends, spouse, home or health, which can produce feelings of helplessness and loneliness worsened by the elderly's decreasing resources for adapting to change.

Other common causes of depression in this age group are drug induced depressions that occur secondary to the administration of drugs (such as reserpine or phenothiazides), metabolic disorders, infections, parkinsonism and organic brain syndrome.

In dealing with depression in the elderly, one should be cognizant that the aged person is a product of unique experiences and lifestyle (Gaitz, 1971). Psychological growth and development, as explained in the theory of disengagement, follows a pattern in which each phase is influenced by the one that preceded it. Thus, the nature of old age is immediately derived from the nature of adulthood, which in turn depends on the nature of adolescence, which is a product of childhood and infancy (Lesse, 1974). In essence, it is imperative to understand the patient's past and present coping mechanisms in order to understand his or her present condition.

Recognition of depression is the most important function of the health care provider, because it is only when the condition has been identified that appropriate therapeutic measures can be instituted to decrease the intensity and duration of the patient's suffering. Unfortunately, depression in the aged often goes unrecognized. The manifestations of illness may have been exhibited by the patient, but overlooked and ignored by the caregiver because of some common misconceptions about the aged (e.g., all elderly have fatigue, constipation and insomnia).

One of the tragic consequences of unrecognized depression is the possibility of suicide. Today, suicide ranks as the eleventh leading cause of death with 70 percent of suicides occurring after the age of 40. It is most likely to occur among individuals who have a past history of suicide attempts, a family history of death by suicide or who live alone and are unemployed or retired. Men are usually more successful at self-destruction than are women, but threats of suicide should be taken seriously in anyone who expresses them. The health care provider should ask specific questions about death wishes, thoughts or plans.

The three current modes of therapy for the treatment of depression are psychotherapy, pharmacological agents and electroshock treatments. If psychotherapy is the treatment of choice, consider the patient's age, type of depression, duration of illness, past history of similar episodes and response to therapy. Mild to moderate depression may be handled by primary health care providers as long as they recognize their limitations. Nevertheless, many types of depression are treated not only with psychotherapy but also with pharmacological agents.

There are two types of antidepressants available: MAO inhibitors and tricyclic antidepressants. Monoamine oxidase is an enzyme that destroys norepinephrine at the synapses of nerve endings. The MAO inhibitors prevent this enzyme from destroying norepinephrine, thus increasing the amount of this transmitter substance. The effect is then to produce an elevation in mood. However, drugs of this type should be used with caution in the elderly because their usage necessitates compliance by avoiding foods high in tyramine (i.e., beer, wine, cheese and pickled herring). In addition, MAO inhibitors should not be given simultaneously with the administration of antihypertensive agents, especially the sympathomimetics, and narcotics. The failure to adhere to these restrictions can produce a hypertensive crisis, headaches and other central nervous system disturbances. In contrast, the tricyclic antidepressants block the reabsorption of norepinephrine at the nerve ending. They are currently the drugs of choice for severe depression. They have been shown to be effective in the treatment of patients who are withdrawn, express a depressed mood or show signs of psychomotor retardation. One distinct advantage of drugs of this type is that they can be administered over long periods of time without tolerance or habituation developing. They should be used with caution in persons with cardiovascular disorders (i.e., arrhythmias, tachycardia or hypertension), and they should not be used in patients who are recovering from a myocardial infarction or who have a history of narrow angle glaucoma or urinary retention. The patient should be told that he or she may not experience an alteration in mood for three weeks after therapy is begun and that drowsiness and/or dryness of the mouth may be experienced. If the patient has previously been treated with an MAO inhibitor, the tricyclics should not be started for at least three weeks after the former drug has been discontinued.

Finally, the third treatment modality available for depression is electroshock treatments. The exact mechanism of action is not known, but it has been proven effective in a large number of cases where other therapeutic agents have failed. It is particularly useful in the treatment of psychotic and endogenous depression.

The purpose of the following protocol is to provide a quick reference guide for the recognition and management of depression. Before a differentiation between a functional and an organic disease can be made, a complete psychosocial and physical assessment of the patient must be done.

The differentiation of depression from an organic illness in the aged is very difficult and time-consuming. Nevertheless, once the diagnosis has been made we can hopefully diminish the patient's suffering and allow him or her to lead as productive and happy a life as possible.

DEPRESSION WORKSHEET

To be used for elderly patients who: 1) complain of a constellation of symptoms (i.e., anorexia, constipation, weight loss, insomnia, fatigue, etc.) for which no organic pathology has been found and which has not responded to normal modes of therapy; or 2) are described as or appear depressed (i.e., crying spells, isolated behavior, gross behavior change, change in mood, etc.)

What you cannot afford to miss: depression of any type; organic brain syndrome, either acute or chronic; metabolic diseases as a cause of depression; brain tumor; anemias; parkinsonism; drug intoxication.

Chief Complaint: _____

SUBJECTIVE DATA: (Describe All Positive Responses)

YES   NO

_____ _____ Onset of difficulties gradual or sudden?_____

_____ _____ Associated with an identifiable loss or event: _____

_____

Duration: _____

Course: _____Constant _____Intermittent

_____Seasonal

Relieved by:_____

Not relieved by: _____

Severity at worst: _____

Getting better or worse:_____

_____ _____ Incapable of managing activities of daily living: ____

RELATED TO:
YES   *NO*

_____ _____ Health: _____

_____ _____ Occupation or retirement: _____

_____ _____ Living situations: _____

_____ _____ Loss of friends and/or spouse by death:_____

ASSOCIATED SYMPTOMS:
YES   *NO*

_____ _____ Fatigue:_____

_____ _____ Sleep disturbances (insomnia, hypersomnia): _____

_____ _____ Appetite changes (increased, decreased):_____

_____ _____ GI problems (i.e., epigastric distress, nausea, vomiting, indigestion, constipation): _____

_____ _____ Weight changes (increased, decreased):_____

_____ _____ Genitourinary symptoms (frequency of urination): _

_____ _____ Cardiovascular symptoms (chest pain, dyspnea, palpitations):_____

_____ _____ Neurologic symptoms (headaches, dizziness, blurred

vision, auditory sensations, paresthesias): _____

_____

_____ _____ Mood alterations (i.e., sadness, despair, hopeless-

ness, helplessness, anxiety, guilt): _____

_____ _____ Psychic symptoms (i.e., impaired ability to concen-

trate, impaired memory, death wishes, delusions): _

_____

_____ _____ Hallucinations (auditory, visual, paranoid ideas): __

_____

PAST MEDICAL HISTORY:
YES   *NO*

_____ _____ Hospitalizations: _____

_____ _____ Serious illnesses: _____

_____ _____ Operations (especially list those without confirmed

organic etiology): _____

_____ _____ Allergies: _____

_____ _____ Medications: _____

_____ _____ Postpartum depression: _____

SEXUAL HISTORY:
YES   *NO*

_____ _____ Impotence: _____

_____ _____ Loss of interest: _____

FAMILY HISTORY:
YES   NO

——— ——— Diabetes: _____

——— ——— Hypertension: _____

——— ——— Heart disease: _____

——— ——— Renal disease: _____

——— ——— Cancer: _____

——— ——— Allergies: _____

——— ——— Mental illness (age of onset, diagnosis, treatment,

cause if known): _____

_____

——— ——— History of suicide in family: _____

PERSONAL AND SOCIAL HISTORY:

Birthplace: _____

Marital status: _____

Occupation: _____

Education: _____

Habits: _____

_____Smoking _____Alcohol _____Sleep _____Coffee

_____Drugs

Financial resources: _____

Religious affiliation: _____

Depression Worksheet

(Describe all positives): _____

_____

_____

_____

_____

_____

OBJECTIVE DATA:

_____Height _____Weight _____Temp.

Pulse: _____Regular _____Irregular

Respirations: _____

Blood Pressure: _____Standing _____Sitting _____Lying

GENERAL APPEARANCE: (Describe All Positive Responses. Any Abnormalities?)
YES   NO

_____ _____ Unkempt:_____

_____ _____ Sadness, crying: _____

_____ _____ Remorseful: _____

_____ _____ Motor activity slow or agitated:_____

_____ _____ Facial expression unchanging, tired, drawn, etc.: ___

_____ _____ Posture nonerect: _____

_____ _____ Speech slow or rapid: _____

SKIN: (Describe All Abnormals)
NORMAL   ABNORMAL

_____ _____   Color (abnormal pigmentation?): _____

_____ _____   Texture (dry and scaly): _____

_____ _____   Hair distribution (alopecia, texture): _____

_____

_____ _____   Scars (location, cause): _____

_____ _____   Inspection (rashes or eruptions?): _____

COMPLETE PHYSICAL EXAM INCLUDING: (Describe All Abnormals)
NORMAL   ABNORMAL

_____ _____   Lymph nodes (enlargement?): _____

_____

_____ _____   Head (signs of trauma?): _____

_____

Eyes:

_____ _____   PERRLA: _____

_____ _____   EOM's: _____

_____ _____   Nystagmus: _____

_____ _____   Ptosis: _____

_____ _____   Visual fields full bilaterally: _____

_____

_____ _____   Fundoscopic exam: _____

Depression Worksheet

Ears:

____ ____ Canals: _____

____ ____ Tympanic membranes: _____

____ ____ Hearing acuity: _____

____ ____ Weber, Rinne: _____

Nose:

____ ____ Septum, mucosa (discharge?): _____

Mouth and Throat:

____ ____ Teeth (present, absent, dentures): _____

____ ____ Tongue, gums: _____

____ ____ Uvula (midline?): _____

Neck:

____ ____ Limitation of motion: _____

____ ____ Auscultation (carotid bruits?): _____

____ ____ Thyroid: _____

____ ____ Trachea position: _____

Back and Thorax:

____ ____ Spine: _____

____ ____ Chest configuration: _____

____ ____ Respiratory movements: _____

____ ____ Auscultation (adventitious sounds?): _____

_____ _____ Breast (tenderness, masses, discharge): _____

Heart:

_____ _____ Inspection and palpitation of precordium: _____

_____ _____ Auscultation (S-1, S-2, S-3, S-4, murmurs?): _____

Abdomen:

_____ _____ Inspection (scars, distention): _____

_____ _____ Palpation (masses, tenderness): _____

_____ _____ Percussion (hepatomegaly, splenomegaly): _____

_____ _____ Auscultation (bowel sounds present): _____

Extremities:

_____ _____ Joints (ROM, redness, warmth, swelling, pain): _____

_____

_____ _____ Pulses (equal?): _____

Genitalia (Rectal):

_____ _____ Sphincter tone: _____

_____ _____ Palpation (masses): _____

_____ _____ Prostate: _____

Neurologic Exam:

_____ _____ Cranial nerves I to XII: _____

_____ _____ Reflexes: _____

_____ _____ Motor strength (muscle strength, tone): _____

Depression Worksheet

———— ———— Sensory:————————————————————

———— ———— Cerebellar function (Romberg, finger to nose): ————

    ————————————————————————————————————

———— ———— Mental status exam (orientation, judgment, recent

    memory, serial 7's, remote memory):————————————

    ————————————————————————————————————

LAB DATA: (Describe All Abnormalities)

NOT   *(Perform the first six tests if not done recently.)*
DONE *DONE*

———— ———— CBC:————————————————————————

———— ———— Urinalysis: ————————————————————

———— ———— EKG:————————————————————————

———— ———— Chest x-ray: ————————————————————

———— ———— Glucose (fasting and 2 hr pc):————————————

———— ———— SMA-12: ————————————————————

    If abnormal neurologic exam (after physician con-
sultation) order:

———— ———— Skull films:————————————————————

———— ———— EEG:————————————————————————

———— ———— Brain scan: ————————————————————

———— ———— VDRL:————————————————————————

    If organic brain syndrome (either acute or chronic)
is suspected, order (after physician consultation):

———— ———— Drug levels: ————————————————————

_____ _____ Arterial blood gases: _____

If blood loss from GI tract is suspected, perform:

_____ _____ Stool hemoccult x 3: _____

If hypothyroidism or hyperthyroidism is suspected, order:

_____ _____ Thyroid function tests: _____

DEPRESSION WORKSHEET RATIONALE

SUBJECTIVE DATA:
Onset
Duration
Course
Severity at Worst
Relieved By
Not Relieved By

These subjective descriptors and the patient's response allow the health care giver to obtain a more complete history of the course of the symptomatology.

Related to:
Health
Occupation
Living situation
Losses

All of these conditions or losses can be a considerable source of stress or grief to the patient. Some authors feel that depression is an extension of the normal grieving process. These questions aid the practitioner in discerning if the symptoms are related to an identifiable event.

Associated Symptoms
Fatigue

Fatigue associated with depression usually occurs early in the disease. It is not related to increased activity or stress and often persists after cessation of work. It is often aggravated by resting, and the patient may say that it follows a diurnal fluctuation as does his or her mood (worse in the A.M. and better in the P.M.). This

423

is in contrast to physiologic fatigue, which usually occurs because of increased stress and is relieved by rest. Psychological fatigue may be associated with nonspecific arthralgias and myalgias.

Sleep disturbances

Insomnia with early morning awakening is the most common complaint recorded in depressed patients. However, the patient may also report hypersomnia and disturbing dreams. Sleep is not restful and is not aided by the use of hypnotics.

Appetite changes

In depressed patients, anorexia is the most commonly reported appetite change, although the patient may complain of an increased appetite. Appetite changes may also exhibit a diurnal variation.

GI problems

Epigastric distress, nausea, vomiting, indigestion and constipation occur frequently with depression. On physical exam, there is no evidence of organic disease.

Weight changes

Weight loss of 5 to 10 pounds is common in the history of depression; some patients, however, will report a weight gain.

Genitourinary symptoms

Depressed patients will frequently complain of dryness of the mouth and will report an increased fluid intake to combat it. The urinalysis is normal, and there is no other evidence of genitourinary pathology.

Cardiovascular symptoms
    Chest pain

In contrast to organic chest pain, pain due to depression is mild, the duration is brief and the intensity is variable. There is lack of clear differentiating symptomatology and abnormal physical findings.

    Dyspnea

The dyspneic episodes associated with depression usually have a sudden onset, variable intensity and are not precipitated by an apparent cause. There are no abnormalities on the physical exam.

    Palpitations

Depressed patients complain of palpitations that are associated with anxiety attacks. These episodes usually occur in the evening and are not associated with a change in pulse.

Neurologic symptoms
    Headaches

Headaches related to depression are usually occipital, temporal or parietal. They may be associated with a pulling sensation of the neck, visual disturbances, and tinnitus. They may fluctuate throughout the day and are usually not relieved by ordinary remedies.

    Dizziness

Dizziness associated with depression may or may not be related to position changes, and is usually not associated with vertigo. Neurologic and ear exams are normal.

    Blurred vision

Blurred vision associated with depression may be associated with photophobia. There is, however, no evidence of neurologic or organic eye disease.

Paresthesias

Depressive associated paresthesias may involve the legs, neck, face and limbs with no physiologic rationale for distribution. Attacks are usually brief and subside without treatment.

Mood alterations

Feelings of sadness, hopelessness, despair, helplessness and guilt are universal components of depression. Anxiety may mask the underlying depression.

Psychic symptoms
Impaired concentration
Impaired memory

These alterations in functioning are secondary to an alteration in cerebral functioning as related to depression.

Death wishes

Ask specifically about suicidal thoughts and plans. The risk of death by suicide is greatly increased in persons who either currently express thoughts, give history of suicide attempts or have a family history of death by suicide.

Delusions

Delusions usually involve a theme of punishment or self-reproachment and are usually indicative of psychotic depression.

Hallucinations

Depressive related hallucinations may either be auditory or visual and are usually indicative of psychotic depression.

Paranoid ideas

Paranoid ideas may also indicate psychotic depression. They may arise, however, from changes in sensory input secondary to hearing deficits in the elderly.

Past Medical History

The patient's past medical history and manner of coping with problems may give you insight into his or her ability to deal with stress (i.e., change and loss). Medications are of particular concern in the elderly, for reserpine and some phenothiazides may induce depressive behavior. Drug intoxication can also present symptoms of organic brain syndrome. A past history of numerous hospitalizations or operations that were performed without any organic evidence of disease or positive pathology report gives significant clues to depression as the cause of past somatic complaints. Also, a history of a postpartum depression is of particular significance.

Sexual History

The depressed male patient may present with a chief complaint of impotence. Both sexes may report a lack of interest in having sexual relations.

Family History

It is helpful to ascertain a history of diseases which have some hereditary predisposition. The history of mental illness, type, etc. is also important because some depressive episodes are believed to have a genetic predisposition.

Personal and Social History

This information is helpful to ascertain a picture of the patient's living environment and available support systems.

Complete Review of Systems

Any positive answer that is not adequately explained or expected from the patient's problem list should be fully investigated to determine an organic etiology. Only after an appropriate accepted medical workup has been performed should a patient's symptom be attributed to a functional etiology.

OBJECTIVE DATA:
General Appearance

The depressed patient usually exhibits slowed speech and/or mentation, and an unkempt appearance. The facies appear tired, drawn, with deep circles under the eyes and very little change in facial expressions. In addition, motor movements may be slow; if anxiety is present the patient may be unable to sit quietly. Crying occurs frequently in depression.

Skin

In hypothyroidism the patient may have slow, slurred speech, dry and scaly skin, and alopecia. Abnormal pigmentation is associated with Addison's disease (which can present as depression).

Complete Physical Exam

An unexplained (i.e., not attributable to a known diagnosis on the problem list) abnormal physical finding should be fully explored (via appropriate protocol, referral, etc.) to rule out the possibility that the patient's depressive complaints/symptoms have an organic basis.

As part of a complete physical, a neurologic exam is done to rule out any organic basis for disease and to help differentiate between organic brain syndrome (OBS) and depression. The depressed patient is oriented to time, date, place, while the patient with OBS may not be. In both acute and chronic brain syndrome, the symptoms are identical. The patient experiences impaired orientation and an impairment of recent memory, but retains the ability to clearly recall events that occurred years previously. In addition, the patient may exhibit poor comprehension, calculation, learning impairment and emotional instability. Recent memory may be impaired in both depression and OBS. Serial 7's or other intelligence tests are normal in depression. Be careful to consider the patient's educational background before assuming that the poor performance in computation is due to OBS.

Laboratory Data

CBC

To rule out anemias or any hematopoietic disorders.

Urinalysis

To rule out renal disease.

EKG

Rule out cardiac disease.

Chest x-ray

Rule out lesions, etc.; secondary metastasis to brain is common in cancer of the lung.

Glucose

Rule out endocrine disorders.

SMA-12

Rule out hepatic, renal disease or electrolyte imbalance.

Skull films

Rule out intracranial masses.

Brain scan, EEG	To rule out lesions if they are suspected because of an abnormal neurologic exam.
VDRL	Rule out syphilis (especially tertiary).
Drug levels	Rule out acute brain syndrome secondary to drug intoxication.
Arterial blood gases	Rule out acute brain syndrome secondary to hypoxia.
Stool hemoccult	Rule out chronic blood loss from GI tract.
Thyroid function tests	Rule out hypo- or hyperthyroidism.
ASSESSMENT:	The complete history and physical will help to differentiate between an organic and a functional basis to the patient's complaints/behavior. The following assessments should be considered if an organic basis has been excluded.
Endogenous Depression	This type of depression occurs without being related to any identifiable event or loss. It is believed that this condition occurs secondarily to internal physiological processes. The symptoms manifested are severe depression, psychomotor retardation, loss of interest in the environment, lack of reactivity to the environment, guilt, suicidal thoughts and physical complaints such as those listed in the subjective data (i.e., early A.M. awakening with an inability to return to sleep, anorexia and weight loss). There tends to be a diurnal variation of

symptoms (the patient feels worse in the morning and better in the evening). There is also a preponderance of somatic complaints.

Neurotic or Reactive Depression

This occurs as a result of an environmental stress or an identified loss. It is believed to be an exaggeration of the normal grieving process. The patient may express sadness and some helplessness. The patient may have difficulty in falling asleep, but once asleep will not awaken until the A.M. Some somatic complaints may be associated with reactive depression; some express suicidal thoughts arising from a loss of hope. This is the most common type of depression seen in the elderly.

Psychotic Depression

The symptoms that the patient manifests in this type of depression are the same as with other depressive illnesses except that the feelings are exaggerated. Not only is the person unable to deal in reality but frequently he or she will have delusions and hallucinations. The delusions tend to have a theme of worthlessness, condemnation and punishment. Suicidal thoughts are not uncommon. The category of psychotic depression includes 1) involutional melancholia and 2) manic depressive illness.

Involutional melancholia

This usually occurs in women in the late 40's or early 50's. In men, it occurs later, usually in the late 50's or early 60's. This implies that involutional melancholia would not occur in the aged population. However, one should remember that people age at different rates. With this type of depression, there is usually no previous history of a depressive illness. The etiology is believed to be secondary to hormonal changes characteristic of this time of life. It is commonly associated with the symptoms of guilt, worthlessness, restlessness, agitation, weight loss and anorexia. The premorbid personality of the person affected is one of a compulsive, passive-aggressive, conforming person who has had an inability to express aggression.

Manic depressive illness

The symptoms associated with this entity are psychomotor retardation, some agitation, delusions, hallucinations and paranoid ideation. The onset of manic depressive illness usually occurs for the first time in the third decade of life. The onset is insidious, and it cannot be linked to any identifiable event. The course is marked by remissions and exacerbations, and the episodes usually have a seasonal variation. The patient may give a history of the episodes always occurring at the same time of year even though they may occur years apart. Typically, the depressive or manic state begins in the spring and ends in the fall; they seldom terminate in either winter or summer. The patients are almost always depressed two to three times longer than they are elated. With increasing age, the manic periods seem to give way to more depression.

PLAN:

Endogenous Depression

In this type of depression, tricyclic antidepressants are indicated. Consultation should be obtained.

Neurotic or Reactive Depression

Psychotherapy and perhaps antidepressants are indicated. Practitioners, if interested in counseling therapy, should be very cognizant of their limitations and ability in this area; they should not be hesitant to consult with and/or refer to a mental health professional if indicated. The therapist should also remember the underlying dynamics of depression; depression is an expression of a repressed anger or suppressed hostility that was internalized. The therapist must be able to deal with the anger and help the patient direct it in such a manner that the main target of the anger can be identified.

Involutional Melancholia

Refer to a psychiatrist.

Manic Depressive Illness

Refer to a psychiatrist. Lithium carbonate has proved helpful in controlling symptoms, but serum lithium levels must be closely monitored to avoid drug intoxication.

REFERENCES

1. Ayd, Frank. *Recognizing the Depressed Patient.* New York: Grune and Stratton, 1961.
2. Burnside, Irene Mortenson. "Recognizing and Reducing Emotional Problems in the Aged." *Nursing 77*, March 1977, pp. 57–59.

References

3. _____. "Loss: A Constant Theme in Group Work with the Aged." *Journal of American Psychiatric Association*, XXI (June 1970), pp. 21–25.
4. Butter, Robert. "The Crisis of Old Age." *RN*, December 1967, pp. 47–50.
5. Claghorn, James. "The Many Faces of Anxiety in Different Age Groups." *New York State Journal of Medicine*, February 1, 1971, pp. 331–334.
6. Cline, Foster. "Dealing with Depression." *Nurse Practitioner*, January–February 1977, pp. 21–24.
7. Cowdry, E. V. and Frank Steinberg, ed. *The Care of the Geriatric Patient*, 4th ed. St. Louis: C.V. Mosby, 1971.
8. Endicott, Noble, and Sidney Jortner. "Objective Measures of Depression." *Archives of General Psychiatry*, XV (September 1970), pp. 249–255.
9. Enelow, Alan. *Depression in Medical Practice*. West Point, Pa.: Merck, Sharpe, Dohme, 1970.
10. Gaitz, Charles. *Theory and Therapeutics of Aging*. New York: Medicom Inc., 1971.
11. Hauens, Anita. "Care of a Depressed Medical-Surgical Patient." *American Journal of Nursing*, LXX (May 1970), pp. 1070–1072.
12. Hoogerbeets, Jacob and John LaWall. "Changing Concepts of Psychiatric Problems in the Aged." *Geriatrics*, August 1975, pp. 83–87.
13. Krakowski, Adam. "Newer Concepts in Office Management of Anxiety and Depression." *New York State Journal of Medicine*, February 1, 1971, pp. 325–330.
14. Lesse, Stanley, ed. *Masked Depression*. New York: Jason Aronson, 1974.
15. Lubin, Bernard. "Fourteen Brief Depression Adjective Checklists." *Archives of General Psychiatry*, XV (August 1966), pp. 205–208.
16. Lyons, D. G. "Endogenous Depression." *Nursing Mirror*, October 17, 1974, pp. 93–94.
17. Moses, Dorothy. "Assessing Behavior in the Elderly." *Nursing Clinics of North America*, VII (June 1972), pp. 225–234.
18. Oberleder, Muriel. "Emotional Breakdowns in Elderly People." *Journal of American Psychiatric Association*, XX (July 1969), pp. 21–26.
19. Parker, Barbara et al. "Finding Medical Reasons for Psychiatric Behavior." *Geriatrics*, June 1976, pp. 87–91.
20. Rosenthal, Saul. "How to Tell If an Old Person is Senile or Depressed." *Consultant*, November–December 1969, pp. 21–23.
21. Schuyler, Dean. *The Depressive Spectrum*. New York: Jason Aronson, 1974.

Chapter 10

Obesity

OVERVIEW

Obesity is defined as an excessive accumulation of fat in the body resulting in the body weight exceeding the desirable weight for the person's height, age and bone structure. An individual who weighs 15 percent or more than the ideal body weight is considered obese. Adiposity is defined as an excess of fat accumulation in the body.

Problems arise in older age groups in deciding what degree of adiposity is normal with advancing age; the fat to muscle proportion increases in both men and women. Frequently the fat proportion is more than 50 percent higher than younger people of comparable build, sex and height. Thus, the elderly may be relatively adipose though not obese. Although it is possible for a person to have adiposity and not be obese, this protocol will deal with those patients whose adiposity causes a 15 percent or greater increase in ideal body weight.

Physiologically, the elderly person's body is experiencing an increase in fat deposition, a demineralization of bone and a decrease in muscle mass. The relative percentage of fat in the body continues to increase in old age even with a decrease in total body weight. In the aged, areas of fat deposition and atrophy differ from the younger individual (Rossman, 1971). Fat deposits in the face and scapular area tend to decrease while fat deposition increases in the abdomen and hips. Perhaps the most marked atrophy (even in average or overweight persons) in the elderly occurs in the arms and legs; most striking is the loss of subcutaneous fat from the forearms.

Because of the changing fat accumulation and deposits, the diagnosis of obesity in the elderly should be made using both Ideal Body Weight tables (appropriate for sex and age) and skinfold measurements. In one study (Hejda, 1963) the thickness of skinfold measurements in males varied from 1.2 cm at ages 25 to 39, to 1.0 cm at ages 65 to 79, to 0.9 cm in those over 80. In females there was relatively little change in skinfold thickness from ages 25 to 39 (1.5 cm) to those over 80 (1.4 cm). In men the most reliable measurement for predicting weight was taken on the right side of the umbilicus and over the hip; in females the most reliable measurement was taken from the umbilicus and upper arm.

Even in rare causes, obesity is almost always the result of an increased food intake in excess of the body needs. Many factors lead to the greater incidence of obesity in the older person. For the elderly, many of whom are retired, food is readily available and enjoyed; physical activity is frequently minimal because of life style and chronic debilitating diseases which limit ability to exercise. The decreased income experienced by many elderly persons causes an inability to buy the proper foods; cost, quick energy, physical limitations on proper food preparation and/or convenience become motivators for the elderly to consume excess empty calories (pastries, candy, etc.). Obesity connected with emotional disturbances such as loss of employment, loss of family or change in friends, home, etc. is common. In addition, knowledge of potential health risks connected with obesity and physical attractiveness are commonly not effective incentives for the elderly to reverse or prevent weight gain.

Total body weights in excess of the ideal range usually indicate an excessive fat content of the body. Underlying organic causes of obesity are rare and total less than 1 percent of all obese patients. The organic causes of obesity have been included in this protocol for the sake of completeness; the organic causes are hypothyroidism, iatrogenic Cushing's syndrome and reactive hypoglycemia. The subjective and objective data requested in this protocol are necessary for the health care provider to: 1) rule out any possible organic causes of obesity and 2) determine the patient's life style, weight history and past history of coping. Organic causes should be appropriately identified and treated; the management of nonorganic obesity will be enhanced by knowing the patient's present and past history.

Weight loss is important for patients because of the hazards of obesity. The actuarial data of life insurance companies demonstrate that even an excess of 10 percent in body weight significantly reduces the life span and that below normal weight increases the life span. The following are some of the complications of obesity: 1) coronary artery disease (due to hyperlipidemia), 2) hypertension (which can result from an increased myocardial workload caused by the heart having to push the blood through an enormously increased number of capillaries), 3) dyspnea (which results from an increased lung work necessary to expand against a fat thorax and abdomen), 4) joint strain, pain and osteoarthritis due to increased weight bearing and 5) an increased surgical risk (from pulmonary atelectasis, thrombotic problem and the increased incidence of wound infections). In addition, obesity unquestionably complicates gallbladder disease, cardiovascular disease, degenerative arthritis, diabetes, gout and lung disease.

The emphasis of the following protocol is on the management plan for those patients deemed to have nonorganic obesity. Initially this protocol is designed to be applied to all elderly patients whose body weight is greater than 15 percent over their Ideal Body Weight. The plan section will apply to the majority of patients (with nonorganic obesity). The protocol may be applied to a very few patients with a total generalized increase in body weight who *do not* have functional obesity; these patients may have either: 1) obesity secondary to organic causes (i.e., hypothyroidism, iatrogenic Cushing's syndrome and reactive hypoglycemia) or 2) a generalized body edema (anasarca). This protocol directs the health provider to refer elsewhere for direction/management of organic obesity and anasarca.

OBESITY WORKSHEET

To be used for patients who have
a total, generalized body
overweight greater than 15 percent
over their Ideal Body Weight.

What you cannot afford to miss: hypothyroidism, iatrogenic Cushing's syndrome, reactive hypoglycemia and anasarca.

Chief Complaint: _____
SUBJECTIVE DATA:

Describe the Following:

SOCIAL HISTORY:

Food preparation—who does this? _____

Patient enjoys cooking? _____

437

Obesity Worksheet

Who does patient eat with?_____

Describe typical (or yesterday's) meals: _____

_____

Describe snack foods, how often eaten: _____

_____

Who does the shopping?_____

Describe finances as they relate to food:_____

_____

Is food preparation area adequate?_____

Where are meals eaten? _____

WEIGHT HISTORY:

What is the most the patient has ever weighed? _____

What is the least the patient has ever weighed? _____

Describe past attempts at weight loss (Has patient attended

weight loss programs, which ones, how successful, etc?): _____

_____

_____

Describe approximate past weights per decade of life beginning at

20: _____ _____ _____ _____

_____ _____ _____ _____

Any permanent weight gain after pregnancies? _____

PERSONAL HABITS HISTORY:

Regular alcohol intake: _____

Medications taken: _____

_____

Exercise (amount and regularity, average 24-hour activity record,

enjoys exercise?) _____

How is leisure time spent? _____

PSYCHOSOCIAL HISTORY:

What is the patient's health/illness rating (scale 1 to 10 with 10 as

highest level of wellness)? _____

Description of patient's feelings toward self (anger, depression,

happiness, etc.): _____

What are patient's life goals? _____

Does patient want to lose weight; if so, why? _____

_____

Patient's goal for weight loss: _____

What does patient think of his or her weight? _____

_____

Describe moods during eating: _____

Manner of coping with anger, depression, boredom, anxiety: _____

_____

What method/system of support for weight loss has patient found successful (structural programs, friendly reminders, strict penalty programs, etc.)? _____

_____

PAST MEDICAL HISTORY:

Was patient a fat baby? _____

Any major illnesses (diabetes mellitus; renal, liver or heart

disease; asthma; hypertension): _____

History of hospitalizations and surgeries (especially thyroid

surgery/irradiation): _____

_____

History of steroid therapy: _____

FAMILY HISTORY:

Strong family history of diabetes mellitus: _____

REVIEW OF SYSTEMS:

A complete review of systems should be done. Particular attention should be made to the following if occurring with the onset of weight gain. (Describe Positives)

YES   *NO*

_____ _____ Dry skin/hair: _____

_____ _____ Alopecia: _____

_____ _____ Cold intolerance: _____

_____ _____ Lethargy/weakness/easy fatigue: _____

_____ _____ Constipation: _____

_____ _____ Mental changes/decreased mental acuity: _____

_____ _____ Hoarseness/dysphagia:_____

_____ _____ Cough/shortness of breath/postural nocturnal dysp-

nea/orthopnea: _____

_____ _____ Constellation of symptoms of: nervousness/anxiety/
hunger/sweating/weakness/confusion/fatigue/nausea/
vomiting/headache/tachycardia that occur about two

hours after eating: _____

_____

OBJECTIVE DATA:

_____Weight _____BP _____Pulse

Skin caliper measurement of umbilical area:_____cm
Describe All Positives

HEAD AND NECK:
YES *NO*

_____ _____ Hair (coarse/dry/alopecia): _____

_____ _____ Face (dull facies, moonface): _____

_____ _____ Enlarged tongue: _____

_____ _____ Abnormal thyroid exam:_____

_____ _____ Increased neck veins: _____

CHEST:
YES *NO*

_____ _____ Rhonchi: _____

_____ _____ Decreased breath sounds: _____

441

Obesity Worksheet

_____	_____	Rales/hydrothorax:_____

HEART:
YES   NO

_____	_____	Slow rate: _____
_____	_____	Arrhythmias: _____
_____	_____	S_3/S_4: _____

ABDOMEN:
YES   NO

_____	_____	Hepatomegaly/splenomegaly:_____
_____	_____	Purple striae: _____
_____	_____	Ascites: _____

EXTREMITIES:
YES   NO

_____	_____	Pitting edema: _____
_____	_____	Loss of visible superficial landmarks under the skin:

_____

_____	_____	Thin extremities: _____

NEUROLOGIC EXAM:
YES   NO

_____	_____	Abnormal reflexes (especially delayed return phase):

_____

_____	_____	Abnormal mental status exam: _____

GENERAL:
YES   NO

_____	_____	High blood pressure:_____

_____ _____ Truncal obesity: _____

_____ _____ Buffalo hump: _____

LAB DATA: (Describe All Results)

If the patient has not had a recent lab screening, the following data should be obtained (as generalized health screening before proceeding with a plan for weight loss): CBC, SMA 18, urinalysis, VDRL, chest x-ray, stool hemoccult × 3.

NOT
DONE   *DONE*

_____ _____ Complete urinalysis (should be done on all patients):

_____

_____ _____ T$_3$, T$_4$, TSH (should be done on patients with sus-

pected hypothyroidism): _____

_____ _____ FBS, 2 hr pc BS (should be done on all patients who have a family history of diabetes or in those patients with suspected reactive hypoglycemia or hypergly-

cemia secondary to Cushing's syndrome): _____

_____

_____ _____ 5 hr GTT (should be done in those patients with sus-

pected reactive hypoglycemia):_____

_____

OBESITY WORKSHEET RATIONALE

SUBJECTIVE DATA:

Social History

Knowing the patient's eating and cooking habits is essential to the development of an adequate weight reduction plan. Behavior modifica-

443

tion programs are based on the knowledge of past habits, with the addition of new ones to foster healthy eating habits. Specifics of food preparation and finances are necessary for the health provider to know; on the basis of this information, the management plan for obesity may need to include such social services as hot food delivery, financial aid, cooking school, etc.

Weight History

Knowledge of the patient's past weight history is essential in the assessment of the probable success rate of the obesity management. For individuals who have been overweight the majority of their adult lives, the long-term cure rate is somewhere between 1 and 5 percent (Ryan, 1975). Frequently the patients have tried many weight loss programs throughout their lifetimes. As a result of these programs, they have an understanding of why they failed and which programs were more successful for which reasons. It is extremely helpful to incorporate the patients' own insights of successful weight watching into the program designed for them at this time. In addition to ascertaining a life-style pattern as a way of estimating the success of a weight loss program, the weight history is helpful in determining possible causes of obesity. Longstanding weight problems tend to be caused by eating habits (e.g., excessive snack food intake, etc.); a recent onset of excessive weight gain is more suggestive of depression, hypothyroidism, a dramatic life-style change, iatrogenic Cushing's syndrome, etc. as possible causes of obesity.

Personal Habits History

Alcohol intake is important to ascertain because the high caloric concentration in alcohol can lead to obesity; the appetite is usually stimulated by moderate amounts of alcohol. In addition, weight gain due to cirrhosis must be suspected if alcohol intake has been substantial.

A generalized history of medication intake is important data to collect; many medications taken for a variety of problems have a high sodium content which can cause edema.

Exercise can play a significant role in reducing or preventing obesity. Knowledge of the patient's exercise and leisure habits helps in the development of an appropriate exercise program to facilitate weight loss.

Psychosocial History

Knowledge of patients' attitudes toward themselves and their health helps in understanding the patients' readiness to change. A very low self-esteem or an unrealistically low assessment of health status may indicate a need for counseling. Patients are much more able to consider weight loss for health reasons or personal attractiveness if negative feelings (e.g., anger, pity, depression, etc.) toward themselves have been removed first.

Determination of the patient's motivation to lose weight is essential. Regardless of how much the health care provider wants the patient to lose weight, if the patient is not interested in weight loss, any program development will be a waste of time. At the very least, the patient *must* be motivated in order for any program to work (short of actual physical food policing, which is impractical in any but the most dependent patient environments). If the patient is not motivated to lose weight (when weight loss is desirable), the health care provider should work on increasing motivation before proceeding with any weight loss plan.

Helping the patient understand the association of moods and food intake helps the patient who begins a behavior modification plan for obesity to correct the stimuli that initiate eating.

Ascertaining the weight loss methods tried in the past helps the practitioner and patient determine any necessary modifications to the behavior therapy (i.e., a technique found helpful to the patient in the past may be added to the weight loss plan).

Past Medical History

Determination that a patient has been grossly overweight since birth will help to set a realistic prognosis: that significant permanent weight loss will be extremely unlikely. The patient is asked about past major illnesses because the practitioner is looking for conditions that could have been treated with steroids (e.g., COPD, asthma, etc.). In addition, ascertaining the past major illnesses will help provide an accurate health status both past, present and future. A history of radiation and/or thyroidectomy for Graves' disease is important; these two treatments are a common cause of hypothyroidism.

Family History

A strong family history of diabetes should alert the practitioner to the possibility of reactive hypoglycemia as the cause for the overweight.

Review of Systems

The listed symptoms are such that if found with a constellation of positives and associated with weight gain, the examiner should be alerted to potential organic causes of general body overweight. A positive symptom should not be considered as a positive if its presence can be explained by a condition on the patient's problem list. If there is no explanation for a symptom from the patient's diagnosis, an explanation for that abnormality should be ascertained in addition to proceeding with this protocol.

The following constellation of symptoms (if associated with the onset of the patient's weight gain) should alert the examiner to the possibility of *hypothyroidism* as an organic cause of the patient's obesity: dry skin or hair, alopecia, cold

447

intolerance, lethargy, easy fatigue, constipation, mental changes, confusion, hoarseness, dysphagia and cough, shortness of breath, (SOB), postural nocturnal dyspnea (PND) and orthopnea.

The following constellation of symptoms (if associated with the onset of the patient's weight gain) should alert the examiner to the possibility of *reactive hypoglycemia* as an organic cause of the patient's obesity: nervousness, anxiety, hunger, nausea, vomiting, sweating, weakness, fatigue, headache and tachycardia occurring approximately two hours after eating.

Symptoms suggestive of congestive heart failure, renal disease and/or liver disease should alert the examiner to the possibility of anasarca as a cause of the patient's excessive weight gain.

OBJECTIVE DATA:

Complete Physical Exam

The listed abnormal physical findings are those that, if found with a constellation of positive abnormalities, should alert the examiner to organic causes of general body overweight. A physical abnormality should not be considered as a positive (to be grouped with a constellation of findings) if its presence can be explained by a condition on the patient's problem list. It is possible that an unexplained abnormal physical finding may be found besides those listed. If there is no explanation (from looking at the patient's list of diagnoses) for the abnormality, the patient should be worked up at least in addition to (if not before) proceeding with the management/ plan section of this protocol.

Finding the following constellation of abnormal physical findings should alert the examiner to the possibility of *hypothyroidism* as an organic cause of the patient's obesity: coarse/ dry hair, alopecia, dull facies, enlarged tongue, abnormal thyroid exam, signs of congestive heart failure (rhonchi, decreased breath sounds, slow heart rate, arrhythmias, S_3 heart sound, hepatomegaly, pitting edema), abnormal reflexes (especially a slowed return phase) and/or an abnormal mental status exam.

Finding the following constellation of abnormal physical findings should alert the examiner to the possibility of *iatrogenic Cushing's syndrome* as an organic cause of the patient's obesity: moon facies, purple abdominal striae, pitting edema, truncal obesity with thin extremities, high blood pressure, and/or a buffalo hump.

Finding the following constellation of abnormal physical findings should alert the examiner to the possibility of anasarca (due to many possible organic entities) as a cause of the patient's overweight: increased neck veins, rales, hydrothorax, organomegaly, ascites, pitting edema and a loss of the visible superficial landmarks under the skin.

Lab Data

General health screening

Unexplained abnormalities should be worked up; depending on the finding, the diagnosis should be made previous to or along with proceeding with this protocol.

Complete urinalysis

Glycosuria may be present in Cushing's syndrome and/or diabetes mellitus. Proteinuria, hematuria, casts, etc. should alert the health care provider to the possibility of renal disease as a cause of a generalized edematous total body weight gain.

Thyroid function tests

Hypothyroidism will show abnormal T_3, T_4 and thyroid stimulating hormone levels.

Blood glucose studies

Hyperglycemia may be present in Cushing's syndrome. If a patient has a reactive hypoglycemia the five hour glucose tolerance test will show a characteristic curve, with the blood sugar dropping to 50 or below between the second and fourth hours; the patient will usually become symptomatic during that drop.

ASSESSMENT:

Anasarca

Anasarca is a massive isometric generalized edema. When edema is generalized, relatively large amounts of water must accumulate in the tissue spaces before swelling can be detected by physical exam. In the adult, extra fluid must accumulate to ten pounds before it is detectable as pitting edema; pitting edema therefore becomes evident when the patient's body weight has increased by approximately 10 percent.

Subjective data that may alert the health care provider to the possibility of generalized body edema as a cause of the overweight may include: 1) a history of liver disease and/or a positive review of systems suggestive of liver disease (e.g., jaundice, dark urine, light stools, leg swelling, easy bruising, and/or a past history of alcohol excess), 2) a history of renal disease and/or a positive review of systems suggestive of renal disease (e.g., hematuria, facial/peripheral puffiness, fever, chills, and/or a history of urinary tract symptoms), 3) a history of cardiac disease and/or a positive review of systems suggestive of heart disease (e.g., cough, chest pain, shortness of breath, postural nocturnal dyspnea, orthopnea, etc.).

On physical exam the patient will have visible generalized edema. Anasarca can be recognized at a glance by the obliteration of the superficial landmarks under the skin. Pitting edema of the arms and legs will be present. In addition, there may be facial puffiness, ascites, S_3 and/or S_4 heart sounds, hepatosplenomegaly, rales, hydrothorax and/or elevated neck veins. Any determination of actual body weight measurements must be made after the abnormal fluid retention has been removed; thus the cause of the patient's anasarca must be diagnosed and managed before considering the patient to be obese and thus proceeding with this protocol.

Organic Obesity
Hypothyroidism

In the adult population, the most common causes of hypothyroidism are Hashimoto's thyroiditis (or irradiation therapy for Graves' disease). The onset of hypothyroidism is insidious. Subjective symptoms may include any of the following constellation of symptoms: dry skin; coarse, dry hair; alopecia; history of weight gain; cold intolerance; lethargy; weakness; constipation; mental changes (decreased mental acuity, confusion, hoarseness); and difficulty in swallowing (due to an enlarged thyroid). In the elderly, however, the classical constellation of symptoms may be absent, thus the disease may progress to the myxedematous state; in this state the presenting symptoms may be those of congestive heart failure.

The objective signs may include: a dry, scaly skin; coarse, dry hair; alopecia and a dull facial expression. If myxedema and congestive heart failure are present, the signs may include: rales, rhonchi, decreased breath sounds (if effusion is present); puffy eyelids and enlarged tongue; bradycardia with or without arrhythmias, S_3 and/or hepatomegaly (depending on degree of cardiac failure); edema; and a decreased return phase of reflexes.

Cushing's syndrome

Cushing's syndrome is an entity characterized by the symptoms of weight gain, truncal obesity, hypertension, hyperglycemia, muscle weakness, fatigability and purple abdominal striae. Extreme obesity is rare. Cushing's syndrome can be secondary to several causes (i.e., bilateral adrenal hyperplasia, adrenal adenomas or iatrogenic causes). In the aged population, the most probable cause of Cushing's syndrome is iatrogenic (i.e., secondary to prolonged administration of glucocorticoids in the treatment of COPD, asthma, etc.). The development of iatrogenic Cushing's syndrome is related not only to the dosage of steroids but also to the duration of therapy.

Subjective data includes a history of steroid therapy for a chronic disease, weight gain, a redistribution of fat deposits to a truncal location, thin arms and legs and/or easy fatigability and/or muscle weakness.

Objective symptoms may include a buffalo hump, moon facies, truncal obesity, abdominal purple striae, hypertension, and/or edema. The lab data may include: x-ray evidence (especially the spine) of osteoporosis, hyperglycemia and glycosuria.

Reactive hypoglycemia

Reactive hypoglycemia may occur secondary to a functional or iatrogenic mild diabetes. Iatrogenic hypoglycemia can occur secondary to insulin or oral hypoglycemic agents. Other causes of hypoglycemia include tumors, liver disease and malnutrition. Obesity secondary to hypoglycemic episodes (though rare as a sole cause of obesity) could be due to the patient's eating to alleviate the symptoms.

The episodes of hypoglycemia usually occur in the early morning or two to five hours after eating. Symptoms include: nervousness, anxiety, hunger, sweating, weakness, fatigue, tachycardia, nausea and/or vomiting. More severe symptoms may include headache and/or mental changes (confusion, loss of consciousness).

The lab tests may include an abnormal glucose tolerance test (with the patient symptomatic during the blood sugar dip below 50). There may also be a low fasting blood sugar.

Nonorganic Functional Obesity   The patient may be considered to have a nonorganic functional obesity if the history and physical do not alert the practitioner to any of the previously discussed causes of generalized total body overweight. Once the presence of obesity has been determined, and organicity has been ruled out, the status and amount of the patient's condition should be determined. The Ideal Body Weight for the patient can be determined from consulting a Desirable Body Weight table for men and women (usually obtained from a life insurance statistical bureau) *or* from using the following calculation:

IBW of Men = 106 lbs (for the first five feet) + 6 lbs (for each additional inch) + [Body Frame Adjustment].

IBW of Women = 105 lbs (for the first five feet) + 5 lbs (for each additional inch) + [Body Frame Adjustment].

Body Frame Adjustment = Add or subtract 10 percent of the IBW depending on the body frame size. A small body frame will allow the patient's thumb and second finger circumference to leave room when surrounding his or her wrist at the radius and ulna. A moderate frame will be a comfortable fit at the radius and ulna circumference (no adjustment in IBW is made for the moderate frame). A large frame does not allow the thumb-second finger circumference to touch when surrounding the radius-ulnar wrist area.

Skin-fold measurement in the elderly is also helpful in determining the degree of obesity. Approximate ideal skin fold thicknesses in the elderly are:

Men: (at the right side of umbilicus and over the hip) 1.0 cm to 0.9 cm.

Women: (at the umbilicus and upper arm) 1.5 cm.

Once the patient's present obesity status has been documented by a weight of at least 15 percent over IBW or a skin-fold thickness much greater than normal, the practitioner should proceed to the plan section for functional obesity.

PLAN:

Anasarca

Anasarca of whatever origin (e.g., kidney disease, liver disease, cardiac disease, etc.) should be referred for a full evaluation. Any patient (suspected of being obese because of significant increased body weight) who has any signs of generalized edema, should be referred for a total diagnostic workup.

Organic Obesity
Hypothyroidism

If the patient's signs and/or symptoms suggest hypothyroidism, draw a T_3, T_4 and TSH and consult/refer the patient. If the patient has signs of myxedema, refer the patient for probable hospitalization.

Iatrogenic Cushing's syndrome

The diagnosis depends on a combination of subjective and objective data. If the patient exhibits a true possible picture of Cushing's syndrome as a cause of obesity, refer to the patient's physician for management.

Reactive hypoglycemia

If hypoglycemia is suspected by information gained from the history, order the appropriate lab tests. If the patient has a documented reactive hypoglycemia, refer to and/or consult with the patient's physician. The patient should receive appropriate diet counseling; this should include an emphasis on frequent small meals and a high protein intake.

Nonorganic Functional Obesity

The practitioner should follow the following steps in managing the patient with obesity (rationale for each step is included):

Step One: Determine whether or not the patient is ready for weight loss.

Step Two: Explain the basis of behavior therapy to the patient.

Step Three: Implement behavior therapy.

Step Four: Provide emotional support.

Step Five: Add shopping/eating cues to the patient's knowledge base.

Step Six: Encourage exercise.

Step Seven: Answer patient questions concerning additional methods of weight loss.

Step I: Whatever the remote causes may be, obesity is almost always the result of increased food intake in excess of the body needs. The practitioner should apply this plan section to the patient if: 1) the patient's overweight is due to functional obesity, 2) the patient's other diagnosed diseases are concurrently being managed and are in reasonable control and 3) the patient's motivation for weight loss is high. It is essential to obtain motivation for weight loss before initiating a plan, because the success rate for obesity correction is low; the long-term cure rate for obesity hovers between 1 and 5 percent (Ryan, 1975).

Understanding the patient's past history of weight loss and attempts at controlling obesity will help the practitioner assess the patient's motivation. A patient who has lost very little weight from numerous attempts can not be expected necessarily to lose great amounts of weight this time. The practitioner should also assess the probability of the patient maintaining a lower body weight after weight reduction. If the history suggests a continual dramatic bouncing weight the practitioner may decide that attempts at weight loss may not be worthwhile.

Motivation assessment also includes an examination of the psychological factors contributing to the obese state. Markedly low self-esteem may be a great detriment to compliance for weight loss; the unhappy person who eats because he or she is unhappy will have difficulty losing weight without supportive adjunctive psychological counseling. The practitioner should remember that obesity for many patients is an attempt at adjustment; dieting may upset the patient's existing psychological balance.

One way to assess the patient's nutritional knowledge, financial ability, food intake habits and motivation is to ask the patient to keep the two-week record of food intake. From this much can be learned about the patient; a poorly balanced diet can be examined to find out if finances, knowledge or environment (physical adeptness, equipment, etc.) is the cause of the problem. Patient management should include correcting deficiencies. In addition (perhaps most important), a patient who keeps an accurate diary for the practitioner can be assessed as being motivated to continue with the program.

Stunkard and McLaren-Hume (1959) have summarized the result of obesity treatment with the observation that most persons will not stay in obesity treatment, and those that do either will not lose weight or will regain the lost weight. Conventional approaches to obesity treatment have emphasized: 1) dieting, 2) the medical aspects of the problem or 3) the inner drive/conflicts which compel the behavior of eating. Many authors (Ryan, 1975, and Stunkard and McLaren-Hume, 1959) have stated that behavioral modification as an approach to weight loss has shown both greater weight loss *during* treatment and superior weight loss maintenance *after* treatment. Standard approaches often ignore important environmental factors in the control of food intake, while behavioral therapy utilizes a habit reformation.

Step II: An important component of

behavior therapy is that behavior is influenced by its consequences. In other words, a stimulus leads to a behavior which results in an event. Concerning obesity, the stimulus can be anything that the patient interprets as a desire to eat (e.g., sight of food, smell of food, hunger, anger, boredom, anxiety, etc.). The behavior concerning obesity is eating; the "event" from eating is frequently relief of negative feelings or prolongation and intensification of pleasure, etc.

In order to break the cycle of emotions or environmental cues initiating eating, the patient must learn to consciously control responses. This technique of controlling the stimulus is directed to the restructuring of the patient's eating environment. Adding a specific stimulus (a new eating environment) will help the patient to think of eating only with that single cue; he or she will therefore gradually become less sensitive to the enormous variety of other stimuli to eat.

Step III: The program consists of helping patients plan a new environment around the following cues:
   1. Patients are directed to obtain a "new" place setting, one that is dramatically different from what they already use. From this point on they should eat only from this different place

setting (dishes, glasses, mat, silverware, etc.).
2. Patients should choose a single eating place in their homes.
3. Patients should remove all visual cues for eating—dishes for cooking, etc.
4. Patients are instructed to isolate eating from all other activities (such as watching TV, listening to music, talking on the phone, etc.)

Restricting eating to this new environment obviously makes eating impulsively (as from a dish in the refrigerator) or in response to an emotional stimulus (talking on the phone to a friend) impossible. The program requires that the patient is not restricted from food but rather is asked to take responsibility for what is eaten before consuming it.

Step IV: The food diary will assist the patient and practitioner in understanding some of the emotions that result in the patient's eating behavior. The practitioner should recognize the underlying emotional state of the patient; if low self-esteem, depression or another problematic emotional state is identified, intervention should be made. If the practitioner has a good counseling technique/ability and a good rapport with the patient, adjunctive supportive counseling should be initiated. If the practitioner ascertains a problem beyond his or her ability, patient referral to an appropriate source should be made.

A positive reinforcement/reward is an important part of the behavior therapy program; tangible rewards designed for the patient's specific needs can help the patient continue to use this plan. The unit of one-half pound (usually detectable on home scales) can be lost between one to four times per week using the behavior therapy program. If patients reward themselves for losing half a pound, they feel increased self-esteem and optimistic about themselves and the program. The reward should be given as close to the time the weight is taken as possible. The practitioner should help the patient select a reward substance: money, trips with supportive friends/relatives, movies, etc. can be selected. The selected reward should be something the patient does or buys for him or herself; for larger items, points can be collected toward a certain reward.

Assistance should be given to the patient in setting a realistic weight loss goal. The patient should not set as a goal any more than one-half pound per week. To expect to lose 30 to 40 pounds in less than a year is not realistic and the patient is likely to fail. The patient should understand that she or he is not going on a diet but instead is learning to plan food intake. The goal weight should be set by the patient; the practitioner may think it too high, but it is the patient's motivation that will lose the weight.

Supportive therapeutic attitudes toward the patient are important. The practitioner should be concerned, nonreproachful, interested in the patient and serious about helping the patient deal with obesity. The practitioner should *never* berate, condemn, show disappointment or disgust when the patient fails to lose weight, because this is in direct opposition to the need for positive reinforcement. Easing feelings of guilt or badness is important; if the patient fails to lose weight it is because the rewards are not sufficiently reinforcing the new eating behavior, *not* because the patient has personally failed.

By accepting the patient's comments and experiences nonjudgmentally, the practitioner is able to show acceptance of the patient. It is likely that the obese patient has never received this type of support and acceptance about his or her weight before; this difference in therapeutic attitude may help the patient stay with the program. The patient realizes that she or he will not be criticized for any failure or reprimanded.

Sometimes a written contract is designed to demonstrate mutual commitment and to provide further motivation for patient compliance. The contract transfers the verbal agreement into explicit written form; the practitioner agrees to provide visits, support and instruction and the patient agrees to keep appointments, conscientiously follow all instructions, follow the reward system, etc.

Step V: When the patient has begun the new eating behavior and has adjusted to the new environment, etc., additional tips toward weight loss can be added to the patient's knowledge base. These include the following:

1. Eat at a leisurely pace. (Rationale: When eating, a certain amount of time must pass before feeling satiated; eating too quickly may add unnecessary calories. Hints: Plan a pause during a meal, put the fork down between bites, do not prepare the next bite while eating the last, etc.)

2. Leave something on the plate. (Rationale: The patient should be reinforced in knowing that cleaning the plate does not signal the end of the meal; instead, food left on the plate is a signal.)

3. The patient should feel comfortable about eating as much as she or he wants of the following foods: artificial sweeteners, clear broth, coffee, tea, herbs, lemon juice, spices, vinegar, low calorie soft drinks. (Rationale: These are low calorie foods; the coffee and/or salt containing foods may need to be modified for other medical reasons.)

4. Favorite high calorie foods should be eaten in smaller amounts and less frequently. (Rationale: Asking a patient to give up favorite foods forever may be impossible, thus giving the program little chance for success. Therefore, suggest that the patient allow him or herself access to favorite foods in reasonable amounts on a schedule.)

5. Always use the new place setting. (Rationale: The patient who frequently eats away from home, in restaurants, etc., may need help in deciding how to continue the program while away from home; taking along a glass, napkin, etc. or any rearrangement of the usual place setting outside the home may serve as a reminder to the patient of the new eating behavior.)

6. Shop correctly. (Rationale: The patient should avoid shopping when hungry; shop only once a week; try to buy only those foods listed on his or her shopping list and buy the majority of foods from the four food groups: meats, fruits/vegetables, bread and milk/cheese.)

Step VI: Exercise is an essential part of weight reduction because most obese persons tend to be more sedentary than thin persons. The following exercise tips should be taught to the patient to increase the patient's motivation to get more exercise:

1. It takes a loss of 3500 calories to lose one pound. The caloric expenditure is proportional to body weight; thus the heavier person does not have to walk as far to burn the same number of calories. Walking is as good as running since it is the distance covered not the power that determines the amount of calories consumed. The following table is helpful in demonstrating these points (Durnin, 1959):

Body Weight in Kilograms (and Pounds)	Calories Expended Per Mile
	(walking, jogging, etc.)
130 kg (286)	147
110 kg (242)	125
90 kg (198)	103
70 kg (154)	80
50 kg (110)	57

2. A moderate increase in activity will not result in an associated rise in appetite. Conversely, appetite may remain higher than necessary after activity has been reduced.

3. Exercise after meals is thought to help food metabolize into heat rather than fat (Ryan, 1975). The obese person who does not engage in mild activity after eating misses an op-

portunity to enhance his or her thermic response.

Step VII: Patients frequently ask about the pros and cons of other forms of weight control. Medications used without an educational program cannot restructure a patient's eating habits. Methylcellulose (expands in the stomach and makes the patient feel full and relieves stomach hunger pains) taken before meals with a full glass of water may be tried; however, satiety is rarely achieved and many patients do not comply for long. The energy boost and appetite effect of anorectics can help the patient eat less, but there is no support when the medication is terminated. In addition, the side effects of anorectics make them undesirable for use in the elderly population. Amphetamines are totally contraindicated for use in the elderly (due to the cardiovascular risks and status in the aging individual).

Fad diets are also contraindicated. Diets very low in carbohydrate and rich in fat have dangers of hyperlipidemia (which can accelerate artherosclerosis). Ketogenic diets may also cause a rise in the blood uric acid concentration. Carbohydrate-free diets have a high incidence of causing fatigue and postural hypotension. In addition, rapid weight loss followed by weight gain (when drug, fad diet, etc. are stopped) leave the patient enduring feelings of failure, guilt, frustration and a loss of dignity.

Dramatic measures such as jaw wiring and/or intestinal bypass surgery are too often associated with severe complications and are definitely contraindicated in the elderly population.

REFERENCES

1. Brightwell, D. R. "Treating Obesity with Behavior Modification." *Postgraduate Medicine*, 55, 1974, pp. 52–58.
2. Brightwell, Dennis R. et al. (ed.) "New Eating Behavior, Practical Management of Obesity" published by Pennwalt Prescription Products, Pennwalt Corporation, Rochester, New York, 14603, 1975.
3. Burley, E. J. et al. "Behavior Modification: Two Nurses Tell It Like It Is." *Journal of Psychiatric Nursing*, 10, January–February 1972. p. 26.
4. _____. "A Critique of Low-Carbohydrate Ketogenic Weight Reduction Regimes." published by the AMA Council on Foods and Nutrition, 535 N. Dearborn St., Chicago 60610, 1973. Reprinted from *JAMA*, 224, 10, June 4, 1973.
5. DeRisi, W. "Writing Behavioral Contracts to Control Problems." *Practical Psychology for Physicians*, 2, 1975, pp. 47–50.
6. Durnin, J. V. G. A. "The Use of Surface Area and of Body-Weight as Standards of Reference in Studies on Human Energy Expenditures." *British Journal of Nutrition*, 13, 1959, pp. 68–71.
7. Hejda, S. "Skinfold in Old and Longlived Individuals." *Gerontologia*, 8, 1963, p. 201.
8. Olson, Verla. "Obesity in the Elderly." Unpublished paper for Geriatric Nurse Practitioner Program, Spring 1976, University of Colorado Continuing Education Services.
9. Rossman, Isadore (ed.). *Clinical Geriatrics*. Philadelphia: J.B. Lippincott Co., 1971.
10. Ryan, Allan J. (moderator). "Round Table, Charting the Factors of Fatness." *The Physician and Sports-Medicine*, July 1975, pp. 57–70.
11. Stunkard A. J., and M. McLaren-Hume. "The Results of Treatment for Obesity." *Archives of Internal Medicine*, 103, 1959, pp. 79–85.

Chapter 11

Dementia

OVERVIEW

For approximately 900,000 people in this country over the age of 65, aging is linked with serious cerebral dysfunction; another 2 million experience mild to moderate cerebral dysfunction (Katzman and Karasu, 1975). Yet there is a dearth of meaningful information available concerning this ongoing and devastating biological process.

Dementia is the progressive loss of higher cerebral function which may involve impaired orientation, memory, judgment, intellectual function, reflective self-awareness, social communication and language. Although disease in several parts of the cerebrum may cause memory impairment, the defects found with dementia are usually related to parts of the cerebral cortex and diencephalon. Any action disturbing the biochemical state of the neurons or changing the morphology of the central nervous system will disturb higher cerebral functions. Since many different structures in the brain are responsible for normal mentation, no accurate description of a specific pathophysiology can be offered.

In those people over 65 who are mentally intact, brain parenchyma has been shown to shrink 10 to 15 percent (Terry and Wisniewski, 1965). This decrease in cerebral substance leads to widening of sulci, narrowing of convolutions and increase in ventricular size. Whether the actual number of neurons change is questionable, and many feel the number remains fairly constant throughout life, decreasing less than 3.5 percent in the ninth and tenth decades (Terry and Wisniewski, 1975). Others feel the decrease in brain parenchyma is significantly greater. In the demented patient, loss of nerve cells is most apparent in the cerebral cortex and has been found to account for approximately 30 percent of the original brain mass (Terry and Wisniewski, 1965).

Microscopically, deposits of amorphous material called "senile plaques" have been found scattered throughout the cerebral cortex.

It has been shown by electron microscopy that the main characteristic of the plaque is the presence of abnormal neural processes. Also seen are neurofibrillary tangles in the cytoplasm of nerve cells. Both the senile plaques and neurofibrillary tangles are seen in older persons with no obvious mental changes but are especially marked in the presenile and senile dementias.

Cognitive changes in the elderly are not usually associated with the vascular stenotic processes of arteriosclerosis, and many senile people have normal vessels in their brains on autopsy. Often a decreased blood flow to the brain is found, which is believed to be not the cause of the dementia but the effect of the regulatory apparatus of the brain which decreases blood flow if cerebral tissue with high metabolic needs is lost (Terry and Wisniewski, 1975).

The overall changes in mental function during the aging process are irregular and seem to depend on genetic and environmental factors specific to each person. It is important to remember that disorientation is not just a psychological phenomenon; some pathology is often the causative factor. I.Q. testing of the elderly has shown that there is little change from tests taken at an earlier age. Often, results are better. The elderly do have difficulty with the speed factor involved in testing, and this must be considered when interpreting test results (Wahl, 1976).

The physiologic aging of the brain is a variable complex of nerve and tissue changes. Neurochemical changes in aging are characterized by impaired transcription of the genetic code for protein synthesis. This disturbed protein synthesis leads to altered metabolic activity and the resultant slowed EEG activity, impaired short-term memory, behavior, sleeping and awareness (Meier-Ruge, 1965). There are, however, limits in quantity and intensity of changes beyond which the condition can no longer be regarded as normal senescence.

Because of the nonspecific nature of the pathology involved and the wide constellation of clinical findings possible, the dementia seen in any patient may be due to a wide variety of clinical pathologies. The primary goal in the work-up of any patient with dementia, regardless of its duration, is to search for a reversible etiology. Every patient with a dementia in whom a treatable cause is not discovered by routine testing, as will be outlined in this protocol, should be seen by a neurologist. When all treatable etiologies have been excluded, the nontreatable dementias are considered.

The etiology of most cases of senile dementia is now thought to be Alzheimer's disease which occurs at a later age. In Alzheimer's disease, fibrillary changes and senile plaques are seen in the major association areas of the cerebral cortex. Loss of neurons is prominent especially in the cerebral cortex, and the brain itself appears shrunken with atrophy of the convolutions and enlargement of the lateral and third ventricle. Changes are especially pronounced in the frontal and temporal lobe with involvement of the basal ganglion.

Pick's disease is seen less frequently than Alzheimer's and is associated with a characteristic pattern of cerebral atrophy. Gross pathologic changes are seen, including severe atrophy of the frontal and temporal lobes as well as atrophy in some subcortical structures. Microscopically, a ballooning out of neurons in the atrophic areas is seen.

The diagnosis of senile dementia is a diagnosis of exclusion, and the data base obtained reflects this. The laboratory tests that will be

TABLE 11-1. Clinical Manifestations of Cerebral Pathology

Frontal Lobe	*Temporal Lobe*
Defects in judgment	Psychomotor seizures
Absurd jocularity	Confabulation
Changes in mood (especially apathy), personality and intellectual functioning	Memory impairment
	Hallucinations and delusions
	Personality changes
Gait disturbance	
Grasp reflex	

Parietal Lobe	*Occipital Lobe*
Problems with spatial relationships	Field defects
Dyspraxia	Visual distortion
Difficulty reading and writing	Color blindness
Neglect or denial of disability	Failure to recognize the familiar

Extrapyramidal Dysfunction	*Pyramidal Dysfunction*
Bradykinesia	Weakness
Rigidity	Clumsiness
Difficulty in maintaining a normal standing position with head upright	Difficulty in initiating voluntary movement
Grasp reflex	Spasticity
Chorea (rapid, involuntary, "dancing" movement), athetosis, dystonia	

proposed for patients with cognitive changes are all searching for a reversible underlying problem. There is no one diagnostic finding, whether it be subjective, objective or laboratory data (other than brain biopsy), which can confirm the diagnosis of a nontreatable dementia; it is only when all other causes have been systematically eliminated that an assessment of senile dementia can be made. Table 1-11 is included to aid in the recognition of localized findings. Although the nurse practitioner may not be involved in ordering or performing all of the tests suggested, they have been included in this protocol so that he or she can look over the entire medical work-up of the patient and be sure that no significant finding was missed through omission of a study.

Another aspect of the assessment of a patient with a loss of higher cerebral function is the evaluation of how the patient is managing in his or her environment, how the patient's behavior is affecting the family and whether or not institutionalization is a viable alternative. The initial assessment provides the practitioner with a baseline from which future evaluations can be compared as well as a basis of formulation of a beginning plan for the patient.

DEMENTIA WORKSHEET

To be used for patients with acute or chronic dementia, e.g. progressive loss of orientation, memory, judgment, intellectual function, reflective self-awareness, social communication or language.

What you cannot afford to miss: tumor, subdural hematoma, normal pressure hydrocephalus (NPH), infection, syphilis, functional disorders, intoxications (drugs, alcohol, metals), endocrinopathies, liver disease, uremia, heart disease, nutritional deficiencies, Wernicke-Korsakoff syndrome, pernicious anemia, metabolic disturbances, collagen disease, cerebrovascular disease (aneurysm), Wilson's disease, porphyria.

Chief Complaint: _____
SUBJECTIVE DATA: (Describe Positive Responses)

ONSET OF DIFFICULTIES:
YES   *NO*

—— —— Gradual/sudden: _____

—— —— Rapidity of progress: _____

—— —— First difficulty encountered: _____

—— —— Precipitating events: _____

MEMORY DEFECT:

—— —— Nature of memory loss: _____

BEHAVIOR:

—— —— Depression/irritability/anger/restlessness:_____

—— —— Personality changes: _____

FAMILY HISTORY:

—— —— Family history of dementia: _____

ASSOCIATED WITH:
YES   *NO*

—— —— Ataxia:_____

—— —— Incontinence: _____

—— —— Drowsiness: _____

—— —— Headache: _____

—— —— Visual problem: _____

—— —— Movement disorders:_____

Dementia Worksheet

_____ _____ Parasthesias:_____

_____ _____ Seizures: _____

PAST MEDICAL HISTORY:

Significant past illnesses: _____

_____

Medications: _____

Dietary history: _____

REVIEW OF SYSTEMS:

_____

_____

_____

_____

OBJECTIVE DATA:

Vital Signs:

_____Temp. _____Pulse _____Resp. _____BP

General Appearance:

Affect: _____

NEUROLOGIC EXAMINATION (Describe Negative Responses):
MENTAL STATUS INTACT:
YES   _NO_

_____ _____ 1. Orientation to person, place, time: _____

_____ _____ 2. Memory

_____ _____   a. Immediate recall (repetition of digit span): __

_____ _____   b. Recent memory (recall of three objects after

                        five minutes):_____

_____ _____   c. Remote:_____

_____ _____   3. General information (name presidents, discuss

                     current events): _____

_____ _____   4. Calculation

_____ _____   a. Serial subtractions (7's; 3's from 20): _____

_____ _____   b. Calculate simple problems: _____

_____ _____   5. Abstraction: _____
                    a. Example: What do a swimming pool and lake
                       have in common?

_____ _____   6. Judgment: _____

_____ _____   a. Example: What would you do if you found an
                       addressed stamped envelope?

_____ _____   7. Language: _____

_____ _____   a. Speech content; naming; repetitions; para-
                       phrase: _____

_____ _____   b. Ability to read; ability to write to dictate:

                   _____

_____ _____   8. Pictures: _____

_____ _____   a. Interpretation: _____

_____ _____   b. Copying and drawing:_____

Dementia Worksheet

_____ _____ *Cranial Nerves I-XII Intact:*_____ _____

_____ _____ *Deep Tendon Reflexes (DTR's) 0-4+ (equal bilater-*

ally): _____

_____

PATHOLOGIC REFLEXES PRESENT: (Describe all positives)
YES   *NO*

_____ _____ 1. Babinski — pathologic plantar response: _____

_____ _____ 2. Snout — puckering of lips in response to gentle

percussion in the oral region:_____

_____ _____ 3. Rooting — turning to a stroking stimulus in the

oral region: _____

_____ _____ 4. Sucking — sucking movements of the lips in response to tactile stimulation on the oral region:

_____

_____ _____ 5. Grasp — stimulation of palm causing grasping

movement:_____

Describe All Negatives

_____ _____ *Motor Strength*: muscle bulk intact and equal bilat-

erally: _____

_____ _____ *Sensory intact* and equal bilaterally: _____

_____ _____ *Cerebellar intact* (rapid alternating movements; heel

to the shin; finger to nose): _____

_____

_____

_____ _____ _Romberg:_ _____

_____ _____ _Gait intact:_ _____

_____ _____ _Speech intact:_ _____

_____ _____ _Complete physical examination_ within normal limits: _____

_____

_____

_____

_____

_____ _____ Absence of local head tenderness: _____

_____ _____ Normal external eye exam: _____

_____ _____ Normal funduscopic exam: _____

LAB DATA:

DONE   _NOT_
       DONE

_____ _____ CBC with RBC indices: _____

_____ _____ Serum glucose: _____

_____ _____ Serum electrolytes: _____

_____ _____ Serum enzymes: _____

_____ _____ Urinalysis: _____

_____ _____ BUN: _____

_____ _____ Thyroid function studies: _____

_____ _____ Serology: _____

_____ _____ Toxicology screen (serum and urine): _____

_____ _____ EKG: _____

_____ _____ EEG: _____

_____ _____ CSF examination: _____

_____ _____ Skull films: _____

_____ _____ Chest x-ray: _____

_____ _____ Brain scan: _____

_____ _____ Computerized tomography (C-T scan): _____

DEMENTIA WORKSHEET RATIONALE

SUBjECT!VE DATA:

Onset of Difficulties
Sudden/gradual

The dementia associated with sub-dural hematomas, Creutzfeldt-Jakob disease, Wernicke's, infection, anoxia, multifocal leuko-encephalopathy and affective causes may present with a great rapidity of onset. Most untreatable and metabolic causes of dementia are marked by slow onset, sometimes to the point that the family cannot pinpoint when the symptoms began.

Rapidity of progress

Subdural hematomas and Creutzfeldt-Jakob disease are marked by a rapidly progressive dementia. Symptoms of Wernicke-Korsakoff's syndrome plateau to a stable level. The majority of patients with other causes of dementia show slow, gradual progression.

First difficulty encountered

In normal pressure hydrocephalus, a gait disturbance is often the first and most disconcerting symptom; subdural hematomas may first present with drowsiness. A speech disturbance may be seen early in Pick's disease.

Precipitating events

Confusion due to anxiety may arise after the removal of familiar landmarks such as what is seen in newly hospitalized patients. Bereavement, isolation or fatigue may precipitate depression. With a history of trauma, a subdural is considered, although this can occur in the elderly with no ascertainable trauma. Changes in personality and behavior have been noted in former boxers.

Memory Defect
Nature of memory loss

In normal senescence, there is a tendency to forget details of an event which itself is recalled. In pathologic dementias, entire portions of the patient's life may be obliterated (Katzman and Karasu, 1975). When the progression is slow, the patient can at first rearrange his or her life to account for faulty memory. This adaptation cannot occur when memory loss is rapid. In progressive memory loss, short-term memory is the first to go. In Wernicke-Korsakoff's syndrome, memory loss is often so marked that the patient is disoriented to time and place; in milder cases, compensatory confabulation is seen.

Behavior

Persons experiencing a decline in cognitive functions often become depressed, irritable, angry and/or restless. In Alzheimer's disease, jealousy and paranoid tendencies are often seen. In the depressed patient who appears demented, there is a decrease in self-esteem and guilt feelings are present.

Family History of Dementia

Huntington's chorea is inherited as a Mendelian dominant which rarely skips generations. Cases of multiple occurrences of Alzheimer's disease and Pick's disease in families have been reported in only a limited number of instances. In dementia due to affective disorders, a high incidence of mental illness has been found in close relatives.

Associated With:
Ataxia

Ataxia is found in both treatable and nontreatable dementias (i.e. Wernicke's; pellegra; bromide, paraldehyde and barbiturate intoxication; liver disease; syphilis; hypothyroidism; Alzheimer's, Pick's, Creutzfeldt-Jakob; pernicious anemia; multiple sclerosis). Ataxia of gait may be the presenting symptom of NPH.

Incontinence

In patients presenting with spastic gait, dementia and urinary incontinence, NPH must be suspected. Incontinence is seen late in most progressive dementias.

Drowsiness

A subdural hematoma should be suspected when drowsiness accompanies a recent personality change.

Drowsiness is also observed in patients with tumors, vitamin B_{12} deficiency, liver disease, uremia and intoxications.

Headache

Headache is an outstanding feature in cerebral abscess, tumor, intracranial aneurysm and subdural hematoma.

Visual problems

In Wernicke's syndrome, sudden onset of ophthalmoparesis occurs. Patients with focal lesions may experience visual disturbances. Oculogyric crises occur in Parkinson's disease and phenothiazine intoxication.

Movement disorders

Extrapyramidal dysfunction is seen in dementia pugilistica; choreiform movements accompany Huntington's chorea; clumsiness of the extremities is seen in multiple sclerosis. Muscular incoordination and involuntary movement is seen in mercury poisoning. Pernicious anemia may be accompanied by spasticity.

Parasthesias

Parasthesias are present in hypothyroidism and folate and B_{12} deficiency.

Seizures

Seizures are found in patients with dementias of focal and diffuse etiology including Alzheimer's, Pick's, systemic lupus erythematosis, trauma, tumor, syphilis and Creutzfeldt-Jakob disease.

Past Medical History
Significant past illnesses

A careful history must be taken to

elicit any previously diagnosed problem which may be contributing to the dementia or possibly causing it.

Medications

It is essential to identify any medication that the patient may be taking. In the elderly, the chance of adverse drug reaction is greater than in the younger population, and careful attention should be given to this aspect of the history. Over-the-counter drugs, especially those containing bromides, should not be overlooked. Patients receiving anti-coagulant therapy are prone to bleeding and should be watched for signs of subdural hematomas.

Dietary history

A history of poor dietary intake might point to a nutritional deficiency. Inadequate diet may be due to insufficient finances, lack of teeth, difficulty with preparation, lack of appetite or alcoholism.

Review of Systems

A meticulous review of systems is necessary to discover systemic disease which may be the primary cause of the dementia, a contributing factor or an incidental finding.

OBJECTIVE DATA:

Temperature

Fever is an indicator of infection. Meningitis, encephalitis and systemic or localized infection should be considered.

Pulse

A rapid pulse is associated with anxiety and hypoglycemia; bradycardia is seen with increased intracranial pressure and hypothyroidism. Irregularities of rate indicate cardiac arrhythmias.

Respiration

Increased rate is seen with anxiety, hypoxia and in liver disease.

Blood Pressure

Hypertension may be secondary to increased intracranial pressure. It is seen in Cushing's disease and arteriosclerotic cardiovascular disease.

General Appearance

A cursory evaluation of the overall status of the patient is necessary in evaluating the severity of the dementia. Depending on the level of impairment and the objectivity of informants, the first visit may be of limited value for anything other than establishing a baseline. Demented patients may have a careless personal appearance, owing to a decline in social standards.

Affect

Most patients with dementia of any etiology have changes in mood, personality and affect. Affect is evaluated to determine if there is a psychiatric component to the picture.

Neurologic Examination
Mental status

Mental status testing is done to determine the severity of the dementia. By eliciting from family, employer and friends the premorbid state of the individual (i.e., level of education, type of employment, interests), appropriate questions can be asked and a baseline established. Since dementia by definition is an alteration in mental status, this exam will demonstrate its presence but will not help with the differential diagnosis except in some cases of functional disorders, such as depressive psychosis.

Cranial nerves I to XII

Abnormalities in olfaction (I) signify pathology in the frontal and temporal lobe. Note, however, that smell becomes diminished through the aging process. Cranial nerve abnormalities often demonstate focal lesions. Disturbance of cranial nerves III, IV and VI are seen in Wernicke's syndrome.

Deep tendon reflexes (DTR's)

Ankle jerks are often absent in the elderly, but absence or asymmetry of upper extremity reflexes is abnormal. Slow return is noted in hypothyroidism. Bilateral hyperreflexia may indicate subdural hematoma, spinal cord compensation, syphilis, multiple sclerosis, liver disease, multiple small strokes, hyperthyroidism and hypoparathyroidism. Areflexia may indicate alcholism with nutritional deficiency, uremia or malignancy.

Pathologic reflexes

Primitive reflexes, normally found early in life, are seen in patients with diffuse bilateral cortical atrophy with higher cortical dysfunction. They are less commonly seen in patients with focal lesions; grasp and suck reflexes have been noted with frontal lobe tumors. A Babinski reflex may be found with subdural hematomas. A pathologically brisk response is seen in Creutzfeldt-Jakob disease.

Motor strength	Elderly persons in general have slight general weakness of the muscles and mildly increased muscle tone which may appear as inconstant action tremors. Muscle weakness is seen in Alzheimer's, Creutzfeldt-Jakob, multiple sclerosis and pellegra. Motor changes vary in atherosclerotic occlusive vascular disease according to the site of involvement.
Sensory	Sensory examination of the aged is generally normal with decreased vibratory sense at the ankles (Paulson, 1971). Peripheral neuropathy is present in uremia metastatic carcinoma, nutritional deficiencies and metabolic-toxic processes. Parasthesias of the distal portion of all four limbs is seen with vitamin B_{12} deficiency.
Cerebellar	Abnormalities in cerebellar function are found in remote metastatic disease and Creutzfeldt-Jakob. Cerebellar testing may be difficult to perform in the demented patient.
Romberg	The Romberg test was originally designed to test proprioception of the ankles. Abnormalities are noted in syphilis, severe peripheral neuropathies, alcoholic liver disease, uremia, cerebellar and brain stem disease.
Gait	The gait seen in the elderly is often slow with less conspicuous movement of head and arms than is seen in younger individuals (Paulson,

1971). The gait seen in demented people is shuffling and distinctly different from that normally observed. The patient who is unable to walk heel-to-toe may be demonstrating an early ataxia of gait.

Speech

Slurred speech is often encountered in Alzheimer's disease accompanied by logoclonia. In early stages, the patient may indulge in small talk of a limited repertoire and only speak when spoken to. Pronounced disturbance of speech and language without pronounced confusion suggests focal lesions in the speech area. Speech and language disturbances are also seen in hypoglycemia, lupus, anoxia, intoxication (drugs or alcohol), trauma, liver disease and myxedema.

Complete Physical Examination

This exam is done in search of abnormalities that would give clues to the presence of metabolic disease with special attention to the heart, kidneys, lungs, thyroid, parathyroid and adrenal glands.

Head

The head is palpated for areas of tenderness indicative of trauma or underlying mass lesion.

Eyes
    External eye exam

Abnormalities of extraocular movement is indicative of Wernicke's syndrome and Parkinson's disease. Anisocoria, decreased visual acuity and abnormalities in peripheral vision are often present with focal lesions. It should be noted that upward gaze is often limited or sluggish in the elderly. Argyll Robertson pupils are seen classically in syphilis but may also be seen with brain tumor, meningitis, chronic alcoholism and arteriosclerosis.

Funduscopic exam	Papilledema is a sign of increased intracranial pressure. Exudates are found in hypertensive encephalopathies. Diabetic changes may be noted.

Laboratory Data

CBC with RBC indices
The CBC can give many clues to the etiology of a dementia. An elevated WBC is indicative of infection. Macrocytic anemia suggests the possibility of pernicious anemia or hypothyroidism. Basophilic stippling occurs in lead poisoning and other toxic states.

Serum glucose
If a low level is discovered at the same time the patient is symptomatic, hypoglycemia should be considered. Elevations are seen in diabetes mellitus, liver and adrenal disease.

Serum electrolytes
Any abnormality of calcium can cause changes in cognitive function; parathyroid disease may cause such alterations. Hypokalemia and hypochloremia are seen in Cushing's syndrome. Electrolyte changes are noted in uremia.

Urinalysis
The presence of protein and casts indicates renal disease.

BUN
Elevations occur in renal disease and dehydration.

Thyroid function studies	Abnormalities indicate hypo- or hyperthyroidism.
Serology	A positive serology may implicate syphilis as the primary cause of the dementia or merely an incidental finding.
Toxicology screen	The toxicology screen is performed to rule out iatrogenic causes of dementias. A heavy metal screen should be included.
EKG	Abnormalities seen in cardiac disease; changes may reflect metabolic disturbances.
EEG	In elderly persons with normal mental status, the EEG shows slowing and occasionally the appearance of focal defects over the left anterior temporal region (Wang and Busse, 1971). Bilateral synchronous slowing is seen in senile dementia with deterioration occurring over time. Diffuse slow rhythms are seen in Alzheimer's disease, normal pressure hydrocephalus (NPH), hypothyroidism, progressive multifocal leukoencephalopathy (PML) and Huntington's chorea. Triphasic waves have been reported in hepatic encephalopathy, anoxia, ketoacidosis, Creutzfeldt-Jakob disease, head trauma, subdural hematoma, cerebral tumor, infarction and hemorrhage. Periodic EEG patterns (bursts of sharp and slow activity) are noted in barbiturate overdose, hepatic and hypoxic encephalopathies, Creutzfeldt-Jakob disease, encephalitis, head injury

and subdural hematomas (Case Records, 1977).

CSF examination

Cerebral spinal fluid obtained on lumbar puncture should be clear, colorless and with no cells. Glucose is normally 50 to 80 mg percent and protein 20 to 50 mg percent. Yellow CSF indicates an increased protein content due to blood or infection, or a high bilirubin content. The presence of cells is seen in infection, metastasis, multiple sclerosis and neurosyphilis. Protein is increased in many CNS and systemic disorders including tumor, hypoglycemia and tubercular meningitis. Increased opening pressure is present in obstructive hydrocephalus, tumor, abscess and infections. A serology should be obtained on the CSF to diagnose syphilis.

Skull films

Any deviation of the pineal body may be indicative of a mass. Fractures should be noted. Erosion of bone is seen in some tumors and abnormal calcification is seen in others. Abnormalities are noted with subdural hematomas.

Chest x-ray

Tuberculosis, lung abscess, fungal disease, as well as tumor can be identified on chest x-rays

Brain scan

Tumors and subdural hematomas are located on brain scan.

C-T scan

The C-T scan delineates cerebral lesions including tumors, hemorrhages and infarctions. It allows for determination of ventricular size, enlargement of sulci and shifts of cranial structures from the middle.

ASSESSMENT:
Tumor

Brain tumors presenting without focal signs are often located in the frontal lobe. The patient may exhibit apathy or slowness in performing tasks, disturbances in attention and indifference to social practices. Smell may be impaired and pathologic reflexes present. In tumors involving other areas of the brain, dementia is seen a variable length of time after the onset of symptoms. Papilledema and focal abnormalities are found. Tumors obstructing the third or fourth ventricles may cause hydrocephalus and subsequent dementia.

In the face of diffuse metastasis to the brain, dementia, headache and cranial nerve palsies are common. The most frequent locations of the primary tumor are the lungs or breasts. Cerebral symptoms may present before clinical manifestations of the primary disease. In some cases, no brain metastasis has been found, but mental changes and cerebellar symptoms have been noted with distant tumors especially of the lung.

Subdural Hematoma

Symptoms include increasing drowsiness, confusion, headache and a recent personality change occurring over a period of days to weeks (occasionally months) and progressing rapidly. In the elderly, especially those with blood dyscrasias or those receiving anticoagulation therapy, trauma may be so mild it is undetected. Anisocoria, hyperreflexia and Babinski sign are often noted. With chronic subdural hematomas, symptoms evolve gradually and may be intermittent. Cerebral spinal fluid is often xanthochromic.

Normal Pressure Hydrocephalus

Normal pressure hydrocephalus (NPH) is a condition in which the usual pathways of absorption of CSF have been blocked and ventricular dilation is maintained by normal CSF pressure. Normal pressure hydrocephalus in most cases is idiopathic but has been noted following a subarachnoid bleed, meningitis and head trauma. A triad of symptoms are characteristic: gait disturbance, memory defects and incontinence. Lower extremity spasticity and Babinski reflex are often seen. Deterioration occurs over 6 to 12 months.

Infection

Encephalitis, when viral in origin, transiently affects mental status, whereas herpes simplex encephalitis has a serious effect on cognitive function. Bacterial meningitis rarely causes a decline in cognitive functions, but impaired intellect, judgment and skills are found in TB and fungal meningitis. Brain abscess produces a psychological and mental picture similar to that seen in brain tumors. Extracranial infections, particularly of the lung and urinary tract, may present with acute confusion with or without fever.

Syphilis

Five to 30 years after transmission of *Treponema pallidum* to the patient, symptoms of neurosyphilis may occur. This begins with confusion and forgetfulness and progresses to apathy, dullness, attrition of intellectual, social and moral capacity, generalized paresis and physical deterioration. A narrow based, unsteady gait is often noted, as is expressionless facies.

Functional Disorders

Often elderly persons with some loss of intellectual capacity are able to function well in an environment with which they have become familiar. This environment offers clues necessary for proper orientation. Anxiety-provoking situations, especially those occurring outside the home, may cause episodes of mental confusion. Depression may present with rapid onset of confusion coupled with guilt feelings, loss of self-esteem, lack of interest, loss of initiative, fatigue, hypochondriasis, urinary retention, tinnitis and walking disabilities (Robinson, 1977).

Intoxication

Prescribed drugs, over-the-counter preparations, chemicals and alcohol all have been implicated as the cause of disturbed mentation in the elderly. Lead poisoning presents with encephalopathy, irritability and impaired memory; signs of mercury intoxication include muscular incoordination, involuntary movements and emotional and intellectual disorders. Exposure to organic compounds causes an acute toxic picture with prolonged mental deterioration. Following the prolonged excessive use of bromides, paraldehyde or barbiturates is a decrease in mental functioning, drowsiness, ataxia, slurred speech and hallucinations. Phenytoin and primidone can cause mental alterations including dementia. Digitalis preparations have also been implicated.

Endocrinopathies

Myxedema is marked by an insidious onset with both mental and physical slowing, cold intolerance, dry coarse skin, constipation and puffy face. Mental slowing progresses to dementia which is not always reversible. Occasionally, hyperthyroidism is accompanied by varying levels of mental dysfunction.

In hyperparathyroidism, neural changes are uncommon but confusion accompanies hypercalcemia. Seizures, papilledema, parathesias, hyperreflexia, tetany, weakness, irritability and dementia are often seen in hypoparathyroidism.

Cushing's syndrome is accompanied by mental changes ranging from fatigability and irritability to severe depression. Mental changes have also been reported in Addision's disease. Signs of alteration in adrenal hormones are present in Cushing's and Addison's disease.

Mental changes have been noted in patients with diabetes mellitus during hypoglycemic episodes and ketoacidosis. Hypoglycemia of any etiology may affect cognitive function. Survivors of prolonged or repeated hypoglycemic episodes may have permanent neurologic damage.

It is particularly characteristic of the dementia associated with endocrinopathies to be precipitated by illness or stress.

Liver Disease

Patients with hepatic encephalopathy often present with dementia, tremor, somnolence, asterixis, ataxia and speech disorders. Impaired attentiveness and consciousness are noted. Signs of hepatic dysfunction are present. There is often a history of alcoholism.

Uremia

The metabolic encephalopathy accompanying uremia presents as a progressive dementia with dysphasia, facial grimacing and myoclonus. Early confusion states progress to short and remote memory impairment. Signs of renal failure are present.

Heart Disease

Myocardial infarctions, cardiac arrhythmias, subacute bacterial endocarditis and congestive heart failure frequently interfere with cognitive function. During transient ischemic attacks or in any situation accompanied by low cardiac output, cerebral hypoperfusion may occur.

Nutritional
Deficiencies

Owing to depression, lack of teeth, lack of finances, etc., elderly persons often have poor dietary habits. Pellegra is a disease of niacin deficiency causing dermatitis, diarrhea and mental changes which progresses to severe dementia with disorientation, confabulation and memory impairment. Neurologic abnormalities are often present. Mental symptomatology may be the first abnormality noted.

Wernicke-Korsakoff syndrome

In the nutritionally deficient alcoholic, Wernicke's disease and Korsakoff's psychosis result from lack of thiamine. The most marked sign in Wernicke's disease is ocular findings of nystagmus (horizontal and vertical) and oculomotor paralysis and palsies. Ataxia and mental changes are also present. Often the ocular manifestations and ataxia precede mental signs by several days to several weeks. Most patients with Wernicke's disease show signs of Korsakoff's psychosis but occasionally a patient may experience the latter first, consisting of distinct impairment in short- and long-term memory out of proportion to other cognitive function. This memory derangement is often covered up by confabulation. The ocular signs of Wernicke's clear dramatically after thiamine administration; some intellectual improvement may also be noted.

Pernicious anemia

The onset of vitamin B_{12} deficiency is insidious over months to years. Megaloblastic anemia is usually present although the blood smear may be normal. Apathy, extreme irritability, confusion, depression and forgetfulness are seen; ataxia occurs late; parathesias, paresis and hyperreflexia are often present.

Metabolic Disturbances

Any metabolic disturbance can cause a picture of dementia. Often implicated are dehydration, nonketotic hyperosmolar states, cardiorespiratory failure, pulmonary insufficiency with hypoxia and hypercalcemia. In some cases of anoxia or carbon monoxide exposure, neurologic disturbances may not be seen for 7 to 21 days. Electrolyte imbalances can cause mental alterations and should be suspected especially in patients on diuretic therapy. It should be kept in mind that any physical illness in the elderly, minor illness included, may cause mental symptoms.

Collagen Disease

Systemic lupus erythematosis, rheumatoid disease, polymyositis and periarteritis nodosa may cause lesions of the arteries and subsequent dementia.

Cerebrovascular Disease
Aneurysms

Rupture of aneurysms of the cerebral vasculature can cause mental deterioration, headache and focal changes. Diagnosis is by angiogram. Onset is sudden since symptoms occur after hemorrhage.

Lacunar state

Multiple small cerebrovascular infarcts produce the lacunar state in which mental deterioration occurs. The patient presents with confusion, emotional lability, bilateral pyramidal signs and a history that suggests previous small focal lesions. Sudden changes are often recalled.

Binswanger's chronic progressive subcortical encephalitis

This rare disease involves atherosclerotic changes and demyelination of the white matter of the cerebral hemispheres. The course is approximately two years, and signs include progressive intellectual deterioration and focal neurologic findings.

Progressive Multifocal Leukoencephalopathy (PML)

Progressive multifocal leukoencephalopathy is a late complication of lymphoproliferative or myeloproliferative disorders, tuberculosis or sarcoidosis and is caused by a virus that multiplies within the CNS in states of altered immunologic responsiveness. The duration of the disease from onset to death is three to six months. Symptoms include dementia, unsteady gait, vertigo, headache and focal signs.

Alzheimer's Disease

Alzheimer's disease is seen after age 40 but usually between 50 and 65 years of age. As previously discussed, it is generally believed that senile dementia is a late manifestation of Alzheimer's disease. Onset is insidious with deterioration of memory, tendency to get lost and language difficulties prominent. Jealousy and paranoid tendencies are often present. Other findings include hyperactivity, difficulty reading and writing, and repetitious speech. Later signs include gait disturbances, weakness, seizures and incontinence.

Pick's Disease

Pick's disease is clinically indistinguishable from Alzheimer's disease. Progression is generally more rapid. Constructional apraxias may be seen early in this disorder.

Creutzfeldt-Jakob Disease (Subacute Spongiform Encephalopathy)

A rare disorder which is transmitted by a slow virus. The disease is rapidly progressive with death occurring within months of onset. Rapidly progressive changes in behavioral and emotional responses, pyramidal and extrapyramidal symptoms are seen. Distinctive EEG changes are present. Creutzfeldt-Jakob disease is a subacute spongiform viral encepalopathy, as is kuru, which is found in New Guinea and is passed on by the practice of cannibalizing brains. It is believed that the scrapies virus found in sheep can be transmitted to humans who eat sheep brains (Gajdnsck, 1977).

Huntington's Chorea

This disorder is transmitted as an autosomal dominant. The disease only rarely skips a generation. The presenting symptom may be choreic movement usually of the upper extremities and neck or intellectual and psychological impairment including neurotic manifestations. Diffuse abnormalities are noted on EEG.

Parkinson's Disease

Patients with Parkinson's disease have their greatest problems with the disturbance of motility. Psychological disturbances and dementia are part of the late clinical picture. Parkinson's disease is usually diagnosed by the slightly retroverted position, adduction and flexion of arms and fingers, slowness of movement, fixed facial expression, tremor of limbs which subsides on purposeful movement, and an accelerating gait with quick shuffling steps.

Multiple Sclerosis (MS)

Although MS generally is a disease of young adults, there have been instances of late onset. In patients with onset late in life, mental symptoms are prominent. Depression is more common than dementia. The disease is marked by remissions and exacerbations with pyramidal tract involvement most prominent.

Dementia Pugilistica (Punch-Drunk Syndrome)

This syndrome is seen in former boxers and is related to the number of head blows and knock-outs received. Dementia, problems with speech and gait and seizures are present. Cerebral atrophy is noted on C-T scan.

Wilson's Disease (Hepato-lenticular Degeneration)

Inherited as an autosomal recessive trait, this disorder usually becomes manifest in the first three decades of life. It is included here because it is treatable and should not be missed. The triad of Kayser-Fleischer rings (brown pigment at corneal margins), cirrhosis of the liver and neurologic signs and symptoms are pathoneumonic of Wilson's disease.

Porphyria

Patients with porphyria have periodic attacks of abdominal colic, severe constipation, neuromuscular disturbances and exhibit neurotic or psychotic behavior. Porphyria is rarely seen in the elderly.

PLAN

In formulating a plan for the patient with dementia, the first thing that must be done is to treat the primary cause, if indeed one has been discovered. Every patient with a decline in higher cerebral functioning for whom a cause has not been found, or any patient for whom standard treatment of the primary cause has not resulted in clearing of the dementia, must have a neurology consultation. Below is a list of the assessments discussed and their respective treatments.

Specific Modes of Therapy

Assessment	*Treatment*
Tumor	
Brain	Surgery; radiotherapy, chemotherapy, Decadron
Metastatic	Surgery; radiotherapy, chemotherapy, Decadron
Subdural Hematoma	Evacuation of clot
NPH	Ventriculoatrial shunting
Infection	Culture and treatment with appropriate agent
Syphilis	Penicillin
Functional Disorders	
Depression	Antidepressants; psychotherapy
Anxiety	Return to familiar environment; reassurance
Intoxications	Withdrawal of toxin; treatment specific to toxin involved
Endocrinopathies	Treat according to established protocols for each disorder
Liver Disease	Decrease in protein intake and routine treatment for liver failure
Uremia	Standard treatment for renal failure
Heart Disease	Treat specific pathology involved

Nutritional Deficiencies

Pelegra	Niacin
Folic acid deficiencies	Folic acid and vitamin B_{12}. (Note: folic acid replacement alone will treat the anemia but not the dementia.)
Wernicke-Korsakoff	Alcohol withdrawal, vitamin B_{12} and B complex vitamins
Pernicious anemia	Vitamin B_{12}
Metabolic Disturbances	Treat according to established protocols for each disorder
Collagen Disease	No specific treatment; steroids may be helpful in SLE

Cerebrovascular Disease

Aneurysms	Medical measures to decrease arterial BP, Amicar, bedrest
Lacunar state	No specific treatment
Binswanger's	No specific treatment
PML	Cytosine arabinoside
Alzheimer's Disease	No specific treatment
Pick's Disease	No specific treatment
Creutzfeldt-Jakob Disease	No specific treatment
Huntington's Chorea	No specific treatment
Parkinson's Disease	No treatment to reverse the process, but drug therapy available to control symptoms
MS	No specific treatment; steroids for exacerbations
Dementia Pugilistica	No specific treatment
Wilson's Disease	Penicillamine
Porphyria	Avoid precipitating drugs (e.g., barbiturates, estrogen); chlorpromazine

Non-specific Modes of Therapy

Psychotherapy	Supportive therapy in the early stages of dementia may be helpful in combating depression which occurs often if the patient has an awareness of his medical course. Some believe that every patient with dementia should receive a trial

of antidepressants to be sure that depression is not the cause (Katzman and Karasu, 1975). Regardless of the etiology of the dementia, it is important to promote the patient's feeling of self-worth.

In advanced dementias several techniques have been useful. Behavior modification, which involves an evaluation of the patient's environment as well as personal resources, aims for changes to promote full use of the patient's ability. Target behaviors are identified; rewards are used for desired behavior and no reward for inappropriate behavior. Behavior modification has been useful in reinstating verbal behavior, improving social interaction and promoting various physical activities (Harris et al., 1977). Reality orientation in which the patient is constantly reminded of essential information (i.e., time, place) and encouraged to constantly use it has been shown to be somewhat effective in improving demented function (Citrin, 1977).

Pharmacologic agents

As dementias progress, behaviors such as agitation, restlessness or depression may develop. Medication to help alleviate symptoms should be used cautiously and with careful monitoring to prevent deterioration of clinical status because of untoward side effects. The use of agents such as warm milk is preferred. Antispasmodic, antiparkinsonism and anticonvulsant medication should be used when clinically indicated.

Genetic counseling

Since the genetic patterns of most senile dementias are unclear, counseling may not be helpful in many cases. For those families with many members suffering from the same disease, genetic counseling should be considered.

Family therapy

The psychological trauma sustained by a family watching the mental deterioration of one of its members is significant. They should be encouraged to verbalize feelings; professional counseling may be helpful.

Diet

The diets of mentally impaired patients tend to be inadequate. Care should be taken to assure that diet is nutritionally sound. Vitamin supplementation may be helpful. Sufficient quantities of fluids should be included to prevent dehydration.

Exercise

Patients should be kept as active as possible to avoid the hazards of immobility and maximize functioning.

Environmental manipulation

The environment of the demented should be as stimulating as possible. Eye glasses and hearing aids should be utilized; night lights are helpful. Familiar objects should be visible and always kept in the same place. Family and friends should be encouraged to visit.

Custodial care

When the family is no longer able to care for the patient at home, custodial care must be considered. The family should be aided in investigating various long-term care facilities and should be encouraged to share their feelings concerning this often guilt-laden decision.

REFERENCES

1. Allison, R. S. *The Senile Brain*. Baltimore: Williams and Wilkins Co., 1962.
2. Bergman, K. "Chronic Brain Failure—Epidemiological Aspects." *Age and Ageing*, Supp. 6, 1977, pp. 4–8.
3. Brocklehurst, J. C. *Textbook of Geriatric Medicine and Gerontology*. London: Churchill-Livingstone, 1973.
4. Caird, F. I. "Computerized Tomography (EMISCAN) in Brain Failure in Old Age." *Age and Ageing*, Supp. 6, 1977, pp. 50–51.
5. Case Records of the Massachusetts General Hospital (Case 43-1977). *New England Journal of Medicine*, 297, 1977, pp. 930–937.
6. Citrin, Dixon D. "Reality Orientation, a Milieu Therapy Used in an Institution for the Aged." *The Gerontologist*, 17, 1977, pp. 39–43.
7. Corsellis, J. A. N. "Observations on the Neuropathology of Dementia." *Age and Ageing*, Supp. 6, 1977, 20–29.
8. Foley, J. M. "Differential Diagnosis of the Organic Mental Disorders in Elderly Patients." *Aging and the Brain*, C. M. Gaitz, ed. New York: Planium Press, 1972.
9. Fox, J. et al. "Dementia in the Elderly—A Search for Treatable Illnesses." *Journal of Gerontology*, 30, 1975, pp. 557–564.
10. Gajdusek, C. "Slow Virus Infections." Talk at 1977 Infectious Disease Society Meeting, Denver, Colorado.
11. Haase, G. R. "Diseases Presenting as Dementia." *Dementia*, C. E. Wells, ed. Philadelphia: F.A. Davis Co., 1971.
12. Harris, S. et al. "Behavior Modification Therapy with Elderly and Demented Patients: Implementation and Ethical Considerations." *Journal of Chronic Diseases*, 30, 1977, pp. 129–134.
13. Horn, J. "Psychometric Studies of Aging and Intelligence." In *Aging*, Vol. II, S. Gershon and A. Raskin, eds. New York: Raven Press, 1965.
14. Judge, T. G. "Drug Treatment in Brain Failure." *Age and Ageing*, Supp. 6, 1977, pp. 70–72.
15. Katzman, R., and T. Karasu. "Differential Diagnosis of Dementia." In *Neurological and Sensory Disorders in the Elderly*, W. S. Fields, ed. New York: Stratton Intercontinental Medical Books Corp., 1975.

16. Lauter, H. and J. E. Meyer. "Clinical and Nosological Concepts of Senile Dementia." *Senile Dementia,* C. H. Muller and L. Ciompi, eds., Switzerland: Hans Huber Publishers, 1968.
17. Livesley, Brian. "The Pathogenesis of Brain Failure in the Aged." *Age and Ageing,* Supp. 6, 1977, pp. 9–13.
18. Manter, J. T. *Essentials of Clinical Neuroanatomy and Neurophysiology,* 5th ed. by F. G. Clark. Philadelphia: F.A. Davis Co., 1975.
19. Meier-Ruge, N. et al. "Experimental Pathology in Brain Research of the Aging Brain." In *Aging,* Vol. II, S. Gershon and A. Roskin, eds. New York: Raven Press, 1965.
20. Miller, E. "The Management of Dementia: A Review of Some Possibilities." *British Journal of Social and Clinical Psychology,* 16, 1977, pp. 17–83.
21. Parker, B. et al. "Finding Medical Reasons for Psychiatric Behavior." *Geriatrics,* 31, 1976, pp. 87–100.
22. Paulson, G. "The Neurological Examination in Dementia." In *Dementia,* C. S. Wells, ed. Philadelphia: F.A. Davis Co., 1971.
23. Robinson, R. A. "Differential Diagnosis and Assessment in Brain Failure." *Age and Ageing,* Supp. 6, 1977, pp. 42–49.
24. Seitelberger, F. "General Neuropathology of Dementia." In *Neurology,* A. Subirana and J. M. Espaddler, eds. Amsterdam: Excerpta Medica, 1974.
25. Slaby, A., and R. Wyatt. *Dementia in the Presenium.* Springfield, Ill.: Charles C Thomas, 1974.
26. Smith, B. *Principles of Clinical Neurology.* Chicago: Year Book Medical Publishers, 1965.
27. Terry, R. and H. Wisniewski. "Pathology and Pathogenesis of Dementia." In *Neurological and Sensory Disorders in the Elderly,* W. S. Fields, ed. New York: Stratton Intercontinental Medical Book Corp., 1975.
28. ————————. "Structural and Chemical Changes of the Aged Human Brain." In *Aging,* Vol. II, S. Gershaw and A. Raskin, eds. New York: Raven Press, 1965.
29. Wahl, P. "Psychosocial Implications of Disorientation in the Elderly." *The Nursing Clinics of North America,* II, 1976, pp. 145–155.
30. Wang, H. S. and E. W. Busse. "Dementia in Our Age." In *Dementia,* C. E. Wells, ed. Philadelphia: F.A. Davis Co., 1971.
31. Weiner, H., and L. Levitt. *Neurology for the House Officer.* Baltimore: Williams and Wilkins Co., 1974.
32. Wells, C. E. "The Clinical Management of the Patient with Dementia." In *Dementia,* C. E. Wells, ed. Philadelphia: F.A. Davis Co., 1971.

Chapter 12

Congestive Heart Failure

OVERVIEW

The incidence of congestive heart failure in the elderly is significantly high. The elderly suffer from cardiac conditions common to their age group and from those heart conditions seen in other age groups. According to most research groups, heart disease has been ranked as the most common cause of death in the aged.

Heart failure is defined as a condition in which the heart cannot pump an adequate volume of blood to supply the tissues with nutrients needed to meet metabolic demands. Failure may occur with or without preexisting cardiac disease. Thus, it is important for the health provider to know changes that occur as a result of the aging process, the pathophysiology of heart failure, the underlying causes (i.e., preexisting myocardial disease, valvular disease or hypertension) and conditions that can precipitate failure.

The heart undergoes changes as a result of the aging process. The process of aging may affect the myocardium, the valves, the vessels or the conduction system of the heart. The myocardium may decrease in both size and efficiency, thus weakening the strength of the contractile force and ultimately causing a decrease in cardiac output. The myocardium responds more slowly to increased demands and reacts poorly to tachycardia (secondary to stress, exercise or metabolic conditions).

The valves become more rigid and thickened secondary to fibrotic and sclerotic changes. These abnormalities render the valves less flexible. These changes may produce murmurs that are difficult to distinguish from those that result from acquired disease. The vessels are also affected by the aging process; there is a decreased elastin content which decreases their resiliency. In addition, there is an increased collagen content of the vessels; this plus the loss of resiliency produces a rise in the peripheral resistance. The conductive system of the heart may also be affected by the aging process. This degeneration is manifested in the form of arrhythmias (i.e., atrioventricular block and/or right and left bundle branch blocks). In addition, the conductive mechanism may be damaged from ischemic heart disease and/or past myocardial infarction damage.

The pathophysiology of congestive heart failure may be discussed in the following ways: 1) increased cardiac output versus decreased cardiac output, 2) acute versus chronic, 3) left-sided versus right-sided and 4) backward versus forward (Wintrobe, 1974). An increase in cardiac output can precipitate failure because the heart is called upon to pump large quantities of blood in order to meet the increased demands of the tissues for oxygen. The physiologic response is an increase in heart rate; the aged myocardium reacts poorly to stress so that under these conditions failure may result. In failure secondary to a decreased cardiac output, the heart has to pump harder to deliver oxygen to the tissues. There may be a decrease in contractile force secondary to aging; this plus the decrease in cardiac output can produce heart failure. Acute cardiac failure (that which occurs with a relatively rapid onset) can occur secondary to an infectious process, increased oxygen demands, increased pulse rate, tachyarrhythmias, pulmonary embolism and/or myocardial infarction; chronic heart failure (either insidious onset or of longstanding duration) can occur secondary to COPD, myocardial disease, chronic anemias, hypertension and renal parenchymal disease. Right-sided failure versus left-sided failure will depend upon the underlying disease process. Left-sided failure may begin first and progress until the right ventricle begins to fail also.

The backward failure theory states that when one of the ventricles cannot efficiently empty its contents, there is an increase in end diastolic volume. The increased volume causes a rise in pressure in the atrium and the vessels behind the failing ventricle. The pressure rise causes fluid to shift into the interstitial spaces. In contrast, forward failure states that the failing heart cannot pump an adequate amount of blood in the peripheral vessels, and this decrease in circulating blood volume causes a decrease in renal perfusion. The decreased renal perfusion results in activation of the renin-angiotensinogen cycle in order to increase the circulating blood volume and promote sodium retention.

Regardless of the mechanism involved when the heart cannot meet the increased demands placed on it, the response eventually is: 1) an increase in the heart rate and 2) hypertrophy of the heart muscle. This increased work effort of the heart uses more oxygen to do less effective work. When these compensatory mechanisms can no longer suffice, the heart begins to fail and the patient exhibits clinical signs and symptoms of failure.

The clinical signs and symptoms of left-sided failure are dyspnea on exertion, orthopnea, paroxsymal nocturnal dyspnea, cough, nocturia, rales and wheezing, etc. Symptoms specifically related to right-sided failure are distended neck veins, peripheral edema (bilateral), hepatic enlargement and tenderness, abdominal distention and ascites.

The practitioner should be skilled in recognizing the signs and symptoms of congestive heart failure; it is important for the nurse to consult and/or refer to the physician those patients with early signs of congestive heart failure. In undetermined causes of heart failure, it is essential that the patient be referred promptly because the primary cause of the failure must be identified. The practitioner should work closely with the patient and family in providing education (about CHF and its treatment), support and counseling.

CONGESTIVE HEART FAILURE WORKSHEET

To be used for patients with *symptoms of a failing heart* (i.e., bilateral pedal edema, dyspnea on exertion, shortness of breath, paroxysmal nocturnal dyspnea, increased cough, orthopnea, chest pain).

What you cannot afford to miss as an underlying etiology of CHF: myocardial infarction, pulmonary embolus, pericarditis, pericardial effusion, arrhythmias.

Chief Complaint: _____

SUBJECTIVE DATA:

Describe all positive responses using all descriptors (i.e., onset, severity, duration, location, frequency, associated symptoms):

CARDIORESPIRATORY:
YES   NO

____ ____   Cough: _____

____ ____   Chest pain: _____

____ ____   Shortness of breath: _____

____ ____   Exertional dyspnea:_____

____ ____   Orthopnea:_____

____ ____   Paroxysmal nocturnal dyspnea: _____

____ ____   Dyspnea at rest: _____

____ ____   Edema: _____

____ ____   Night sweats: _____

____ ____   Palpitations: _____

PAST MEDICAL HISTORY:
YES   NO

____ ____   Hospitalizations, operations:_____

____ ____   Medications (especially digitalis, diuretics, anti-ar-

rhythmia drugs): _____

____ ____   History of: asthma, murmurs, rheumatic disease, COPD, hypertension, renal disease, cancer, diabetes

mellitus, cardiac disease, pacemaker implant:_____

Congestive Heart Failure Worksheet

_____ _____ History of smoking, alcohol intake: _____

Complete review of systems: (Describe All Positive Responses)

GENITOURINARY:
YES   *NO*

_____ _____ Nocturia: _____

_____ _____ Oliguria: _____

_____ _____ History of recurrent urinary tract infections or renal

pathology: _____

GASTROINTESTINAL:
YES   *NO*

_____ _____ Nausea, vomiting: _____

_____ _____ Abdominal pain: _____

_____ _____ Anorexia: _____

_____ _____ Diarrhea/constipation: _____

CONSTITUTIONAL:
YES   *NO*

_____ _____ Insomnia:_____

_____ _____ Weakness/fatigue: _____

_____ _____ Vision changes: _____

_____ _____ Epistaxis:_____

_____ _____ Vertigo/syncope: _____

GENERAL:
Ask these questions in the absence of preexisting cardiac disease and in instances where no causative agent for CHF can be identified.

YES   *NO*

____ ____ Weight gain/loss: _____

____ ____ Hoarseness/dysphagia:_____

____ ____ Skin/hair changes:_____

____ ____ Lethargy/nervousness: _____

OBJECTIVE DATA:

VITAL SIGNS:

_____Wt _____ Resp. (note rate and rhythm) _____Temp.
_____ Pulse (one full minute—note rate and rhythm apical and radial) BP (right and left): _____ lying _____standing _____sitting

Are the following present? (If So Describe Positives)

SKIN:
YES   *NO*

____ ____ Jaundice: _____

____ ____ Cyanosis: _____

____ ____ Pallor: _____

____ ____ Diaphoresis:_____

RESPIRATORY SYSTEM:
YES   *NO*

____ ____ Chest deformities:_____

____ ____ Increased AP diameter: _____

____ ____ Palpation/percussion abnormalities (dullness, hyper-

resonance, increased or decreased fremitus): _____

_____

Congestive Heart Failure Worksheet

_____ _____ Rales/rhonchi (clear with coughing?): _____

_____ _____ Wheezing: _____

CARDIOVASCULAR SYSTEM:
YES   NO

_____ _____ Distended neck veins:_____

_____ _____ Precordial pulsations/thrills/heaves:_____

_____ _____ Abnormal PMI:_____

_____ _____ Arrhythmias: _____

_____ _____ Murmurs, abnormal 1st or 2nd heart sounds: _____

_____ _____ S_3/S_4: _____

_____ _____ Abnormal pulses (check carotids, brachial, radial,

femoral, popliteal, posterior tibial, dorsalis pedis):

_____

EXTREMITIES:
YES   NO

_____ _____ Edema: _____

_____ _____ Calf tenderness, warmth, swelling: _____

ABDOMINAL SYSTEM:
YES   NO

_____ _____ Abdominal distention: _____

_____ _____ Ascites: _____

_____ _____ Pulsatile mass: _____

_____ _____ Hepatomegaly, splenomegaly, palpable masses: ___

_____ _____ Bruits: _____

MENTAL STATUS:

Is there an abnormality in the following? (If So, Describe)
YES   *NO*

_____ _____ Alertness, orientation (to time, place, person): _____

_____ _____ Serial 7's: _____

_____ _____ Memory (recent and remote): _____

_____ _____ Judgment: _____

LAB DATA:

These tests should be initially performed on all patients with suspected or known CHF. Describe all test results.
      NOT
DONE *DONE*

_____ _____ CBC: _____

_____ _____ Sedimentation rate: _____

_____ _____ BUN/creatinine: _____

_____ _____ Electrolytes: _____

_____ _____ SMA 12: _____

_____ _____ Urinalysis (micro and macro): _____

_____ _____ Thyroid panel: _____

_____ _____ Chest x-ray: _____

_____ _____ EKG: _____

The following tests should be performed in the following specific conditions:

DONE	NOT DONE	
_____	_____	Stool hemoccult × 3 (if the patient has an anemia or a history of GI bleeding, or any positive GI symptoms): _____
_____	_____	VDRL (if the patient has a suspicious history for syphilis or if there is no documented VDRL in the patient's record):_____
_____	_____	Digoxin levels (if the patient is taking a digitalis preparation):_____
_____	_____	Blood culture (if the patient is toxic, has a fever, etc.):

CONGESTIVE HEART FAILURE WORKSHEET RATIONALE

SUBJECTIVE DATA:

Cough

The presence of a complaint of cough in a patient who has not previously experienced this, or an increase in production of cough, may be an early sign of CHF. Ascertain the quantity and quality of the sputum production. A frothy white productive cough is indicative of left ventricular failure; a pink or bloody productive cough is indicative of tuberculosis, bronchiectasis, pulmonary embolus or lung cancer. In the absence of other signs of congestive heart failure, the differential diagnosis of a cough includes: cough secondary to smoking, pulmonary disease, asthma, neoplasms, allergic disorders, nervous disorders, inflammation, physical agents causing a cough, sinus problems and/or tuberculosis.

Chest Pain

In the aged, diagnosing chest pain can be difficult due to such things as memory impairments and diminished pain thresholds. A myocardial infarction may sometimes present as acute dyspnea rather than chest pain. Myocardial infarction should be suspected when angina-like pain persists.

Pulmonary embolism as a cause of chest pain should be suspected if there is a calf tenderness, hemoptysis, tachycardia or evidence of right-sided heart failure.

If the patient presents with a difference in blood pressure in the arms, apprehension, pain in the epigastrium radiating to between the scapula, and severe sweating, a dissecting aortic aneurysm should be suspected as a cause of the chest pain.

Cardiac origins of pain include angina, myocardial infarction; respiratory origins of pain include pneumonia, pleurisy, tumors and pulmonary embolism. Gastrointestinal origins of pain include hiatal hernia, perforating ulcer, esophagitis and gallbladder disease.

Shortness of Breath

Shortness of breath is one of the primary signs and symptoms of congestive failure. In the early stages, the breathlessness may occur only on exertion (DOE) or with increased activity, but if the failure progresses, the dyspnea becomes increasingly present with decreasing activity until it occurs at rest. The breathlessness occurs as a result of less oxygen being delivered to the tissues to meet metabolic demands. Acute dyspnea may be the first sign of an acute myocardial infarction in the aged. Breathlessness may, however, be due to pulmonary disease, obesity, the symptoms of CHF, or (occurring at night) hiatal hernia. In addition, all of the following may also produce SOB: abdominal distention from GI disease, ascites from any cause, bronchial asthma or COPD. Dyspnea may be observed in those patients whose anxiety causes them to sigh frequently.

Types of Dyspnea
Exertional

Dyspnea on exertion may be one of the first signs of left-sided failure; it is caused by pulmonary venous engorgement which produces a decreased compliance of the lungs.

Orthopnea

Orthopnea, defined as a shortness of breath in the recumbent position, occurs when the blood and fluid from the lower extremities are redistributed and returned to the lungs and the right side of the heart. As a result the intrathoracic blood volume increases, which reduces the vital capacity of the lung and increases the pulmonary and capillary vessel pressure. The breathlessness awakens the patient who sits upright causing alterations in pulmonary pressure and blood volume with a resultant relief of breathlessness. As CHF continues, the patient is unable to recline at all and must sit upright to breathe.

Paroxysmal nocturnal dyspnea

Paroxysmal nocturnal dyspnea usually occurs from one to two hours after the patient retires in the recumbent position. Paroxysmal nocturnal dyspnea results from the overloading of the left ventricle (it receives an increased fluid volume from the reabsorption of fluid accumulated during the day). The increased fluid causes lung congestion and dyspnea from a rise in pulmonary pressure. The patient complains of a suffocating feeling, with resultant anxiety. He or she may become cyanotic, pale and/or perspire heavily. This condition is indicative of pulmonary edema; the patient, in sitting up, prevents this by temporarily relieving the pulmonary congestion.

At rest dyspnea

Dyspnea at rest occurs as pulmonary congestion progresses. In failure progressively smaller amounts of activity can provoke the dyspnea.

Edema

Edema or the accumulation of fluid in interstitial spaces may be explained by the backward failure theory (i.e., the ventricles fail to empty efficiently, causing a back-up of the pressure in the atrium and the vessels; this increase in pressure causes fluid to go into the tissues). The forward failure theory explains edema on the basis that the decrease in cardiac output causes a decrease in kidney perfusion, which causes an activation of the renin-angiotensin system.

Initially the dependent edema from heart failure subsides overnight; however, as the heart failure continues untreated, the dependent edema persists and increases. Especially in bedridden patients, subcutaneous edema may collect in sacral areas, flank, pretibial, pedal and thighs and abdomen (as seen in RHF).

The edema from congestive heart failure is usually symmetrical; therefore, unequal edema suggests a noncardiac cause. Noncardiac causes of edema include: malnutrition, varicose veins, anemia, pelvic or intraabdominal masses, neurologic conditions, inactivity, kidney disease and/or lymphatic obstruction.

Night Sweats

Profuse cold sweats may occur with the patient who is experiencing paroxysmal nocturnal dyspnea because the patient becomes anxious in struggling for the air. Night sweats are also seen in tubercular disease.

Palpitations

Palpitations may be a sign of arrhythmias secondary to early cardiac symptoms of hyperthyroidism, supraventricular tachycardias, etc. The conditions may precipitate failure either on the basis of an increased cardiac output (hyperthyroidism) or a decreased cardiac output (supraventicular arrhythmias).

Past Medical History
Hospitalizations, medications, asthma, COPD, high BP, renal disease, cancer, diabetes mellitus, cardiac disease

It is important to ascertain any history of these illnesses as well as the nature of past hospitalizations because this information might give clues to the causes that have precipitated the current condition of CHF.

Unfortunately, it may be difficult to obtain an accurate history of past cardiac illnesses in the patient which may have contributed to the heart failure. Memory deficits may prevent obtainment of the needed information. In the aged, pacemakers are often present and information concerning the implant time, battery change time and reasons for the need are important facts to gather. With battery failure and the resultant bradycardia, CHF can result from a decreased cardiac output.

Nocturia

Nocturia results from the reabsorption of edema from the day being excreted at night because of the increased renal perfusion in the recumbent position.

Nocturia in the absence of other signs and symptoms of CHF should bring to mind renal pathology, benign prostatic hypertrophy or adult onset diabetes mellitus.

Oliguria

Oliguria from right-sided failure may

be present in the day, with polyuria occurring in the night. Although it is more common in right heart failure, it may occur with left-side failure. This is a late sign of CHF and an ominous one.

In the presence of oliguria potassium supplements should be withheld or carefully monitored.

Recurrent UTI or Renal Pathology

Recurrent UTI's may cause renal parenchymal disease with the resultant development of high blood pressure; high blood pressure may be present first and cause resultant renal parenchymal disease. Either of these situations can lead to congestive heart failure.

Gastrointestinal
Nausea, vomiting, abdominal pain, anorexia, diarrhea, constipation

Anorexia, nausea and/or abdominal pain may be symptoms associated with CHF because of an enlargement and congestion of the liver seen in RHF. However, in this age group digitalis toxicity must also be considered as a cause of nausea and vomiting; other associated symptoms of digitalis toxicity (e.g., visual disturbances) must be ascertained. Diarrhea can be a symptom of digitalis toxicity or hyperthyroidism; constipation can indicate hypothyroidism. Digitalis toxicity may precipitate CHF because of the associated arrhythmias and resultant decrease in cardiac output.

Insomnia

Insomnia may be secondary to breathlessness (i.e., orthopnea, paroxysmal nocturnal dyspnea, or

Cheyne-Stokes respirations). Other causes may include depression or nervousness, particularly as associated with hyperthyroidism.

Weakness/Fatigue

Although these symptoms may be vague and involve many systems, they may be associated with congestive heart failure. In CHF fatigue is caused by the following: the oxygen supply to the tissues may be lacking as impaired circulation slows the removal of the waste products; the muscles are thus unable to regain their strength.

Late symptoms of CHF (due to the decreased cardiac output) may include weakness and fatigue upon exertion. Some possible causes of fatigue other than CHF include: anemia of any origin, renal disease, cancer, hypokalemia of any origin (but particularly secondary to diuretics), hypothyroidism, depression, mitral stenosis from underlying rheumatic heart disease, tachycardia, extreme weight loss, anorexia, malabsorption syndrome, diarrhea, excess sedation, drug toxicity or hyperthyroidism. Fatigue which presents in the early A.M. and clears in the afternoon may be a symptom of depression.

Vision Changes

Blurred vision may be secondary to a hypertensive crisis. Patients complaining of yellow flickering lights or halos in association with diarrhea, etc. may be suffering from digitalis intoxication.

Epistaxis

Nosebleeds may be seen in malignant hypertension, anemia, rheumatic fever, changes in atmospheric pressure, and salicylism.

Vertigo/Syncope

Vertigo and syncope may occur secondary to the following (signs of congestive heart failure may or may not be present): heart block with bradycardia, myocardial infarction with arrhythmias, aortic valvular disease after exercise, Stokes-Adams syndrome or carotid sinus syndrome. Digitalis toxicity and electrolyte imbalance may also cause vertigo/syncope secondary to arrhythmias.

General

If the patient has several complaints within the following symptom complex, consider hypothyroidism as perhaps the underlying etiology of the CHF: weight gain, hoarseness, dry skin or hair, alopecia, cold intolerance, constipation, dysphagia and/or lethargy. The following symptom complex may indicate hyperthyroidism as a cause of CHF: weight loss, nervousness, hair or skin changes, insomnia, diarrhea, tachycardia or eye changes—exophthalmos.

OBJECTIVE DATA:

Vital Signs

The vital signs should always be taken on *any* patient but particularly in the elderly because of their numerous medications, etc.

The blood pressure should be taken in several positions in order to ascertain any positional BP changes.

There is much controversy over the definition of hypertension. However, it is fairly commonly agreed that hypertension may be said to exist if the elderly patient has a diastolic pressure greater than 100 mm Hg. One of the effects of sustained hypertension is hypertrophy of the left ventricle and eventually the development of heart failure when the overtaxed heart can no longer compensate.

The temperature should be taken because any increase in temperature can be enough of an increased demand to cause CHF in the aged. Respirations (rate, rhythm, quality) help ascertain SOB, apnea, etc. The pulse should be taken both apically and radially simultaneously to rule out any disparity. The pulse rate and rhythm should be noted to rule out arrhythmias and/or tachycardias.

Skin

In right-sided heart failure, jaundice may be seen in conjunction with tenderness and/or enlargement of the liver. In addition, cyanosis may be seen in the peripheral nail beds. This and a decreased temperature in the extremities occurs as a result of the shunting of blood from the extremities to the vital organs. Cyanosis may also be seen in any condition that causes a decreased oxygen saturation of the blood. Pallor may be present with anemia; anemia may be the cause of heart failure.

Because of increased demands, the skin may be diaphoretic with a pulmonary embolism, myocardial infarction; it may be warm in hyperthyroidism or cool, dry and scaly with hypothyroidism.

Respiratory System

Kyphoscoliosis, which is commonly seen in the elderly, may cause compromised functioning of the heart and lungs. In addition, the patient who has an increase in his anterior-posterior chest diameter secondary to emphysema, may have very distant breath sounds. Adventitious sounds such as rales and rhonchi may be indicative of congestive failure; however, they may also be heard in infectious processes. Unilateral rales may present with pulmonary emboli or pneumonia.

Cardiovascular System
Inspection

Look for distended neck veins and an increase in jugular venous pressure. Both are indicative of right-sided failure. Precordial pulsations from heart disease may be difficult to visualize because of a shift in the point of maximal cardiac impulse (PMI) secondary to skeletal changes of aging or because of an increased AP chest diameter secondary to COPD.

Palpation/percussion

In the aged, the PMI may be displaced secondary to kyphoscoliosis, COPD or thoracic cage deformities. However, in the absence of these conditions a displaced PMI may be indicative of LVH. Left ventricular hypertrophy is evidenced by the presence of a strong and prolonged impulse. In left ventricular dilation, the impulse will be very diffuse. Cardiomegaly may be secondary to an underlying cardiomyopathy of different origins.

Auscultation

Auscultation of the apical pulse should be done for one full minute to detect not only the rate but also the rhythm. Arrhythmias (i.e., secondary to conduction defects or digitalis toxicity) may be the underlying cause of CHF. Systolic murmurs may be functional or organic (e.g., aortic stenosis is a loud systolic murmur which radiates to the neck and may be accompanied by a thrill, while the murmur of mitral insufficiency is an apical systolic murmur that may radiate to the axilla).

Diastolic murmurs are always abnormal (e.g., mitral stenosis secondary to rheumatic heart disease or aortic insufficiency secondary to untreated tertiary syphilis). Valvular disease may be the underlying cause of CHF. An S_3 gallop is usually indicative of left ventricular failure. This is best heard at the apex, and may be increased during expiration. An audible S_4 may be indicative of a noncompliant left ventricle.

Check all the pulses to ascertain that they are present and of an equal quality. An absent pulse may indicate a thrombus or embolus. If unequal, there may be some obstruction or aneurysm. Apical and radial pulses should be taken simultaneously to ascertain any disparities.

Extremities

Check the extremities for excessive warmth, calf tenderness, presence of pulses and/or edema. Edema secondary to cardiac problems is bilateral.

Abdominal System

Inspect for abdominal distention which can be indicative of right-sided heart failure. Emphysema and/or kyphoscoliosis may cause a downward shift of the liver edge which could be interpreted as hepatomegaly. However, percussion of the liver span should be normal.

A pulsatile mass associated with a bruit (particularly if accompanied by a complaint of midabdominal pain radiating to the back) may indicate an aneurysm and must be referred immediately. However, right-sided heart failure in association with tricuspid insufficiency may simulate a pulsatile abdominal mass because the liver may pulsate with each beat of the heart. Splenomegaly may be present with some anemias.

Mental Status

A complete mental status exam including testing for alertness, orientation, intelligence, recent and remote memory and judgment is essential in determining any abnormality in mental functioning.

Changes in the mental status exam are usually not present in uncomplicated heart failure. However, in chronic heart failure complicated by dyspnea, symptoms of cerebral impairment are common. This confusion is attributed to the hypoxia that may result from a poor cardiac output. In addition, mental changes in the aged may be seen in digitalis toxicity, electrolyte imbalance, renal insufficiency, cerebral vascular insufficiency, cerebral arteriosclerosis and pulmonary edema. Other causes to consider for increasing mental confusion may be: digitalis delirium, diuretic toxicity (due to elevating blood urea nitrogen), lack of fluid intake, organic brain syndrome, depression, fever, trauma, use of sedatives, morphine or barbiturates. Transition from home to a nursing home or hospital may also cause confusion and/or disorientation.

Laboratory Procedures
CBC

A CBC should be done to rule out anemia, infection or polycythemia secondary to COPD. An increased white blood cell count may indicate an infection; an infection may be the precipitating cause of the CHF.

Sed rate

The sedimentation rate may be slightly elevated because of an increase in serum fibrinogen and/or any infectious process.

BUN/creatinine

The BUN/CR may be elevated in renal disease; resultant high blood pressure may be the cause of the CHF. If the BUN is elevated (due to decreased blood flow) frequent monitoring is necessary when diuretics and digitalis are administered jointly.

Electrolytes

The electrolytes should be monitored to rule out an imbalance secondary to metabolic causes or to diuretic therapy.

SMA 18

A low serum albumin may be seen in conditions in which liver damage has impaired its formation. Hypoproteinemia may also be seen in malnutrition and in entities involving the GI tract. The CPK, SGOT and LDH may all be elevated enzymes in myocardial infarction. The SGOT may be elevated from cirrhosis, the intake of many drugs, acute infections, liver neoplasms, muscular dystrophy, etc. The CPK and LDH may also be elevated from right-sided heart failure, injections, bruises, muscular dystrophies, severe muscular exertion, cerebral infarction, hypothyroidism, muscle trauma, etc.

Urinalysis

The urinalysis should be studied to look for evidence of renal parenchymal disease (blood, casts, etc.). Renal disease can cause high blood pressure which can cause CHF.

Thyroid tests

The thyroid panel should be drawn to rule out a hypo- or hyperthyroidism as an underlying cause of CHF.

Chest x-ray

The chest x-ray is taken to evaluate an increased or decreased heart size and to ascertain its configuration, the appearance of the great vessels and lung fields.

EKG

The EKG is obtained to look for abnormalities in rate (bradycardia, tachycardia), rhythm (arrhythmias), and the length of the PR or QRS interval. The EKG should also be examined for voltage problems, evidence of hypokalemia or hyperkalemia, signs of ischemic damage and/or axis deviations.

Additional Tests

A stool hemoccult should be done to rule out gastrointestinal bleeding as a cause of any anemia or possibly CHF. The VDRL should be drawn if indicated because of the association between untreated tertiary syphilis and valvular disease that can cause CHF. Digoxin levels should be drawn in order to determine patient compliance, appropriate therapeutic levels and/or any potential toxicity. Blood cultures should be drawn on the toxic patient to rule out septicemia with fever as a cause of the CHF.

ASSESSMENT:

The nurse practitioner should consult with and/or refer to a physician when the initial assessment of congestive heart failure is made. *Prompt* referral and/or hospitalization must be made if any of the following are found: severe chest pain, pulsating mid/upper abdominal mass, bradycardia (below 50), tachycardia (above 120), arrhythmias not before documented, severely elevated blood pressure, delirium, shock, continued cyanosis despite oxygen therapy or suspected digitalis toxicity.

The following is provided to assist in diagnosing a left or right heart failure. The cause for the failure must always be determined:

Left Ventricular Failure
Signs and symptoms

Signs and symptoms include: exertional dyspnea, paroxysmal nocturnal dyspnea, orthopnea, cough, nocturia, exertional fatigue and weakness, pulmonary congestion, wheezing, rales, pleural effusion, acute pulmonary edema (hemoptysis), cyanosis, Cheyne-Stokes respirations, and gallop rhythm.

Causes

Causes of LVF include: 1) hypertension, 2) valvular heart disease (usually aortic valvular disease), 3) coronary heart disease.

Less common causes are congestive cardiomyopathies, mitral valvular disease, hypertrophic cardiomyopathy, and infective endocarditis.

Right Ventricular Failure
Signs and symptoms

Signs and symptoms include: edema—peripheral or central; hepatic enlargement and tenderness; distended neck veins; abdominal distention; anorexia, nausea, vomiting; ascites; renal insufficiency/oliguria.

Causes

All causes of LVF also cause RVF. In addition, the following also cause RVF: tricuspid valvular disease, pulmonary parenchymal or vascular disease, and infective endocarditis.

Common Precipitating Factors/ Diseases

Common precipitating factors/diseases that cause congestive heart failure include: 1) myxedema, 2) anemia, 3) pneumonia or infections, 4) thyrotoxicosis, 5) COPD with cor pulmonale, 6) respiratory infections, 7) arrhythmias, 8) myocardial infarctions, 9) rheumatic carditis, 10) pulmonary embolism, 11) excessive salt intake (sodium), 12) subacute bacterial endocarditis, 13) rapid administration of parenteral fluids, 14) corticosteroid administration (promotes sodium retention), 15) atherosclerosis, 16) hemorrhage, 17) environmental heat and humidity, and 18) discontinuation of digitalis.

PLAN:

The plan for the patient with congestive heart failure should be initially determined by the physician with whom the nurse made the assessment of CHF. The following guidelines are presented to help monitor the patient's progress and provide the optimum in ongoing health management.

Overall Objectives of Therapy

A. To prevent the following possible stasis complications of CHF:
1. thrombophlebitis
2. pneumonia
3. pulmonary embolism

B. To prevent the following complication of CHF:
1. pulmonary edema, peripheral edema
2. hypokalemia secondary to diuretic therapy

3. digitalis toxicity
4. cardiac arrhythmias
5. infections

C. To decrease the workload of the myocardium.

D. To support the patient physically and emotionally.

E. To provide patient/family education concerning the disease process/therapy.

F. To conduct an ongoing physical assessment to ascertain status changes and patient progress.

Implementation of Therapy	*Objectives*
Prevent stasis complications	Passive and active leg exercises should be done daily to promote circulation. Some authors prefer the use of elastic stockings in the phlebitis-prone patient to prevent thrombophlebitis and/or emboli. However, some favor the use of anticoagulants. Examine the lower legs routinely for signs of redness, tenderness, etc. and look for positive Homan's sign. Change bed patients' position every two hours in the elderly to avoid stasis, decubiti and/or pneumonia.
	In addition, the development of pneumonia may be prevented by encouraging the elderly patient to periodically cough and deep breathe. This helps to aerate the lungs more completely.

Prevent pulmonary edema and peripheral edema	Elevation of the head of the bed is important to decrease the pulmonary venous congestion. Maintenance of fluid balance is extremely important and must be carefully monitored by a daily weight check (same time daily) and a low sodium diet (up to 2 gm sodium is usually allowed daily). Potent diuretics help allow this amount.
	Sodium retention is responsible for the major complications in congestive heart failure.
Prevent hypokalemia	Potassium levels must be monitored in the patient taking digitalis and/or thiazide diuretics. If renal failure should occur, suspect possible potassium retention. In this instance supplemental potassium should be withdrawn until electrolyte levels have been obtained. Spironolactone may be used in conjunction with thiazide diuretics to avert hypokalemia. With the use of these drugs, potassium salts must not be given because of the threat of hyperkalemia. These combinations should only be given in the presence of good renal function. In addition, potassium salts should not be given in conjunction with potassium-sparing agents because of the danger of developing hyperkalemia.
Prevent digitalis toxicity	Digitalis, a preparation which increases cardiac output may be used in elderly patients for congestive heart failure. However, this drug should not be used in patients who

have ventricular tachycardias. Digoxin is the most commonly used preparation because of its shorter half life which tends to diminish the duration of toxicity if it should occur. However, in any patient taking digitalis preparations a periodic serum digitalis level should be ascertained. The maintenance dosage of this preparation will depend on the patient's therapeutic response and renal function.

Prevent cardiac arrhythmias

Regular frequent assessments of cardiac rhythm will allow immediate referral if the onset of arrhythmias should occur.

Prevent infections

Prompt assessments with immediate treatment/referral should be done on illnesses that could precipitate congestive heart failure (e.g., URI's, UTI's, etc.). Infections that result from breakdown of skin in bedridden patients may be thwarted by the use of water beds or sheepskin as well as frequent position changes to prevent the development of pressure areas.

Decrease Workload of the Heart

The workload of the heart can be decreased by the promotion of rest. At first this is best achieved by placing the patient on absolute bedrest. However, as the failure improves the patient's activity may be gradually increased as long as this can be accomplished without precipitating dyspnea or tachycardia.

Adequate rest until some compensation has occurred is necessary.

Subsequently, progressive activity as tolerated may be added. Close observation is necessary to determine the levels at which the patient can function without symptoms of dyspnea, weakness, tachycardia, etc.

Using a commode by the side of the bed, if the patient is bedridden, is often less taxing than using a bedpan. Oxygen therapy is usually indicated for the patient in CHF with respiratory distress, pulmonary edema or severe dyspnea. The oxygen flow liter control should be kept at from two to three liters.

Emotional Support

Emotional stress probably taxes the heart as much as does physical stress. Patients should be reassured about their prognosis. Advice should be given to follow normal habits and to avoid undue physical exertion and/or emotional worries. Explanations of needed procedures and treatments as well as explanations of their disease may well help to alleviate some fears for the aged. Family support and staff understanding are important for the aged, particularly those who may have to make a transition from home to a hospital/nursing home setting for further care.

Patient/Family Education

The adequate management of congestive heart failure depends upon the combined efforts of the physician/provider and the patient. In addition, the cooperation of the patient's family is imperative to prevent the recurrence of the process. This can only be accomplished if the patient and his family have a clear understanding of the disease process and its long-term implications.

Diet: Instruction should include the reasons for sodium restriction and potassium supplements, the caloric and sodium content of snack and processed foods, the importance of taking vitamins and iron if indicated, and the need for limited fluid intake and a normal balanced diet. If the patient is taking a diuretic, he or she should be aware of the importance of eating foods high in potassium.

Medications: The side effects, warning symptoms of toxicity and implications of drug noncompliance should be taught to the patient. If on digitalis therapy, the patient should be taught to take his or her pulse before taking the medication and should learn not to take the medicine and notify the physician if the pulse is below 60.

Disease Process: Comprehensible explanations of the physiology of CHF are important. Explaining why the symptoms present may improve compliance and thus may help keep the patient from a crisis in disease management.

General Health Maintenance: Rest, physical activity within tolerance, and the avoidance of emotional upsets are vital for maintaining an individual's well-being.

Ongoing Assessment of Patient with CHF

Subjective and objective assessments of the patient should be done on a routine basis, depending on the clinical signs and symptoms. In addition, yearly health maintenance examinations are mandatory. Regular observations should include: 1) complete ROS to determine any new symptoms and status of original symptoms, 2) determination of drug compliance, 3) examination of heart, pulses, blood pressure, weight and extremities, and 4) routine lab depending on the clinical signs and symptoms, (to include digoxin levels, electrolytes, urinalysis, kidney function tests, chest x-ray and EKG).

Based on the patient's status, determination should be recorded of how often exam and/or lab tests should be performed. The following flow sheet may be helpful in following the patient's status:

Flow Sheet for the Ongoing Assessment of the Patient with Congestive Heart Failure

How Often to Be Performed Date:				
Blood Pressure				
Weight				
Temperature				
Cardiac Exam (note presence of M, S_3, S_4)				
Heart Rate, Rhythm				

Chest (note presence of rales/ rhonchi/wheezing)				
Edema (1 to 4 scale) right pedal left pedal right pretibial left pretibial				
Skin Condition (note cyanosis, pallor, broken skin, temperature)				
Note Medications Being Taken (Record numbers that correspond to the key)				
Mental Status Exam (check if intact)				
Complete ROS (if any change)				
Lab Tests (list and record results) 1. _____ 2. _____ 3. _____ 4. _____ 5. _____				

Key for Medications

Note Medications Being Taken
1. _____
2. _____
3. _____
4. _____
5. _____

REFERENCES

1. Beeson, Paul and Walsh McDermott. "Cardiovascular Diseases—Heart Failure." In *Textbook of Medicine*, 14th ed. Philadelphia: W.B. Saunders Company, 1975, pp. 878–904.
2. Chinn, Austin, ed. "Clinical Aspects of Aging, Special Features of Heart Disease in the Elderly Patient." In *Working with Older*

People, Vol. IV. U.S. Dept. of Health, Education and Welfare, Public Health Service Publication No. 1459, July 1971.

3. Conn, M.D. "Congestive Heart Failure." In *Current Therapy 1975*. Philadelphia: W.B. Saunders Company, 1975, pp. 176–182.

4. Freidberg, Charles. *Diseases of the Heart*, 3rd ed. Philadelphia: W.B. Saunders Company, 1966, pp. 195–279.

5. Krupp, Marcus and Milton Chatton. *Current Medical Diagnosis*, 16th annual ed. Los Altos, Calif: Lange Medical Publications, 1977, pp. 215–224.

6. MacBryde, Cyril and Robert S. Blacklow. *Signs and Symptoms*, 5th ed. Philadelphia: J.B. Lippincott Co., 1970, pp. 378,599–614, 723–742, 804–830.

7. Rossman, Isadore. "Heart Disease in the Aged." In *Clinical Geriatrics*. Philadelphia: J.B. Lippincott Co., 1971, pp. 143–162.

8. Steinberg, Franz U. *Cowdry's The Care of the Geriatric Patient*, 5th ed. St. Louis: C.V. Mosby, 1976, pp. 66–78.

9. Wintrobe, Maxwell M. et al. *Harrison's Textbook of Medicine*, 7th ed. New York: McGraw-Hill Book Co., 1974.

Chapter 13

Hypertension

OVERVIEW

Hypertension is a significant health problem that affects one in five Americans. It is the most common preventable cause of myocardial infarction, congestive heart failure, stroke and renal failure.

Among the chief pathophysiological changes that contribute to the development of hypertension in the elderly are increased peripheral vascular resistance (especially from loss of vascular elasticity), decreased cardiac output (and other changes in cardiac function), and compromised renal function (that can be worsened by recurrent urinary tract infections).

Changes in blood vessels start to occur after age 25; these changes lead to a loss of elasticity (involving both the intimal and medial layers of vessels) and a loss in the distensibility of the arteries. In addition, the ratio of collagen to elastin (which gives resiliency) increases in the aorta and large muscular arteries, making them less elastic and more tortuous. There is also medial atrophy and sclerosis with calcification. Vessels may become dilated and elongated and aneurysms may form.

Arteriosclerosis is a thickening and hardening of the arterial walls. This thickening of the arterial walls and narrowing of the lumen is a process associated with hypertension. The smallest arterioles are affected throughout the body. In the afferent arterioles of the kidneys, this process leads to nephrosclerosis. It affects the arterioles of the retina and the vasculature of other viscera as well. The effect of arteriosclerosis is to sustain hypertension.

Atherosclerosis is a common and important form of arteriosclerosis. After menopause, it occurs at an equal rate in men and women. The large and medium-sized arteries (aorta, coronary, cerebral and arteries of the lower extremities) are chiefly affected. The evident cause of atherosclerosis is the deposit of lipoprotein containing plaques in arteries. This most often occurs at the mouth of a vessel and at vessel bifurcations. Increasing levels of serum cholesterol with age are associated with increasing incidence of atherosclerosis; a significantly increased risk of vascular accidents is present in those with moderate to severe hypercholesterolemia; hypertension both aggravates and accelerates this process.

Changes in cardiac function occur because of alterations in the heart and blood vessels. There is a general decrease in cardiac muscle cell size and a loss of muscle fibers with some focal hypertrophy of muscle tissue. There is a progressive decrease in the strength and efficiency of contraction and in the cardiac output and stroke volume (the cardiac output decreases about 30 to 40 percent between ages 25 to 65) as well as delayed recovery of contractile ability. At the cellular level, there are metabolic changes in the myocardium, increased myocardial irritability, and conduction system changes, from ischemia and prior myocardial infarctions. Chemical changes involve the increased binding of calcium ions in the vessels, which contributes to a greater tortuosity and stiffness of the aorta and other vessels; this makes them become less distensible to blood flow. Atrial atrophy occurs along with decreased aortic elasticity and a rise in resistance to diastolic filling. The time necessary for contraction of the chambers is prolonged.

Remember the formula, $BP = CO \times PR$ (blood pressure equals cardiac output times the peripheral resistance). Because of the decreased vascular compliance (i.e., increased peripheral resistance) and the diminished cardiac output, the two factors of the blood pressure formula have been altered. Therefore, for a given amount of work, there is less cardiac power and a resulting greater energy expenditure. As a result, performance and functional reserve have diminished.

To overcome this structural increase in peripheral resistance and concomitant difficulty in filling and emptying the left ventricle, the arterial pressure increases and left ventricular hypertrophy can follow. This leads to a further increase in systolic pressure which causes increased myocardial work and increased oxygen consumption.

The rigidity of the aorta with aging can increase the systolic pressure and decrease the diastolic pressure; this leads to systolic hypertension and the widened pulse pressure often seen in the elderly. Eventually, if the functional demands of the heart are not met, congestive heart failure or symptomatic coronary artery insufficiency develops.

Once hypertension is established, it also tends to accelerate the atherosclerotic process by which intimal and subintimal deposits of lipids in major arteries occur, further aggravating the situation. Reducing arterial pressure eases these complications and retards the progression of disease, resulting in fewer cardiovascular complications.

With atherosclerotic changes in the vessels of the brain, the blood pressure must increase to provide adequate perfusion. Impaired cerebral blood flow alters the function of vital centers of cerebral function and of autonomic reflexes, especially baroreceptor reflexes. For example, memory can be impaired and positional changes can lead to hypotension and fainting when blood flow is inadequate. Two significant events associated with hypertension in the elderly are transient ischemic attacks and focal or large cerebrovascular infarcts and hemorrhages.

There is up to a 50 percent loss of renal function over a 50-year span. This means that renal blood flow is decreased along with a decreased glomerulofiltration rate. Renal tubular changes can result in an impaired ability to concentrate urine or a decreased ability to respond to sudden changes in acid-base equilibrium. The nephrosclerosis associated with hypertension in the elderly may thus be added to a preexisting loss of renal function. In addition, the elderly are at risk for renal problems; this is because of their increased likelihood of developing obstructive urinary tract disease and their increased susceptibility to infection, both of which can lead to further renal parenchymal damage and loss of function. Antihypertensive treatment is aimed at decreasing or delaying further loss of function.

One definition of systemic hypertension is sustained elevated arterial pressure involving both systolic and diastolic pressures. Sustained hypertension is generally associated with target organ damage, whereas borderline or labile hypertension (which does not become sustained) is generally not. Systolic hypertension with a normal diastolic pressure is also much less likely to be responsible for organ damage.

There is no sharp dividing line between normal and abnormal blood pressure; however, with information from actuarial studies, many consider any blood pressure over $\frac{140}{90}$ to be abnormally high for any young, middle-aged or older adult. The Framingham study showed that, in a person with a blood pressure elevated to a consistent level of $\frac{160}{95}$, there was a higher incidence of sudden death, heart attack and angina. It was also found that there was equal risk to both sexes (despite previous findings that females tolerated untreated hypertension with fewer complications than males) and that the risks of untreated hypertension were as great to those over 50 years of age as to those under 50. In the Veteran's Administration Cooperative study, the severe complications of a group of patients with untreated diastolic blood pressures from 115 to 129 mmHg were eventually so striking that treatment of the elevated pressure could not justifiably be withheld from this group of patients so that portion of the study was halted. In the same study's conclusions, the benefits of treatment to those with diastolic blood pressures from 90 to 114 mmHg were also evident.

In addition, hypertension is especially prevalent and virulent in blacks of both sexes. Excessive salt intake seems to play a role in the development of hypertension in humans. Studies have shown that rats can be made hypertensive with excessive salt, and there is much clinical and empirical evidence to show that this may be the case with humans.

Hypertension, especially some degree of systolic hypertension, is quite prevalent in the elderly (e.g., it is estimated that 40 percent to 65 percent of males over 70 years of age have hypertension). There is a steady rise in the average systolic and diastolic pressure up to age 65 to 70 in both sexes. After that age, the average systolic BP is stable in males and may decrease in females; the diastolic pressure is generally stable in both. There are differing opinions as to what level of blood pressure indicates a need for treatment in the elderly. Some feel that a BP greater than $\frac{160 \text{ to } 170}{95}$ in this group needs treatment unless there is some compelling reason not to treat. Others feel that there is adequate evidence that a BP of $\frac{195}{105}$ is the upper limit of normal for a male aged 70 to 79, and that $\frac{210}{110}$ is the upper limit of normal for a female aged 70 to 79. Thus, the level at which treatment should be instituted undoubtedly continues to be individualized according to the cause, severity of hypertension and the condition of the patient.

Essential hypertension (which has no definitive cause, affects 90 percent of patients and characteristically has no symptoms) is different from secondary hypertension (for which a definite cause can be determined). Renal disease is a chief cause of secondary hypertension. Renal artery stenosis causes a decreased renal perfusion and activation of the renin-angiotensin system. This system is activated when the kidney secretes renin which results in the formation of angiotensin I, which is converted to angiotensin II (a potent pressor substance). Angiotensin II also stimulates aldosterone secretion by the adrenal cortex, resulting in sodium reabsorption, fluid retention and increased plasma volume. Renal parenchymal disease includes acute and chronic glomerulonephritis, chronic pyelonephritis and obstructive uropathy (e.g., renal stones and benign prostatic hypertrophy). Therefore, hypertension may result from an injury to the renal blood vessels (from inflammation and fibrosis) which leads to a decreased perfusion followed by an activation of the renin-angiotensin system.

Secondary endocrine causes of hypertension include: primary aldosteronism (aldosterone-induced sodium retention leads to hypertension), Cushing's syndrome (excess glucocorticoids lead to sodium retention with a resultant increased BP), pheochromocytoma (increased secretion of epinephrine and norepinephrine by a tumor of the adrenal medulla results in an excess stimulation of adrenergic receptors which cause peripheral vasoconstriction), and hyperthyroidism (a general hypermetabolic state results in hypertension and diabetes mellitus which is associated with an accelerated arteriosclerosis including nephrosclerosis). Coarctation or constriction of the aorta may cause hypertension directly or secondarily because of accompanying changes in the renal circulation. Hypercalcemia with resultant renal parenchymal damage from renal stones and nephrocalcinosis may also cause secondary hypertension.

HYPERTENSION WORKSHEET

To be used in patients with consistently elevated blood pressure.

Chief Complaint: _____

Age: _____

SUBJECTIVE DATA: (Describe All Positive Responses)

REVIEW OF SYSTEMS:
CARDIORESPIRATORY
YES   *NO*

_____ _____ Cough: _____

_____ _____ Chest pain: _____

_____ _____ SOB: _____

_____ _____ PND:_____

_____ _____ Orthopnea:_____

_____ _____ Wheezing: _____

_____ _____ Edema: _____

ENDOCRINE
YES   *NO*

_____ _____ Polyuria: _____

_____ _____ Polyphagia: _____

_____ _____ Polydipsia:_____

_____ _____ Diaphoresis:_____

_____ _____ Headache: _____

_____ _____ Palpitations:_____

_____ _____ Weakness: _____

_____ _____ Fatigue:_____

_____ _____ Muscle cramps: _____

_____ _____ Weight changes (give amount gained or lost):_____

_____ _____ Skin/hair/eye changes:_____

_____ _____ Nervousness, temperature intolerance, frequent

stools: _____

_____

CENTRAL NERVOUS SYSTEM
YES   *NO*

_____ _____ Visual disturbances, dizziness: _____

Hypertension Worksheet

_____	_____	Numbness, tingling: _____
_____	_____	Weakness, paralysis, incontinence: _____

GENITOURINARY

YES	NO	
_____	_____	Dysuria: _____
_____	_____	Hematuria: _____
_____	_____	Nocturia: _____
_____	_____	Urgency: _____
_____	_____	Back pain: _____
_____	_____	Hesitancy, dribbling: _____

PAST MEDICAL HISTORY:

YES	NO	
_____	_____	Previous history of high BP: _____
_____	_____	High BP associated with pregnancy: _____
_____	_____	Treatment (specify): _____
_____	_____	Excessive salt intake: _____
_____	_____	Diabetes mellitus: _____
_____	_____	COPD: _____
_____	_____	Rheumatic heart disease: _____
_____	_____	Murmur: _____
_____	_____	Heart disease: _____
_____	_____	Frequent UTI (frequency, treatment, etc.): _____
_____	_____	IVP, cysto (result): _____

_____	_____	Renal stones: _____
_____	_____	BPH: _____
_____	_____	Trauma to flank: _____
_____	_____	Drugs, medications: _____
_____	_____	Drug allergies/adverse reactions: _____

FAMILY HISTORY:
YES   _NO_

_____	_____	High BP: _____
_____	_____	CVA: _____
_____	_____	Myocardial infarction: _____
_____	_____	Renal disease: _____
_____	_____	Diabetes mellitus: _____
_____	_____	Other: _____

SOCIAL HISTORY—HABITS:
YES   _NO_

_____	_____	Significant life changes/stress: _____
_____	_____	Smoking: _____
_____	_____	Exercise: _____

OBJECTIVE DATA: (Describe All Findings)

Vital Signs: Height_____   Weight_____   Pulse_____

Respirations_____   BP (right arm and left arm): _____

lying_____   sitting_____   standing_____

General appearance: _____

Skin, body development: _____

Describe All Positives:

FUNDI:
YES　　*NO*

_____ _____ AV nicking/narrowing: _____

_____ _____ Hemorrhages: _____

_____ _____ Exudates: _____

_____ _____ Papilledema: _____

NECK:
YES　　*NO*

_____ _____ Elevated JVP: _____

_____ _____ Increased thyroid size: _____

_____ _____ Thyroid nodule: _____

_____ _____ Carotid bruit: _____

_____ _____ Transmitted murmurs: _____

THORAX/LUNGS:
YES　　*NO*

_____ _____ Kyphoscoliosis: _____

_____ _____ Increased AP diameter: _____

_____ _____ Decreased expansion: _____

_____ _____ Decreased breath sounds: _____

—— —— Rales: _____

—— —— Rhonchi: _____

—— —— Dullness: _____

HEART:
YES   *NO*

—— —— Displaced PMI: _____

—— —— S_1 abnormality: _____

—— —— S_2 abnormality: _____

—— —— S_3: _____

—— —— S_4: _____

—— —— Murmur: (systolic):_____ (diastolic):_____

ABDOMEN:
YES   *NO*

—— —— Hepatosplenomegaly: _____

—— —— Masses: _____

—— —— Bruits: _____

GENITOURINARY:
YES   *NO*

—— —— Prostate hypertrophy/nodule: _____

EXTREMITIES:
YES   *NO*

—— —— Edema: _____

—— —— Carotid pulse abnormality: _____

—— —— Radial pulse abnormality: _____

Hypertension Worksheet

_____ _____ Brachial pulse abnormality: _____

_____ _____ Femoral pulse abnormality: _____

_____ _____ Popliteal pulse abnormality:_____

_____ _____ Posterior tibial pulse abnormality: _____

_____ _____ Dorsalis pedis pulse abnormality:_____

_____ _____ Radiofemoral lag: _____

NEUROLOGIC—ABNORMALITY OF:
YES   _NO_

_____ _____ Cranial nerve: _____

_____ _____ Strength: _____

_____ _____ Motor:_____

_____ _____ Sensation: _____

_____ _____ Deep tendon reflexes: _____

_____ _____ Mental status:_____

LAB DATA (Describe All Test Results):
_____ _NOT_
DONE   _DONE_

_____ _____ Urinalysis (macro and micro):_____

_____ _____ Urine culture:_____

_____ _____ BUN/creatinine: _____

_____ _____ Electrolytes:_____

_____ _____ Glucose: _____

_____ _____ Uric acid:_____

_____ _____ EKG: _____

_____ _____ Chest x-ray: _____

_____ _____ CBC: _____

_____ _____ Albumin: _____

_____ _____ Calcium/phosphorus: _____

_____ _____ Cholesterol/triglycerides (if the patient has a history

of lipid abnormalities or early xanthelasmas): _____

_____ _____ Thyroid function tests (if the history of physical is

suspect for hyperthyroidism as the cause of the hy-

pertension): _____

ADDITIONAL LAB:

A detailed work-up for secondary hypertension is reserved for those patients with severe hypertension or with definite clinical features suggestive of secondary causes (the patient's care should then be primarily managed by the physician). The following should be ordered (only after physician referral/consultation in those patients with unresponsive hypertension):

VMA, catecholamines
Hypertensive IVP
Renal scan

The following should be ordered (only after physican referral/consultation) in the patient with clinical features or an abnormal IVP that makes one suspect renal artery stenosis as the secondary cause of the hypertension:

Renal scan
Renal arteriogram
Renal vein renin study

The following should be performed (only with physician referral/consultation) as indicated to rule out a secondary cause of hypertension in the patient with clinical evidence of Cushing's syndrome:

A.M. and P.M. plasma cortisol
24-hour urine for 17 hydroxysteroid or 17 ketogenic steroids
Dexamethasone suppression test

The following should be ordered (only after physician referral/consultation) in the patient whose hypokalemia suggests primary aldosteronism:

Plasma renin activity during sodium restriction
Plasma aldosterone or 24-hour urine aldosterone during sodium loading
Adrenal venography
Adrenal vein aldosterone levels

HYPERTENSION WORKSHEET RATIONALE

SUBJECTIVE DATA:

Chief Complaint

The majority of patients with hypertension present with few, if any, symptoms referrable to hypertension unless there has been specific target organ damage; in that case, the symptoms will be referrable to the involved organ systems.

Age

Secondary hypertension often develops before age 35 or after age 55. Essential hypertension may become evident in the 20s or 30s, but more often between the ages of 30 and 55.

Review of Systems
Cardiorespiratory
Cough

The symptom of cough may be associated with early left heart failure (though it can be a sign of an acute or chronic infection or pulmonary congestion).

Chest pain

Anginal chest pain can be a sign of coronary artery insufficiency, which may occur secondary to hypertension. The presence of angina is a contraindication to the use of several antihypertensive medications. Cardiac pain is often less severe in the elderly though the site, radiation and other characteristics of the pain are the same as in younger patients.

SOB, PND, orthopnea

Shortness of breath (SOB), postural nocturnal dyspnea (PND), and orthopnea are common symptoms of congestive heart failure which can be a complication of untreated or inadequately treated hypertension.

Wheezing

Wheezing is sometimes associated with congestive heart failure, asthma, and COPD with a bronchospastic component.

Edema

Edema is sometimes associated with congestive heart failure, renal disease or cirrhosis.

Endocrine
Polyuria, polyphagia, polydipsia

This triad classically presents in uncontrolled diabetes mellitus. Polyuria is also seen in potassium depletion, hypercalcemia and renal failure.

Diaphoresis, headache, palpitations

These symptoms together can suggest the presence of pheochromocytoma. This is a rare cause of secondary hypertension. The symptoms are secondary to the catecholamine release associated with this tumor; the symptoms can also occur with menopause, anxiety (associated with essential hypertension) or with the use of sympathomimetic drugs. Occasionally a morning occipital headache can be seen in severe or longstanding high blood pressure.

Weakness, fatigue, muscle cramps	These symptoms may suggest hypokalemia secondary to primary aldosteronism or diuretic therapy.

Weight changes

Weight gain (classically truncal obesity) may be seen in Cushing's syndrome. Weight loss may be associated with pheochromocytoma and hyperthyroidism. Weight gain or loss can be seen in diabetes mellitus. There is also a strong association between obesity and hypertension.

Skin/hair/eye changes

Purple striae are often seen on the trunk in Cushing's syndrome. Smooth, warm, moist skin, fine hair and exophthalmus are seen in hyperthyroidism.

Nervousness, frequent stools, temperature intolerance

These symptoms may be associated with hyperthyroidism.

Central nervous system
Visual disturbances, numbness, tingling, dizziness

Transient episodes of visual disturbances, dizziness, tingling, and numbness can be secondary to transient ischemia of cerebral tissue.

Weakness, paralysis, incontinence

These symptoms may be the sequelae of a cerebrovascular accident from uncontrolled hypertension.

Genitourinary
Dysuria

Dysuria is often a sign of infection or inflammation of the urethra, bladder or prostate gland. An untreated cystitis may cause a retrograde infection to the kidneys and result in renal parenchymal damage.

Hematuria

Hematuria is a possible sign of urinary tract infection or renal disease.

Nocturia

Nocturia may be associated with infections, edema, chronic renal insufficiency or a partial obstruction. In addition, it may be an early sign of congestive heart failure or uncontrolled diabetes mellitus.

Urgency

Urgency may result from an irritation of the trigone or posterior urethra (from infection, inflammation, stones or a tumor).

Back pain

The pain of prostate disease is sometimes felt as low back pain. The enlarged prostate may cause some obstruction and predispose to the development of an infection with resultant parenchymal damage to the kidney.

Hesitancy, dribbling

Hesitancy may be associated with benign prostatic hypertrophy. Benign prostatic hypertrophy may be the contributory cause of the development of high BP; the obstruction sets up a good medium for chronic UTI's and this may result in renal parenchymal damage.

Past Medical History
Previous history of high BP associated with pregnancy; past treatment details

This information can be helpful in determining a possible cause of hypertension and in uncovering any past treatment problem. There is an unclear but possible association be-

	tween the toxemia of pregnancy and the later development of sustained hypertension.
Dietary history, salt intake	An excessive salt intake (causing an increased plasma volume) may lead to the development of hypertension. Salt intake from the history should be described as mild, moderate or excessive.
Diabetes mellitus	Diabetes mellitus is associated with accelerated vascular disease from arteriosclerosis since diabetes mellitus is often associated with lipid abnormalities.
COPD	The presence of COPD may be associated with pulmonary hypertension.
Rheumatic heart disease	The patient with a history of rheumatic heart disease may have had some contributory degree of heart failure.
Murmur	Previous knowledge of a murmur can be an indicator of cardiac disease.
Heart disease	Angina or previous myocardial infarctions can be indicators of coronary insufficiency from hypertension.
Frequent UTI's	A history of urinary tract infections is important because of possible renal parenchymal damage secondary to repeated infections. Chronic pyelonephritis with resultant renal parenchymal damage may be completely asymptomatic.

IVP, cysto results	Urological procedures are helpful in determining the etiology of renal problems and may establish the cause of hypertension. The procedures are done to ascertain any evidence of renal artery stenosis, obstructive uropathy, or renal parenchymal disease.
Renal stones	Renal stones cause obstructive uropathy which can lead to hypertension secondary to renal parenchymal damage. A history of calcium renal stones is strongly suggestive of hypercalcemia which may also be associated with hypertension.
BPH	Benign prostatic hypertrophy may be associated with obstructive uropathy and repeated UTI's; these conditions can lead to renal parenchymal damage.
Trauma to flank	A history of flank trauma can be a cause of renal injury and a precursor to hypertension.
Current meds	Estrogens, thyroid preparations, steroids, amphetamines, licorice and over-the-counter cold remedies are among the drugs associated with an elevated blood pressure (secondary to sodium retention or vasoconstriction).
Drug allergies/adverse reactions	Knowledge of this will help avoid contraindicated medications in planning a treatment program.

Family History
High BP
CVA
Myocardial infarctions
Renal disease
Diabetes mellitus
Other

The majority of patients with essential hypertension will have a family history of hypertension or hypertensive complications, such as CVA's or myocardial infarctions. Renal disease may be a cause of the patient's hypertension. There is a familial association of diabetes mellitus and some types of renal disease.

Social History—Habits
Significant life changes/
stress

These are associated with hypertension, though sometimes temporary.

Smoking

A risk factor for the development of cardiovascular and pulmonary disease.

Exercise

Helps in controlling weight; physical conditioning may actually lower the blood pressure.

OBJECTIVE DATA:

Vital Signs
Height/weight

Height and weight measurements are necessary to compute ideal body weight. There is a well-recognized association between being overweight (or obese) and hypertension. As obese patients lose weight and approach their ideal body weight, the blood pressure is often lowered significantly and may occasionally become normal (assuming there is not a secondary cause for both the obesity and the hypertension). Sudden increases in weight can be due to the development of congestive heart failure or renal disease. Often mild weight loss is seen when diuretic therapy is begun because of a decrease in plasma volume. Weight loss may also be seen in hyperthyroidism and pheochromocytoma.

Pulse

Check the rhythm, character, quality and rate of the pulse bilaterally. The pulse may be slow if the patient is taking digitalis or a therapeutic dose of propranolal, or if the patient has some conduction defect. Rapid, regular rhythm in the elderly is often due to supraventricular or ventricular tachycardia or may be secondary to an undetected infections. In the patient with hypertension, a rapid pulse may point to hyperthyroidism, anxiety or pheochromocytoma. In the latter, the pulse is usually intermittently rapid.

Respiration

Check the rate and effort of the respiration.

Blood pressure

It is important to use the appropriate size sphygmomanometer cuff. It is generally agreed that serial blood pressure determinations at weekly intervals for three weeks are necessary before determining that treatment is indicated (unless the systolic or diastolic level initially is dangerously elevated or there is evidence of target organ damage).

Positional blood pressure readings are recommended to determine if significant orthostatic changes are present prior to treatment; after treatment is begun, this is a way of monitoring the effect of medications known to produce a lowering of the BP with positional changes.

Postural hypotension is a common finding in the elderly because of normal autonomic changes. A paradoxical rise in diastolic BP on standing is often seen in essential hypertension, but orthostatic changes (generally a decrease in BP) can be seen in secondary causes because of excessive vasoconstriction.

Check the BP in both arms; (some experts suggest a single leg BP reading with a thigh-sized cuff as well). Significant circulatory abnormalities are associated with a difference of greater than 20 mm Hg between left and right arm BP readings. Coarctation of the aorta, which is occasionally discovered in the elderly, is suspected if the thigh BP reading is significantly lower than the arm BP reading or if the bilateral arm readings vary more than 20 mm Hg.

General Appearance

The main purposes of objective assessment in the patient with hypertension are to detect signs of secondary causes of hypertension and to assess the patient's general condition.

Skin, Body Development

The following signs are suggestive of a hormonal or secondary cause of hypertension: 1) increased fat distribution on face (moon facies) and/ or neck, shoulders and trunk (seen in Cushing's syndrome); 2) muscular development of the upper portion of the body out of proportion to the lower and/or collateral vessels on the chest (seen in coarctation); 3) plethora, malar rash, neurofibromata or striae (seen with some secondary causes).

Fundi

The eye is a target organ; the funduscopic exam provides an early indicator of the stage of the disease in this and other target organs. The retina is the only tissue in which arteries and arterioles can be examined directly; thus, it provides a check on the progress of the vascular effects of hypertension. A sequence of damage to the retina occurs; initially present is arteriolar narrowing and a decrease in the caliber of vessels distal to the disc. Focal spasm, hemorrhages and exudates may occur in further advanced stages, but these may be reversible. Loss of venous pulsations, loss of the disc margins are signs of papilledema. This is seen in malignant hypertension.

Neck

Elevated jugular venous pressure is a sign of congestive heart failure. Check for thyromegaly or nodules, since hyperthyroidism may be associated with an elevated blood pressure. Examine the neck for carotid artery pulsations and listen for bruits (secondary to atherosclerotic plaques). Transmitted cardiac murmurs can sometimes be heard while auscultating the carotid arteries.

Thorax/Lungs

The presence of kyphoscoliosis can distort the normal cardiac and pulmonary sounds or the location of the PMI. Rales are lung sounds secondary to fluid or exudate movement in the alveoli. Medium or coarse rales (rhonchi) are heard at the lung bases in congestive failure. Wheezes represent airway obstruction secondary to mucus or spasm, etc. In emphysema, loss of elasticity and air trapping gives hyperresonant, sometimes distant or harsh breath sounds. The extra air volume in emphysema holds the thoracic walls in an inspiratory position (causing an increased anterior-posterior diameter); the kyphoscoliosis seen in the elderly produces a barrel chest without the typical auscultatory findings of emphysema.

Dullness in the lung fields may be indicative of pleural effusion, fibrosis or pneumonia.

Heart

Check for evidence of left ventricular enlargement as evidenced by a left shift of the PMI and a prominent left ventricular impulse (since a hypertrophied left ventricle strikes the precordium with an increased force). Precordial pulsations and thrills may be less prominent or absent, secondary to emphysema or kyphoscoliosis. S_1 and S_2 should be normal; normal heart sounds in the elderly are identical to normal heart sounds in the young. An accentuated aortic second sound may be heard in hypertension. A third heart sound is usually indicative of failure. A fourth heart sound is an atrial filling sound; it is indicative of a decreased ventricular compliance.

In the elderly with hypertension, a soft systolic ejection murmur (aortic insufficiency) is often heard; it is probably secondary to changes in the aorta, aortic valve, or its supporting structures. A diastolic murmur is always abnormal.

Left ventricular hypertrophy represents cardiac compensation for an increased workload from increased systemic pressure. In this situation, initially there is a diminished left ventricular function, progressing to ventricular dilatation, resulting in left ventricular failure. Left ventricular hypertrophy, S_3 and S_4 are all evidence of cardiac decompensation from hypertension.

Abdomen

A tender, congested liver can be felt in right-sided congestive heart failure. Splenomegaly can occur because of massive congestion, as in longstanding cardiac failure. The liver edge may also be down because of emphysema or kyphoscoliosis. (In this instance the liver span should be normal.) Occasionally, large kidneys (due to a mass or polycystic disease) can be palpated. Renal artery bruits must be listened for. The bruit will have a diastolic component and be heard just to the right or left of the midline, above the umbilicus or in the flanks. A bruit can sometimes be heard with stenosis of the artery (from fibromuscular dysplasia) and can be heard about half the time with significant stenosis (from athero- or arteriosclerosis).

Genitourinary

Prostatic hypertrophy (detectable as a rubbery or firm symmetrical enlargement of the lateral lobes of the prostate) can play a role in the development of obstructive uropathy; an associated infection or reflux can increase the risk of renal parenchymal disease. The incidental findings of a hard, nontender prostatic nodule in an elderly male raises the suspicion of a carcinoma of the prostate.

Extremities

Check for edema which is seen in congestive heart failure, renal problems or with sodium and water retention from certain antihypertensive drugs. The edema of CHF is usually bilateral. Unilateral edema may be a result of venous lymphatic obstruction or any number of causes. Check for adequacy of the peripheral pulses. Pulses will be diminished with generalized arteriosclerotic vascular disease or with atheromatous vascular disease causing an obstruction to the flow.

Radiofemoral lag (discovered with a simultaneous palpation of the radial pulse and femoral pulse unilaterally) or a diminished femoral pulse may suggest coarctation of the aorta.

Neurologic

Neurologic symptoms of damage from hypertension can be secondary to a stroke, TIA's, or a series of small brain tissue infarcts resulting in limited motor or sensory deficits. A stroke can be associated with specific cranial nerve abnormalities, varied degrees of loss of motor and sensory function and hyper-reflexia. There is usually no neurologic abnormality between episodes of transient cerebral ischemia. Altered frontal lobe function, cognitive impairment, poor memory and dull personality may be the result of years of ETOH intake or uncontrolled hypertension.

Lab Data

Lab data are gathered to help rule out secondary causes, or complications of hypertension, to provide baseline data before starting drug therapy, to assess the patient's general health status and to find any evidence of risk factors for the development of cardiovascular disease, etc.

Urinalysis/culture

Macroscopic examination of the urine includes the dipstick which is a simple means of checking for the presence of protein, blood, and glucose (which can indicate the presence of diabetes and/or renal parenchymal disease). On the microscopic urinalysis, look for evidence of infection, inflammation (WBC, RBC, bacteria) and diseases of the kidney (cellular casts, tubular casts and granular casts). A urine culture is done if the history of the urinalysis provides suspicion of an underlying infection.

BUN/creatinine

A BUN/creatinine and/or a creatinine clearance test help to assess kidney function. Decreased renal function and diminished renal blood flow are often present in the elderly (since arteriosclerosis of the renal arterioles and capillaries commonly leads to diminished function). Therefore, medications that avoid compromise of suboptimally functioning kidneys can be important to elderly patients with hypertension. It often remains unclear whether renal parenchymal damage is the cause or effect of hypertension.

Electrolytes

Electrolyte abnormalities of serum sodium and potassium are found in primary aldosteronism (increased sodium and decreased potassium). Hyponatremia is seen in the inappropriate use of diuretics.

Glucose

The glucose should be checked since diabetes mellitus is associated with an accelerated arteriosclerosis with resultant nephrosclerosis. Cushing's syndrome and pheochromocytoma can be associated with hyperglycemia. An initial serum glucose serves as a baseline for later comparison, because thiazide diuretics may cause a slight rise in serum glucose levels.

Uric acid

There is an increased incidence of hyperuricemia in both renal and essential hypertension. An initial uric acid level serves as baseline; thiazide diuretics can elevate the serum uric acid level.

EKG

An electrocardiogram provides information about the heart size, hypertrophied chambers and the condition of the myocardium. Minor ST-T wave changes are often seen but are of no great clinical significance. Changes of left ventricular hypertrophy (including axis deviation and increased voltage) are sometimes found in hypertension. Hypokalemic EKG changes include T wave depression, prolongation of the Q-S interval, and U waves. Hyperkalemic EKG wave changes are evidenced by the presence of narrow high peaked T waves.

Chest x-ray

The chest x-ray gives information about the heart size, degree of tortuosity and condition of the great vessels, calcification of the aorta, evidence of CHF, and the presence or absence of disease of the lungs. Aortic dilatation and rib notching are seen with coarctation of the aorta.

In the elderly, an increase in the cardiothoracic ratio sometimes reflects a decreased chest diameter rather than absolute cardiomegaly.

CBC

A CBC gives information regarding the general hematologic status of the patient. Anemia is common in chronic renal disease. An increased hematocrit is seen in some renal diseases and COPD.

Albumin

A decreased serum albumin may be seen in liver disease, renal diseases (nephrotic syndrome) and gastrointestinal enteropathies.

Calcium/phosphorus

One-third of patients with hyperparathyroidism (an outstanding feature of which is hypercalcemia), have hypertension. Elevated calcium can also suggest renal disease or neoplasm. In addition, serum calcium may become elevated in those on thiazide diuretic therapy.

Cholesterol/triglycerides

Cholesterol/triglycerides measurements are collected because hyperlipidemia, like hypertension, is a risk factor for the development of atherosclerotic heart disease. Lipid abnormalities are often seen in diabetes. There is some controversy as to the reversibility of increased lipids after age 70.

Thyroid function tests

Thyroid function tests are done where indicated to rule out hyperthyroidism as a cause of elevated BP.

Additional Tests
VMA/catecholamines/
metanephrine

A 24-hour urine collection of VMA, catecholamines, and metanephrine is done to screen for the presence of increased amounts of the metabolites of epinephrine and norepinephrine (found in the presence of pheochromocytoma). These tests are not performed as a routine screening measure, but only if suggested by features of the history and examination of the patient.

Hypertensive IVP/renal scan/arteriogram/renal vein renin determinations

These tests show evidence of renal artery stenosis, obstruction or other unilateral or parenchymal disease. Abnormal results are: delayed dye excretion, a kidney size difference of greater than 1.5 cm, or an irregular contour of the renal silhouette suggesting renal infarction or atrophy. If an abdominal flank bruit (suggestive of renal disease) is heard, then an IVP or renal scan is done. If one is abnormal, then the other is done as well. If both are positive, then renal vein renin determinations and renal arteriograms can be done. There is a small false negative rate of both the IVP and the renal scan.

Renal arteriograms can establish the presence of a lesion in the renal arteries and determine whether it is atheromatous or fibromuscular However, before these studies are undertaken in the elderly, the risks and benefits and likelihood that knowledge from the outcome of the study will alter treatment should be thoroughly considered. Some experts feel that the sudden appearance of hypertension after age 55 is an indication for these radiologic diagnostic studies to be undertaken.

Plasma cortisol/17 hydroxysteroid/17 ketogenic steroid

The plasma cortisol level is tested to rule out Cushing's syndrome as a cause of secondary hypertension. The plasma cortisol level is elevated in Cushing's. Increased 17 hydroxysteroid levels in the urine may be associated with Cushing's as a secondary cause of high blood pressure.

Plasma renin activity/ plasma aldosterone/ adrenal venography/ adrenal vein aldosterone levels

The plasma renin is elevated in hypertension secondary to renal artery stenosis. In hypertension secondary to primary aldosteronism, the plasma renin is decreased while the serum aldosterone is elevated. The plasma aldosterone is taken to rule out primary aldosteronism as a cause of hypertension; the levels will be high. The adrenal venography is done to measure the renin and aldosterone levels; the results are compared bilaterally. The adrenal vein aldosterone levels and the renal vein renins are done to rule out primary aldosteronism as a cause of hypertension; the aldosterone levels will be elevated while the renins are decreased.

ASSESSMENT:

Primary Cause of Hypertension/ Essential Hypertension

The majority of patients will have no symptoms from essential hypertension (unless there is specific target organ damage, in which case there will often be symptoms referable to that system). Objectively, in mild to moderate hypertension, there can be a slight left ventricular lift or left ventricular hypertrophy and prominent S_4, narrowing of the retinal arterioles, and sometimes retinal exudates. In more severe hypertension, there will be signs of left ventricular failure, papilledema and retinal hemorrhages and exudates. Common late findings are left ventricular hypertrophy on chest x-ray and EKG with left axis deviation; sometimes proteinuria and microscopic hematuria is present.

Secondary Causes of Hypertension
  Coarctation of the aorta

There are often no symptoms. Sometimes fatigue of legs is seen in coarctation of the aorta. Objectively, the BP in the legs is lower than in arms, with diminished or delayed femoral pulses. Also found is a systolic murmur, intercostal pulsations and aortic vascular disease. The chest x-ray shows rib notching by collateral vessels, and left ventricular hypertrophy.

Primary hyperaldosteronism

Subjectively, these frequently are episodes of muscular weakness, paresthesias, tetany, polyuria, polydipsia, nocturia, and headaches. This condition can occur in the elderly, but it is more common in the 30 to 50 year age group. Objectively, one sees a mild to moderate hypertension, and occasionally peripheral edema.

Lab results show low serum potassium (best screening measure), increasing urinary potassium loss, an elevated serum aldosterone (on a high sodium diet), and a low plasma renin unresponsive to restricted sodium intake. Electrocardiogram changes include a slightly prolonged PR interval, sagging ST segment, inverted T waves, and prominent U waves. In the urinalysis proteinuria may sometimes be found.

Cushing's syndrome

Subjectively, the patient may complain of weakness, alteration of sexual function (amenorrhea or impotence) changes in appearance, polyuria, polyphagia, polydipsia, backache (osteoporosis), and emotional lability. Objectively, one may see truncal obesity, acne, hirsutism, striae, purpura, muscle wasting, edema, and plethora. The lab results may show polycythemia, hyperglycemia, glucosuria, increased urinary excretion of 17 ketosteroids and 11 oxysteroids, and a low dexamethasone suppression test.

Pheochromocytoma

The patient may present with palpitation, headache, nervousness, diaphoresis, tachycardia, and weight loss; this lesion accounts for 0.5 percent of the hypertensive population. It is more common in young adults, though it can occur at any age.

Objectively, the patient may have intermittent hypertension, orthostatic hypotension, fever, and cafe-au-lait spots. Abnormal lab results seen may include hyperglycemia and glucosuria, increased urinary catecholamines and the metabolites of epinephrine and norepinephrine and increased serum levels of catecholamines.

Hypercalcemia

One-third of the patients with hyperparathyroidism have hypertension which is attributed to renal parenchymal damage from renal stones and nephrocalcinosis. An increased calcium level may have direct vasoconstrictive effects. The hypertension is sometimes reversible when calcium returns to normal unless there has been irreparable renal damage.

Subjectively, the patient will complain of constipation, vomiting, malaise, behavior disturbances, polyuria, nocturia, pruritus, weakness and a history of renal stones and hematuria.

Objectively, the patient may present with signs of hyperparathyroidism; look also for band keratopathy (opacities around limbus), ectopic calcifications in the conjunctiva, an elevated serum calcium, ectopic calcification subcutaneously (rare), a prolonged QT interval in the EKG, and hypertension. There may be calcium crystals in the urine sediment.

Renal disease

In renal arterial hypertension (with obstructive lesions of the renal arteries due usually to atherosclerotic plaques or fibromuscular hyperplasia), decreased perfusion of the renal tissue from stenosis of a main or major renal artery is thought to activate the renin-angiotensin system. The presence of angiotensin II results in direct vasoconstriction. The stimulation of aldosterone secretion leads to sodium retention and stimulation of the adrenergic nervous system.

In renal parenchymal disease (loss of tissue function from inflammation or fibrosis), the activation of the renin-angiotensin system is also postulated as a factor in both acute and chronic renal parenchymal disease. In this case, a decreased perfusion results from the fibrotic and inflammatory changes of the small renal vessels. The damaged kidneys may also: 1) produce another unidentified pressor substance besides renin; 2) fail to produce a vasodilating agent; 3) fail to dispose of circulating pressors, and/or 4) fail to effectively dispose of sodium leading to sodium retention and hypertension.

Subjectively, the patient may complain of flank pain, a history of flank trauma or recurrent UTI's, polyuria, dysuria, an onset of hypertension after age 55, and an abrupt rise in longstanding hypertension.

Objectively, the practitioner may find a bruit in the flank or abdomen, hypertension, rapidly progressive hypertensive retinopathy, proteinuria, reduced urine specific gravity and a microscopic urinalysis showing RBC's, WBC's, granular casts, hematuria and/or bacteriuria. An enlarged kidney or mass discrepancy in size or excretory function between the kidneys may be found on IVP and/or renal scan. A reduction in the volume and sodium excretion between the two kidneys may be found on retrograde ureteral catheterization; there may be arteriographic evidence of unilateral obstructive renal arterial lesions and there may be an increased plasma renin activity.

PLAN:

Section I
Essential hypertension

For established essential hypertension, implement a sodium restriction and weight reduction diet where indicated. The first line drug in mild to moderate hypertension is usually a thiazide diuretic.

Transient elevations of blood pressure can be due to anxiety, discomfort, activity or stress; hence, the need for serial BPs before the assessment of hypertension is established. Serial blood pressures are not necessary where the blood pressure initially is dangerously high or where there is evidence of target organ damage. Labile or fluctuating blood pressure may develop into sustained hypertension, so it should be checked every several months. In the controversy about the need for treatment of isolated systolic hypertension, there is no good evidence to suggest it is advisable, so it is generally not recommended. These patients should have regular follow-up (every three to six months) to screen for the development of electrolyte imbalances or hyperuricemia.

See Section II for additional plan guidelines.

Secondary causes of hypertension

Coarctation of the aorta

Conservative (i.e., nonsurgical) management is appropriate in the asymptomatic, elderly patient. Referral of the patient to a physician is indicated.

Primary aldosteronism

The patient should be referred to his or her physician. Therapy of choice is surgical removal of the aldosteronoma. In some cases, particularly when symptoms are not severe, moderate salt restriction and the administration of aldosterone antagonists can be effective therapy.

Cushing's syndrome

Cushing's syndrome usually presents in a much younger age group; although rare in the elderly, if present it is usually due to an iatrogenic cause. The patient should be referred to his or her physician. If the cause of glucocorticoid excess is an adrenal lesion, then a unilateral adrenalectomy is performed. If bilateral adrenal hyperplasia is present, there may be need for a subtotal bilateral adrenalectomy and/or pituitary irradiation. This is a serious disorder with about 50 percent mortality in five years if untreated.

Pheochromocytoma

Pheochromocytoma is a rare cause of hypertension; it accounts for about 0.1 percent of the causes of secondary hypertension. Referral of the patient should be made to the patient's physician. Ninety percent of pheochromocyte tumors arise from the adrenal tissue, so radiologic evidence of the tumor is sought in the suprarenal area. Surgery is the first choice of treatment since the lesion can be lethal.

Pharmacologic adrenergic blockade is carried out before surgery is undertaken. Medical management of pheochromocytoma may include phenoxybenzamine for inoperable tumors; this is an alpha-adrenergic

blocking agent. Inhibitors of catecholamine synthesis (alpha-methyl-
para-tyrosine) has also been used
recently.

Hypercalcemia

The patient should be referred to
his or her physician. In hypercalcemia, there may be possible primary or secondary hyperparathyroidism. Definitive therapy of
hyperparathyroidism is removal of
the parathyroid tumor. This is
strongly recommended if the patient is symptomatic, the calcium is
greater than 13 mg, or there is evidence of renal damage. Nonopera-
tive treatment is the administration
of thyrocalcitonin or the antitumor
agent nithramycin (both are thought
to work by inhibiting the bone resorption of calcium).

Renal disease

The patient should be referred to
his or her physician. The demon-
stration of a pyelographic lesion in
a hypertensive patient is not sufficient indication for surgical correction. (Pyelography and renal scan
have a 15 percent false negative
rate.) There should be a degree of
certainty that the demonstrated lesion is responsible for the hypertension and that its removal would be
followed by a reduction in blood
pressure. Significant renal ischemia
may be demonstrated by: 1) abnormal excretion of urine contents and
diminished urine volume on bilateral retrograde ureteral catheterization, 2) renal vein renins, and/or
3) renal arteriograms. Such documentation of renal ischemia can be

additional indication for surgical correction.

With parenchymal lesions, if the patient is a surgical candidate, nephrectomy is sometimes performed. In renal artery stenosis with very diseased arteries, endarterectomy or nephrectomy can be carried out. But, in patients with renal artery stenosis caused by athero-arteriosclerosis, there is no evidence that repair of the stenosis improves life expectancy.

Section II

MEDICATIONS

Drug therapy in the elderly must be carried out with a number of special considerations. The first is the possibility of alterations in drug absorption, metabolism and elimination in the elderly (because of characteristic pathophysiologic changes). The second is that of the variation in effectiveness of prescribed drugs (because of coexisting conditions and concomitant drug therapy).

Factors that affect absorption of drugs include gastric motility, intestinal motility, mesenteric blood flow and gastric pH. Conditions in which these factors are altered are pyloric stenosis, gastric ulcer, vagotomy, diabetic gastroparesis, severe malabsorption syndrome and achlorhydria. Generally, the absorption of acidic and neutral drugs is not significantly impaired in the elderly.

The distribution of drugs in the elderly can be affected by changes in body composition (i.e., there is a decrease in the percentage of fat and muscle in the elderly). In CHF, drugs can be inadequately distributed to some parts of the body, exposing the heart and brain to excessive drug concentrations. Low serum protein and dehydration are also factors in altered distribution of drugs.

The liver is the major site of drug metabolism. Impairment of liver function (as with declines in function of other organ systems) may allow toxic levels of a drug to accumulate.

The elimination of drugs is dependent on the liver and kidney function. Renal excretion is a chief means by which drugs and metabolites are removed from the body. A normal serum creatinine and normal BUN are not necessarily indicators of adequate renal function, since creatinine is affected by the decline in muscle mass seen in aging, and a decrease in the rate of creatinine excretion can result in a normal serum creatinine when clearance is reduced. BUN is affected by a number of nonrenal factors such as the dietary intake of protein, hepatic disease, an existing catabolic state, the degree of dehydration, and the presence of GI bleeding.

Chapron and Dennis (Reichel, 1978) recommend an estimate of renal function (i.e., creatinine clearance) before starting new drugs in the elderly; in addition, they recommend starting with the lowest recommended dosage of a drug followed by titration according to clinical response or measured blood levels.

The aim of treatment of hypertension is to retard or stop the damage to secondary organs. In certain cases, the cure of a primary etiology can be achieved (e.g., the surgical correction of renal artery stenosis or the removal of a tumor secreting pressor substances). However, for the overwhelming majority of patients, the control of blood pressure will be a lifelong effort aimed at lowering the blood pressure. The lowering mechanism aims to directly or indirectly lower the peripheral vascular resistance and/or plasma volume by reducing intravascular volume and by interfering with vasoconstricting factors in the CNS.

The therapeutic plan with respect to antihypertensive medications always follows a steplike progression in the addition and combination of medications. When several drugs are used, they are chosen because of their synergetic effect and the fact that drugs with different sites of action can maximize the effect of all drugs given.

The aim of antihypertensive therapy in the elderly is to lower the blood presure without aggravating: 1) brain function (from diminished cerebral blood flow); 2) renal function; 3) cardiac function, and/or 4) without causing symptoms of orthostatic hypotension or other incapacitating side effects. The sudden reduction of BP from hypertensive to more normal levels may result in acute cerebral, coronary or renal insufficiency.

It is, therefore, critical initially to lower the blood pressure moderately and to frequently monitor the BP level and symptoms of possible side effects.

The nurse should consult with the physician before initiating drug therapy. As the need for additional step medications becomes evident, physician consultation/referral is advised. Before recommending any drug therapy, the practitioner should be thoroughly familiar with dosages, contraindications, and side effects of the medicine; complete drug information can be found in many currently available drug manuals/texts.

Hypertension drug management is approached using a series of steps:

Step I is the administration of a thiazide diuretic (unless there are contraindications). In the great majority of patients with mild to moderate hypertension, the BP can be controlled with this single agent which is well-tolerated. It reduces plasma volume and also on a long-term basis probably decreases peripheral vascular resistance.

If an adequate response is not seen in BP, then one of the Step II medications is added.

Step II medications are antiadrenergic agents that inhibit adrenergic nerves and the structures innervated by them. They selectively inhibit certain responses to adrenergic nerve activity and epinephrine. They chiefly work in the central nervous system to interfere with constriction which contributes to hypertension. These medications are methyldopa, clonidine, propranolol and reserpine.

Reserpine, although it is inexpensive, is largely avoided in the elderly because severe depression is a possible side effect. Methyldopa is widely used and generally well tolerated (though drowsiness is a common side effect). It should not be used in active liver disease, but is quite useful in renal disease with hypertension, since it does not compromise renal blood flow.

Clonidine is a powerful drug that can be effective in very small doses; it is useful in patients who reliably take medications since a sudden stoppage of this drug without tapering can result in dangerous rebound hypertension. Propranolol is an antiadrenergic agent that produces a specific blockade of beta-adrenergic receptors. It should be avoided in those patients with diabetes mellitus, asthma or congestive heart failure, since heart failure can be caused slowly or suddenly by the drug. Six weeks should be allowed before fully evaluating the drug's effectiveness.

If control is not achieved after four to eight weeks on a diuretic plus a Step II drug, then a Step III drug is added.

Step III drugs are vasodilators. They lower the BP by dilating the arterioles and thus decreasing the peripheral vascular resistance. Hydralazine mocks the sympathetic nervous system and cardiac output increasing the heart rate. For this reason, it is often combined with propranolol which blocks this effect. Hydralazine can also increase plasma volume so it is always used with a diuretic.

Prazosin is another arterial dilator that does not increase the stroke volume as hydralazine does. It can be hazardous in those with cerebral arteriosclerosis since it causes syncope in about 1 percent of patients.

Step IV—when a patient seems to be complying with the medication regimen and his or her BP is not yet controlled, the step IV drug, guanethidine is sometimes added. However, patients unresponsive to previous treatment are often reevaluated for secondary causes of hypertension or for factors that are interfering with the drug therapy.

DIET

A no-added-salt (NAS) diet is often recommended for patients with hypertension because of the strong association between excessive salt intake and the development of hypertension. Salt restriction is sometimes the sole treatment in patients with labile hypertension or is used with a weight reduction plan in obese patients with mild BP elevations. No added salt means no salt at the table with small to reasonable amounts used in cooking. Patients should avoid large quantities of obviously salty food (pickles, chips, etc.) and should also avoid substances with hidden salt (cold cuts, meat tenderizers, sodium bicarbonate, antacids high in salt, soy sauce and other prepared sauces). Some patients use "light salt" because it has one-half the sodium content and some potassium.

Patients with normal serum potassium prior to drug treatment are usually placed on thiazide diuretics without a potassium supplement. When or if the potassium level starts to fall, patients may then be placed on a 20 to 40 mg supplement every day. However, some patients can maintain an adequate potassium level by consuming several high potassium foods daily (bananas, orange juice, potatoes, dried fruit). Most prefer this because of the very bitter taste of liquid or powdered effervescent potassium substitutes. The slow release potassium supplement tablets are avoided by some clinicians because of the possibilty of GI ulceration associated with this form of supplement.

ACTIVITY

Activity must be individualized. Increased activity often needs to be encouraged, especially as part of a weight reduction plan. Physical conditioning seems to help lower the blood pressure.

PATIENT EDUCATION

Patient education is very important in hypertension management because compliance is so critical. The education program designed for the patient should ensure the patient understanding of the following:

1. That "high blood pressure" is hypertension.

2. The asymptomatic but lifelong and serious nature of essential hypertension.

3. The risks of untreated hypertension and likely target organ damage (i.e., CNS, retina, renal and cardiac).

4. Their pretreatment blood pressure level and the goal of treatment.

5. The importance of taking medications regularly, every day, and an understanding of the notion of control versus cure for the majority of cases.

6. The name and dosage schedule of each of their medications; it is desirable for patients to carry a card listing their medications in case of an emergency.

7. Individualized information about the possible side effects of each medication in their regimen.

8. The importance of follow-up examinations to determine the efficacy of therapy.

9. The importance of diet, cessation of smoking, and exercise.

Hypertension is generally a silent disease. In patients without symptoms, the prescribed treatment may be expensive or may cause side effects which are unpleasant or uncomfortable. The notion of a silent but lifelong-life-threatening disease is a difficult one for many to accept. Patients must be dealt with in a firm but understanding manner and the benefits of treatment must also be reinforced.

FOLLOW-UP CARE

Once the blood pressure is controlled and stabilized, the patient should be monitored at least every three months, or as indicated by the presence of other ongoing problems. At every visit, a cardiorespiratory review of systems and exam, extremities exam, inquiry about problems with medications, and vital signs (weight, BP, P) should be done. The potassium level should be checked several times a year. Other exams and laboratory work should be repeated as indicated by the patient's other conditions or by medications.

At yearly intervals, generally, the patient should receive a chest x-ray, EKG, urinalysis, BUN, creatinine, potassium, uric acid, CBC and fasting blood sugar (FBS). Funduscopic exam and, by some, a complete physical examination is also done at yearly intervals.

At return visits, patients should be counseled about their role in minimizing risk factors for the development of cardiovascular disease to the extent feasible (e.g., discontinuing smoking, following a regular exercise program three times weekly and achieving and maintaining an ideal body weight).

REFERENCES

1. Caird F. I. and T. G. Judge. *Assessment of the Elderly Patient.* Tunbridge Wells, Kent, Eng.: Pitman Medical Publishing Co., 1974.
2. Cappell, Peter T. and David B. Case. *Ambulatory Care Manual for Nurse Practitioners.* Philadelphia: J. B. Lippincott Co., 1976.
3. Chrysant, Steven, Edward Frohlich, and Solomon Pepper. "Why Hypertension Is so Prevalent." *Geriatrics*, October 1976.
4. _____, ed. *Clinical Principles and Drugs in Aging.* Springfield, Ill.: Charles C Thomas, 1963.
5. Freeman, Joseph T. *Clinical Features of the Older Patient.* Springfield, Ill.: Charles C Thomas, 1965.
6. Joint National Committee on Detection, Evaluation and Treatment of High Blood Pressure, Report of "A Cooperative Study." *JAMA*, 237, January 1977, 225–261.
7. Moore, Michael A. "Hypertension in the Ambulatory Patient." *American Family Physician*, 16, 5, November 1977, 188–197.
8. Reichel, William, ed. *Clinical Aspects of Aging.* Baltimore: Williams and Wilkins Co., 1978, chapter by Chapron and Dennis.
9. Rossman, Isadore, ed. *Clinical Geriatrics.* Philadelphia: J.B. Lippincott Co., 1977.
10. Thorn, George W. et al., eds. *Harrison's Principles of Internal Medicine*, 8th ed. New York: McGraw-Hill Book Co., 1977.

Index

Numerals in *italics* indicate a figure or table concerning the subject.

Abdomen and edema, 293-295
Acrochordon, 347
Adenoma, senile sebaceous, 351, 364
Aging process, 4
Aldosteronism, 575-576
Alzheimer's disease, 497-498
Anasarca, 450-452, 456
Anemia, pernicious, 495-496
Angiokeratoma, 350
Angioma, senile (cherry), 346-347
Aorta, coarctation of, 570-571, 575
Arthritis
  of acute rheumatic fever, 49-50
  degenerative joint, 43-46
  episodic rheumatoid, 36-37
  gonococcal, 48-49
  psoriatic, 47-48
  rheumatoid, 46-47
  septic (infectious), 32-34
  tuberculous, 38-39
Arthropathy, neurogenic, 40
Athlete's foot, 353, 368-369
Audiogram, 146-154, *113, 149, 151-153*
  conduction hearing loss and, 151, *152*
  mixed hearing loss and, 151, *153*
  sensorineural hearing loss and, 150, *151*
Audiometric data, 146-162
  audiogram in, 146-154, *149, 151-153*
  impedance audiometry in, 158-162, *160-161*
  speech audiometry in, 154-156
  speech discrimination score in, 156-158
Auditory canal, 136-137
Auditory training, 180-181
Aural rehabilitation history, 134-135
Auricle, 135-136

Bing test, 146
Bones, 4

Bowel diseases, inflammatory, 41-42
Bowel flow sheet, 404

Cancers, cutaneous, 355-360
Carcinoma
  basal cell, 359, 372-373
  squamous cell, 359-360, 373
Cartilage, 4
Cellulitis, 355, 370-371
Cerebral pathology, *471*
Cerebrovascular disease and dementia, 496-497
Chondrocalcinosis, 39
Coarctation of aorta, 570-571, 575
Cochlear pathologies, 167-170
Collagen, 3-4
Collagen vascular disease, 50-51, 496
Congestive heart failure, 506-539
  edema and, 307-308
  flow sheet for assessment in, 537-538
  laboratory procedures in, 527-529
  left ventricular failure in, 530
  objective data and, 522-531
  patient/family education in, 535-537
  plan in, 531-538
  right ventricular failure in, 530
  subjective data and, 514-522
  worksheet in, 508-514
Connective tissue and rheumatic disease, 3-4
Constipation, 381-409
  assessment in, 394-398
  bowel flow sheet in, 404
  food diary check list in, 404
  laboratory data in, 393-394
  laxatives and, 405-407
  objective data in, 392-394
  patient education and, 407-408
  plan in, 398-403
  subjective data in, 387-392
  worksheet in, 382-387

Index

Creutzfeldt-Jakob disease, 498
Cushing's syndrome, 453, 456, 571-572, 576
Cystitis
  female, 260-261
  male, 258-259

Dementia, 469-505
  Alzheimer's disease and, 497-498
  assessment in, 490-500
  cerebrovascular disease and, 496-497
  collagen disease and, 496
  Creutzfeldt-Jakob disease and, 498
  dementia pugilistica and, 499
  endocrinopathies and, 493-494
  functional disorders and, 492
  heart disease and, 494
  Huntington's chorea and, 498
  infection in, 491
  intoxication and, 492-493
  laboratory data in, 487-490
  liver disease and, 494
  metabolic disturbances and, 496
  multiple sclerosis and, 499
  neurologic examination in, 483-486
  normal pressure hydrocephalus and, 491
  nutritional deficiencies and, 494-496
  objective data in, 482-490
  Parkinson's disease and, 498-499
  pernicious anemia and, 495-496
  physical examination in, 486-487
  Pick's disease and, 498
  plan in, 500-504
  porphyria and, 500
  progressive multifocal leukoencephalopathy and, 497
  subdural hematoma and, 490-491
  subjective data in, 478-482
  syphilis and, 492
  tumor and, 490
  uremia and, 494
  Wernicke-Korsakoff syndrome and, 495
  Wilson's disease and, 499
  worksheet in, 472-478
Dementia pugilistica, 499
Depression, 410-434
  assessment in, 430-433
  laboratory data in, 429-430
  objective data in, 428-430
  plan in, 433
  subjective data in, 423-428
  worksheet in, 414-423
Dermatitis
  contact, 361
  senile seborrheic, 351-352, 365
  stasis, 362

Diuretics and edema, 317
Drug eruptions, 360
Drug exposure and hearing loss, 127-129
Dysuria, 203

Ear and ear canal, 163
Edema, peripheral, 270-324
  abdomen in, 293-295
  assessment in, 302-316
  bilateral, 290
  brawny, 290
  chest in, 291-292
  congestive heart failure in, 307-308
  generalized, 306-308, 322-324
  glomerulonephritis and, 311-312
  heart and, 292-293
  hepatomegaly in, 294-295
  iatrogenic, 315
  lab data in, 297-302
  liver disease and, 313-314
  localized, 302-306, 319-322
  myxedema and, 314-315
  neck veins in, 291
  nephrotic syndrome and, 312-313
  objective data in, 289-297
  past medical history in, 285-288
  pitting, 290
  plan in, 317-324
    diuretics in, 317
    flow sheet and, 318-319
    patient education in, 318
    staff education and, 317-318
  protein deficiency and, 316
  renal disease and, 308-310
  sodium excess and, 316
  splenomegaly in, 295
  subjective data in, 279-289
  unilateral/localized, 289-290
  vital signs in, 289
  worksheet in, 272-279
Education
  patient
    congestive heart failure and, 535-537
    constipation and, 407-408
    edema and, 318
    hypertension and, 581-582
    urinary incontinence and, 230-231
    urinary tract infection and, 267-268
  staff
    edema and, 317-318
    urinary incontinence and, 229-230
Elderly, chronic conditions common to, 379-583
Endocrinopathies, 493-494
Enuresis, 205-206
Environmental hazards
  falls and hip injury and, 92-94

586

Environmental hazards (Continued)
  history of falls and, 87-88
Epithelioma, 359
Eustachian tube, 137-138

Falls and hip injury, 63-94
  hip pain secondary to fall and, 65-70
  history of falls and, 73-88
    assessment in, 79-88
    cardiovascular conditions in, 84-85
    complete exam in, 76-78
    environmental hazards in, 87-88
    lab data in, 78-79
    neurologic problems and, 85-86
    objective data in, 76
    pathological fractures in, 79-84
    subjective data in, 73-76
  physiology and, 63-64
  prevention of, 63, 88-94
  worksheet in, 64, 70-73
Female
  distribution of skin disease in, 376
  hearing deficit and, 97
  ideal body weight of, 455
  urinary incontinence and, 208
  urinary tract infection and, 247
Food diary check list, 404
Fractures, pathological, 79-84
Frequency response of hearing aid, 183

Genital data in urinary tract infection,
    242-243, 246-247
Glomerulonephritis, 311-312
Gout, 34-36

Hearing aids, 182-190
  candidacy determination for, 185
  frequency response of, 183
  gain and, 183
  geriatric patient and, 185-189
  history in, 131-134
  range of amplification of, 182-183
  troubleshooting and, 189-190, 188
  types of, 183, 184
Hearing deficit, 95-191
  assessment in, 163-174
  audiogram in, 113
  audiometric data in, 146-162
  aural rehabilitation history in, 134-135
  cochlear pathologies in, 167-170
  conduction, 151, 152
  difficult listening situations and, 120-
    135
  drug exposure in, 127-129
  external ear and ear canal in, 163

Hearing deficit (Continued)
  family history in, 129-130
  females of different ages and, 97
  hearing aid history in, 131-134
  lesion testing in, 162
  males of different ages and, 96
  management of, 179-190
    auditory training in, 180-181
    hearing aids in, 182-190
    speech conservation in, 182
    speechreading in, 181-182
  mixed, 151, 153
  noise exposure in, 130-131
  objective data in, 135-162
  otologic medical history in, 124-125
  otoscopic exam in, 135-138
  plan in, 174-179
  related medical history in, 125-126
  retrocochlear pathology in, 170-174,
    172, 174, 175
  sensorineural, 150, 151
  subjective data and, 114-120
  tinnitus and, 117
  tuning fork tests in, 138-146
  tympanic membrane in, 164-167
  tympanogram in, 113
  worksheet for, 98-114
Heart
  dementia and, 494
  edema and, 292-293
Hematoma, subdural, 490-491
Hematuria, 203-204
Hepatomegaly, 294-295
Herpes zoster, 360-361
Hip injury, falls and, 63-94
Huntington's chorea, 498
Hydrocephalus, normal pressure, 491
Hyperaldosteronism, 571
Hypercalcemia, 572-573, 577
Hypertension, 540-583
  activity in, 581
  assessment in, 570-574
  coarctation of aorta and, 570-571, 575
  Cushing's syndrome and, 571-572, 576
  diet in, 581
  follow-up care and, 582-583
  hyperaldosteronism and, 571
  hypercalcemia and, 572-573, 577
  lab data in, 565-568
  medication in, 578-581
  objective data in, 558-570
  patient education in, 581-582
  pheochromocytoma, 572, 576-577
  plan in, 574-578
  primary aldosteronism and, 575-576
  renal disease and, 573-574, 577-578
  subjective data in, 552-558
  worksheet in, 544-552

Index

Hypoglycemia, 453-454, 456-457
Hypothyroidism, 51, 452, 456

Impedance audiometry, 158-162, *160-161*
Incontinence, urinary, 192-231
Infection and dementia, 491
Intoxication, 492-493

Joints
  cartilaginous, 4
  fibrous, 4
  mono- and polyarticular pain in, 26-28
  synovial, 4

Keratoacanthoma, 357-358, 372
Keratoses
  actinic (solar), 356-357, 371-372
  seborrheic, 355-356, 371

Laxatives, 405-407
Left ventricular failure, 530
Lentigines, 345-346
Leukoencephalopathy, progressive
  multifocal, 497
Leukoplakia, 358, 372
Lichen simplex chronicus, 348-349, 365-
  366
Liver disease
  dementia and, 494
  edema and, 313-314
Liver spots, 345-346

Male
  distribution of skin disease in, 377
  hearing deficit and, *96*
  ideal body weight of, 455
  urinary incontinence in, 208-209
  urinary tract infection and, 246-247,
    256-260
Melanoma, malignant, 360, 373
Metabolic disturbances, 496
Monoarticular disease, 32-43. *See also*
  individual diseases.
Mono- and polyarticular pain, 3-62
  assessment in, 32-55
  family history in, 25
  gastrointestinal symptoms in, 20-21
  general physical examination in, 28-29
  genitourinary symptoms in, 21
  hypothyroidism in, 51
  involved joint examination in, 26-28
  lab data in, 30-32
  local symptoms in, 18-19

Mono- *(Continued)*
  monoarticular disease and, 32-43. *See*
    also individual diseases.
  monoarticular x-ray changes in, 52-54
  neurologic symptoms in, 24
  objective data in, 25-32
  overview of, 3-5
  past medical history in, 21-24
  patient management plan in, 55-61
  periarticular rheumatic disorders in,
    51-52
  polyarticular disease in, 43-51. *See also*
    individual diseases.
  polyarticular x-ray changes in, 54-55
  respiratory symptoms in, 20
  subjective data in, 14-25
  systemic symptoms in, 19-20
  worksheet for, 5-14
Multiple sclerosis, 499
Myxedema, 314-315

Neck veins and edema, 291
Nephrotic syndrome, 312-313
Neurodermatoses, 361
Neurologic problems
  history of falls and, 85-86
  mono- and polyarticular pain and, 24
Nocturia, 204
Noise exposure and hearing loss, 130-131
Nutritional deficiencies, 494-496

Obesity, 435-468
  anasarca and, 450-452, 456
  assessment in, 450-456
  Cushing's syndrome and, 453, 456
  hypoglycemia and, 456-457
  hypothyroidism and, 452, 456
  nonorganic functional obesity and, 454-
    456, 457-468
  objective data in, 448-450
  plan in, 456-468
  reactive hypoglycemia and, 453-454
  subjective data in, 443-448
  worksheet in, 437-443
Osteoarthritis, 43-46
Osteoporosis, 42-43
Otoscopic exam, 135-138
  auricle in, 135-136
  eustachian tube in, 137-138
  external auditory canal in, 136-137
  tympanic membrane in, 137

Parkinson's disease, 498-499
Perlèche, 349-350, 367
Pheochromocytoma, 572, 576-577

Pick's disease, 498
Polyarticular disease, 43-51. *See also individual diseases.*
Polyarticular pain. *See* Mono- and polyarticular pain.
Polymyalgia rheumatica, 50
Porphyria, 500
Presbycusis, 95, 171-174, *172, 174, 175*
Presenting complaints, protocols for, 1-378
Prostatitis, 259-260
Protein deficiency, 316
Pruritus vulvae and ani, 354-355, 370
Pseudogout, 39
Psoriasis, 361-363
Purpura, senile, 346
Pyelonephritis, 261-263

Rehabilitation, aural, 134-135
Renal disease
  edema and, 308-310
  hypertension and, 573-574, 577-578
Retrocochlear pathology, 170-174, *172, 174, 175*
Rheumatic disease
  connective tissue types in, 3-4
  definition of, 3
  joint types in, 4
  manifestations of, 3
  periarticular, 51-52
Rheumatic fever, 49-50
Right ventricular failure, 530
Rinne test, 144-145
Rosacea, 349, 366-367

Schwabach test, 142-143
Serum sickness, 40-41
Skin diseases, 325-378
  acrochordon (skin tag) and, 347
  actinic (solar) keratoses and, 356-357, 371-372
  angiokeratoma and, 350
  assessment in, 345-362
  basal cell carcinoma and, 359, 372-373
  cellulitis and, 355, 370-371
  contact dermatitis and, 361
  cutaneous cancers and, 355-360, 371-373
  distribution of, 376-377
  drug eruptions and, 360
  herpes zoster and, 360-361
  incidental-inveterate conditions and, 360-362, 373
  keratoacanthoma and, 357-358, 372
  lab data in, 343-345
  lentigines (liver spots) and, 345-346

Skin diseases *(Continued)*
  leukoplakia and, 358, 372
  lichen simplex chronicus and, 348-349, 365-366
  malignant melanoma and, 360, 373
  neurodermatoses and, 361
  objective data in, 340-343
  perlèche and, 349-350, 367
  plan in, 362-373
  primary lesions in, *374*
  pruritus vulvae and ani and, 354-355, 370
  psoriasis and, 361-363
  rosacea and, 349, 366-367
  seborrheic keratoses, 355-356, 371
  secondary lesions in, *375*
  senile (cherry) angioma in, 346-347
  senile purpura and, 346
  senile sebaceous adenoma and, 351, 364
  senile seborrheic dermatitis and, 351-352, 365
  squamous cell carcinoma and, 359-360, 373
  stasis dermatitis and, 362
  subjective data in, 335-340
  syphilis and, 362
  tinea onychomycosis and, 352-353, 367-368
  tinea pedis and, 353, 368-369
  venous lakes and, 347
  venous star in, 347-348
  verruca and, 353-354, 369-370
  worksheet in, 327-335
  xerosis and, 350, 363-364
Skin tag, 347
Sodium excess, 316
Speech audiometry, 154-156
Speech conservation, 182
Speech discrimination scores, 156-158
Speechreading, 181-182
Splenomegaly, 295
Spondylosis, cervical, 49
Syphilis
  dementia and, 492
  skin disease and, 362

Tinea onychomycosis, 352-353, 367-368
Tinea pedis, 353, 368-369
Tinnitus, 117
Tumor
  dementia and, 490
  monoarticular disease and, 42
Tuning fork tests, 138-146
  Bing test, 146
  Rinne test, 144-145
  Schwabach test, 142-143

Index

Tuning fork tests *(Continued)*
  Weber test, 143-144
Tympanic membrane
  assessment of, 164-167
  examination of, 137
Tympanograms, 159, *113, 160-161*

Uremia, 494
Urethritis
  female, 261
  male, 256-258
Urinary incontinence, 192-231
  assessment in, 215-224
  continuous, 219-224
  dysuria and, 203
  enuresis and, 205-206
  episodic, 215-219
  females and, 208
  hematuria in, 203-204
  laboratory data in, 212-215
  males and, 208-209
  neurogenic, 227-229
  nocturia and, 204
  objective data in, 210-215
  patient education in, 230-231
  plan in, 224-227
  staff education goals in, 229-230
  subjective data in, 202-210
  worksheet in, 194-202
Urinary tract infection, 232-269
  abdominal exam in, 247-248
  assessment in, 256-263
  back examination in, 248
  cystitis in, 258-259, 260-261
  female assessment in, 260-261

Urinary infection *(Continued)*
  genital data in, 242-243
  lab data in, 248-256
  lower, 256-261
  male assessment in, 256-260
  male genital exam in, 246-247
  objective data in, 246-256
  past medical history in, 244-246
  patient education and, 267-268
  plan in, 263-267
  prostatitis in, 259-260
  pyelonephritis in, 261-263
  social history in, 246
  subjective data in, 238-246
  systemic data in, 243-244
  upper, 261-263
  urethritis in, 256-258, 261
  worksheet in, 233-238

Venous lakes, 347
Venous star, 347-348
Verruca, 353-354, 369-370

Warts, 353-354, 369-370
Weber test, 143-144
Wernicke-Korsakoff syndrome, 495
Wilson's disease, 499

Xerosis, 350, 363-364
X-ray changes
  monoarticular, 52-54
  polyarticular, 54-55